THE HOME OFFICE AND THE DANGEROUS TRADES

REGULATING OCCUPATIONAL DISEASE IN VICTORIAN AND EDWARDIAN BRITAIN

THE WELLCOME SERIES IN THE HISTORY OF MEDICINE

Forthcoming Titles:

The Regius Chair of Military Surgery in the University of Edinburgh, 1806-55
By Matthew H. Kaufman

Cultures of Child Health in Britain and the Netherlands in the Twentieth Century
Edited by Marijke Gijswijt-Hofstra and Hilary Marland

Dental Practice in Europe at the End of the Eighteenth Century
Edited by Christine Hillam

For Fear of Pain: British Surgery 1790–1850
By Peter Stanley

The Wellcome Series in the History of Medicine editors are C. J. Lawrence, M. Neve and V. Nutton.
Please send all queries regarding the series to Michael Laycock, The Wellcome Trust Centre for the History of Medicine at UCL, 24 Eversholt Street, London NW1 1AD, UK.

THE HOME OFFICE AND THE DANGEROUS TRADES

REGULATING OCCUPATIONAL DISEASE IN VICTORIAN AND EDWARDIAN BRITAIN

P. W. J. Bartrip

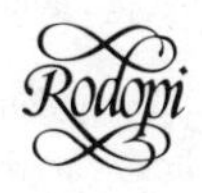

Amsterdam – New York, NY 2002

First published in 2002
by Editions Rodopi B. V., Amsterdam – New York, NY 2002.

Design and Typesetting by Michael Laycock,
The Wellcome Trust Centre for the History of Medicine at UCL.
Printed and bound in The Netherlands by Editions Rodopi B. V.,
Amsterdam – New York, NY 2002.

Index by Dr. Laurence Errington.

British Library Cataloguing in Publication Data
A catalogue record for this book is available from the
British Library
ISBN 90-420-1218-8 (Paper)
ISBN 90-420-1228-5 (Bound)

The Home Office and the Dangerous Trades:
Regulating Occupational Disease in
Victorian and Edwardian Britain
Amsterdam – New York, NY:
Rodopi. – ill.
(Clio Medica 68 / ISSN 0045-7183;
The Wellcome Series in the History of Medicine)

Front cover:
Skull with jaw affected by phosphorous poisoning. Courtesy, *Wellcome Library,* London. The Potteries looking towards Burslem from the tower of Hanley Parish Church, Stoke-on-Trent. Courtesy: *The Times* Newspaper.
Montage by Michael Laycock.

Printed in The Netherlands
All titles in the Clio Medica series (from 1999 onwards) are available to
download from the CatchWord website: http://www.catchword.co.uk

Contents

List of Tables

Acknowledgements

Research for this book began many years ago and has been delayed by the intervention of several other projects. It is, therefore, both a pleasure and a relief to see its final publication. At some points I feared that I would never reach this point. In researching and writing the volume I have, at least metaphorically speaking, incurred numerous debts. Work on it began when I was Senior Research Officer at the ESRC's Oxford Centre for Socio-Legal Studies in Oxford. Initial funding for the research was derived from ESRC. Subsequently, I received further financial assistance from the Health and Safety Executive as part of an HSE-funded project on socio-legal aspects of the regulation of health and safety at work. I am extremely grateful to ESRC and the HSE for their support. I am also grateful to University College Northampton for the generous provision of sabbatical leave. Much of the work on the book was undertaken at the Centre for Socio-Legal Studies, Wolfson College, Oxford and I owe much to that institution and its staff, academic, administrative, and secretarial. I would particularly like to thank the current director, Professor Denis Galligan, and his predecessor, Donald Harris for their support. When not engaged on this work at a desk in the Centre I was often to be found doing the same in a library or an archive somewhere in England. I wish to acknowledge the assistance provided by the Public Record Office, West Yorkshire Archives, Bodleian, Rockingham (UCN), and University of North London Libraries. At the Bodleian, where I consulted most of my printed sources, I would like to highlight the splendid service provided by the staff of the Official Paper Room and the Radcliffe Science Library. All pagination in references to parliamentary papers conforms to the set housed in the basement of the Radcliffe Camera, at the Bodleian Library, Oxford. All references to PRO files conform to usage at the time the records were consulted.

Parts of the manuscript have been 'tried out' at conferences – including at Oriel College, Oxford, University College Swansea and Midhurst in Sussex – teaching sessions, and in print. I am grateful to the conference organisers, students and editors for providing me with opportunities for test 'runs'. Finally, I thank the following individuals for having assisted me in various ways: Pam Bartrip, Jenny Dix, Paul Fenn, Keith Hawkins and Judith Knelman.

1

Introduction

Aims and contexts

This book is less a history of occupational health and medicine, more a study of the regulation of the so-called 'dangerous trades' in Victorian and Edwardian Britain. It makes no claim to comprehensiveness for it pays no attention to, for example, mining diseases (an important omission). It aims to open up and develop a subject that historians, in the United Kingdom at least, have tended to neglect. By focusing on the first hazards and trades to come under regulation it charts the origins, nature, consequences and significance of a series of parliamentary, bureaucratic and other steps which sought to eliminate, or at least to control, the four diseases (lead, phosphorus and arsenic poisoning and anthrax) that were the first to be officially recognised as constituting occupational hazards of manufacturing industry. It aspires to do this by interweaving social, political, economic, medical and cultural history. So while it recognises the importance of scientific discovery and legislative enactment, it also seeks to place such events within a context that takes account of the experiences of workers, employers, factory inspectors, trade unionists and others with personal knowledge of the 'dangerous trades'.

The recent historiography of occupational health is discussed in more detail below but anyone acquainted with labour and medical history in nineteenth and twentieth centuries will surely acknowledge that these sub-disciplines do little more than touch upon diseases of the workplace. In contrast, such themes as radicalism, trades union organisation, medical quackery and medical discovery are well tilled, perhaps over-exploited, fields. In some ways such neglect is surprising for, as Adam Smith observed in 1776, 'some peculiar infirmity' was associated with almost every trade and over exertion reduced the working lives of many.[1] In other words occupational disease and disability were commonplace – the almost inevitable corollary of employment. Hence, historical neglect of occupational health reflects not the rarity of workplace disease but the priorities of a society in which neither medical practitioners nor labour leaders or politicians placed much emphasis upon improving occupational health. Such limited interest is well illustrated by the fact that there was no English translation of Bernardino Ramazzini's final version of *Diseases of Workers*, a classic study of occupational ill health dating from the early eighteenth century, until 1940. As one of the pioneers of British occupational medicine, Charles Turner Thackrah, wrote in the 1830s, with only slight exaggeration: 'we find volumes on the symptoms, character and treatment of diseases, but rarely a line on the causes as produced by employments and habits and this line as frequently erroneous as correct'.[2]

In seeking to explain why occupational diseases gained the attention of medical scientists, politicians and regulators at a comparatively 'late' stage, it must be acknowledged that in several respects, these diseases were 'different'. Their victims did not perish in the epidemic devastations that might have claimed public sympathy, awakened public fears and prompted political action. Instead, workplace illness and death tended to affect individuals or comparatively small groups of workers. Collectively, the numbers involved could be large but it was a case, to paraphrase John Benson (see below), of epidemic by instalment. Neither did occupational ill health, in contrast with sexually transmitted diseases, set off any religious or moral 'alarm bells' which might have given them priority in the eyes of middle-class reformers. The single most important distinguishing feature of the victims of workplace disease was their socio-economic status. Almost exclusively, it was the poor, the unenfranchised, the unorganised, the politically impotent and the inarticulate who suffered trade-related illness. Indeed, as a generalisation, the unhealthiest occupations were pursued by the poorest, least educated sectors of the population, with women and juveniles being heavily represented in the dangerous trades.[3] In contrast those whose involvement in industry occurred off the shop floor, for example, as investors, proprietors, directors and managers were seldom afflicted by the health hazards of work. In effect, wealth and social position conferred immunity. What all this means is that occupational diseases, alongside deficiency diseases such as malnutrition and rickets, had a strong tendency to social class specificity in their choice of victims. In this respect they differed from the water-borne diseases such as cholera or typhoid that attracted such great attention from Victorian politicians, social reformers, medical practitioners, journalists and novelists.[4] These were diseases that exacted a toll, albeit an unequal one, on all socio-economic groups. Even those at the pinnacle of society were susceptible. Thus, in 1861 typhoid killed the Prince Consort; ten years later it nearly accounted for his eldest son, the future Edward VII. Other members of the Royal Family, including Victoria herself, were also typhoid victims.[5]

Once afflicted, occupational disease victims tended to suffer with resignation and in silence and anonymity. Hidden from public view in unnumbered factories, collieries, mining villages and slum districts of industrial cities and towns, their ranks were swelled not by sudden catastrophes but by a process of relentless accumulation. Such a pattern was present in other areas of health. Thus, whereas the cholera epidemics of the 1830s, 1840s, 1850s and 1860s generated widespread alarm and attracted huge publicity, the numerically more devastating endemic disease of tuberculosis was accepted as a fact of life (and death). As F.B. Smith points out in relation to tuberculosis:

> As a fundamental destructive force it was rivalled among illnesses only by the venereal diseases and insanity; but until about 1890 sufferers' kin, philanthropists and legislators were resigned to it as a morally neutral, ubiquitous affliction beyond official intervention.[6]

While occupational disease (almost certainly) did not claim as many lives as tuberculosis, there were other similarities, especially in terms of victims' acceptance of their fate and of official neglect.[7]

Society's neglect of occupational diseases and their victims was not simply a reflection either of numbers or of the superior claims for attention of the epidemic over the endemic. The poverty and powerlessness of industrial disease victims does much to explain the medical profession's relative lack of interest. Victorian and Edwardian medical practitioners were, to a considerable degree, businessmen intent on building solid, lucrative practices.[8] Notwithstanding the profession's rhetoric about relieving the suffering of all sections of the community, or the fact that many practitioners did provide their services free or at reduced rates for those unable to pay for medical attention, no young practitioner in search of riches, fame or social preferment would have contemplated specialising in occupational medicine. As a result the best medical brains, with some notable exceptions, were attracted into more rewarding and glamorous areas of practice. It follows that occupational health was something of a 'Cinderella', even a 'ghetto', field of medicine in which the deprived and the destitute were treated by relatively deprived and destitute practitioners. Meanwhile, the leaders of the profession plied their trade elsewhere. By the same token, those doyens of Victorian and Edwardian occupational medicine: Charles Thackrah and the three Thomases (Arlidge, Oliver and Legge) were not only few in number but, decidedly, members of the second rank of the medical pantheon. This, perhaps, reflects less on their intrinsic abilities than on public and professional receptiveness to their writings.[9]

In view of the medical profession's long neglect of occupational illness, it is ironic that one of the few middle-class groups that faced a significant occupational health risk was the medical profession itself. Obviously, this was mainly owing to practitioners' regular contact with infectious disease. The early-nineteenth century occupational health pioneer, John Darwall, author of *Diseases of Artisans with Particular Reference to the Inhabitants of Birmingham*, died in 1833, at the age of 37 when, as a result of performing a post-mortem examination, a hand wound was infected with pus from the cadaver. The susceptibility of Darwall and, presumably, of other medical practitioners to contract illness from the patients they treated raises a question of definition. Darwall clearly succumbed to an occupational disease but, during the period covered by this study, occupational illness was viewed as a condition of manual labour or (given that surgery undoubtedly comprises manual work) of manual labourers who belonged to the lower socio-economic groups. Clearly, it is necessary to decide what constitutes occupational illness and how victims of such diseases are to be defined. This is important in terms of indicating the extent of occupational ill health in society. But the question arises: is it possible to quantify the amount of occupational illness among British workers of the nineteenth century?

Since the early 1800s, if not earlier, government and society have sought to quantify all manner of phenomena as a prelude to the making of public policy.[10] The census is the prime example, while Thomas Malthus's projections about famine were founded on statistical speculations about population growth. Much of this enthusiasm for quantification centred upon commercial matters, but it also involved questions of social policy. Malthusian concerns influenced the decisions to conduct the early censuses. They also provided the backdrop to the *Poor Law Amendment Act, 1834* which, arguably, was the single most important piece of social policy legislation in the whole of the nineteenth century. Notwithstanding the passion for counting, for much of the nineteenth century and well beyond, information about the incidence of occupational ill health is scanty. Factory inspectors, who, from 1845, recorded statistics of accidents, had no obligation to collect occupational disease data for another fifty years. As a result, there are few official indications (and less hard data) of the connections between work and ill health. When calculations were made, usually in respect of a particular trade in the course of an isolated investigation, the results were generally fragmentary, inconclusive and unsatisfactory. As a result we are heavily reliant on anecdotal evidence of the sort provided by Charles Shaw. In his autobiography, first published in the early-twentieth century, Shaw reflected on the unhealthy state of the North Staffordshire pottery industry of the early-Victorian period. There was, he said:

> heavy sickness and mortality in those days. If I was to ask the question, 'Where are the friends of my youth?' with comparatively few exceptions, I should have to say, 'They have long been lying in their graves.' What holocausts have been offered to our great but badly-managed industry?[11]

Victorian mortality tables indicate that innkeepers and licensed victuallers ran a particularly high risk of premature death while Thackrah considered them 'generally unhealthy', not least because they were 'almost universally addicted to unnecessary drinking' as a result either of addiction or of yielding to customers' solicitation.[12] Thomas Oliver referred to them as 'notoriously a short-lived class' whose life styles involved 'considerable danger'. They took little exercise, worked long hours in an atmosphere 'reeking with the odour of spirits, tobacco smoke [and] emanations from the men and women who lounge at the bar'.[13] They also ate irregular meals, faced recurrent temptation to drink and experienced a state of constant stress both in endeavouring to maintain order among their customers and in avoiding breaches of the licensing laws. Were such men, when they contracted alcoholism, gout, urinary or liver disease, victims of occupational ill health? Since the incidence of alcoholism among publicans, innkeepers and their servants was many times higher than for all occupied males, common sense suggests that they were. Officially, they were not. When, in 1906, the 'no fault' system of workmen's compensation was extended to victims of specified occupational illness (initially, lead, mercury, arsenic and phosphorus poisoning, anthrax and ankylostomiasis), the act specified that for ill health to be compensable it had to arise 'out of and in the course of employment'.[14] Publicans were not covered (and neither were surgeons). The act's framers were intent on excluding claims for any condition which might be contracted by the general population. Cirrhosis of the liver could afflict any heavy drinker; inn keeping may have been a high-risk occupation but as far as parliament and the courts were concerned alcoholic publicans were not victims of an occupational disease. If logic suggests otherwise, it may also underline the impossibility of arriving at any realistic appreciation of the 'true' extent of occupational ill health. Indeed, it should be noted that that ubiquitous 'occupational disease' of the early-twenty-first century: stress, is now deemed to afflict at least 30% of the population.[15] It follows, therefore, that on some definitions at least, occupational illness is an extremely widespread phenomenon. If this seems to beg the questions as regards quantification, it is worth quoting from a 1995 government report in which the Department of Health's Chief Medical Officer observed that the 'amount of harm caused by accidents and health risks in the workplace is notoriously difficult to quantify'.[16]

There is another point to be made here. Those who worked long hours in unwholesome atmospheres or performed heavy work in extremes of temperature, or stood for long periods in damp conditions often received poor pay. As a result they also endured sub-standard housing in unsanitary neighbourhoods and ate inadequate meals. To what extent were their health problems the consequence of work? To put it another way, which contributed more to ill health: Manchester or the mill? Except in the most general terms, such questions are unanswerable. Indeed they are largely meaningless; social class and place of residence, in other words, accident of birth, were the main determinants of where people worked just as it was accident of birth that mainly determined the sort of food they ate and the kind of residence in which they lived. Hence the reality is that, leaving aside specific diseases that were unarguably contracted 'out of and in the course of employment', occupation was, routinely, but one factor in an unhealthy lifestyle.[17]

In any case, it might be asked, even if we possessed official statistics, what would they reveal about 'real' incidence? Evidence from recent years suggests that these may grossly underestimate shop-floor realities. During the 1980s the annual number of occupational disease fatalities reported to the Health and Safety Executive was about 750. In 1978 the Royal Commission on Civil Liability estimated that only some 20% of occupationally-related illness was reported. If this were so then the annual number of fatalities would have been in the region of 3750. Yet trade union estimates paint a still grimmer picture, that is, some 20,000 occupational ill-health fatalities each year. Even the official statistics are impressive: 1.6m accidents at work annually and 2.2m cases of work-related illness. Each year 30m work days are lost and 20,000 people forced to give up work at an estimated total cost of between £11bn-£16bn per year (2-3% of GDP).[18] So it is worth repeating that society's traditional neglect of occupational ill health should not be assumed to indicate the small scale of the problem.

For the nineteenth century we have very little knowledge of morbidity and mortality rates even for single industrial diseases, let alone all work-related ailments. As we have seen, defining occupational ill health is highly subjective, so much so that there are few illnesses of which it can be stated categorically that workplace conditions have played no part. But even if occupational ill health is so narrowly defined as to make it a comparatively small-scale problem, it should be recognised that some diseases that were, numerically, less significant than others – cholera is again the obvious example – helped spawn large-scale state intervention. In the case of cholera it was not the scale of its depredations but the fact that it was a 'shock disease'. Its inexorable progress towards Britain's shores, its rapid onset, its horrible symptoms and the speed with which it could kill roused both the individual and the collective imagination, inspiring a mixture of fear and loathing on the part of its potential victims. Of all occupational diseases only anthrax, which was rare, awakened similar emotions – gaining it, as we shall see, an undeserved 'eminence' (in relation to the number of its victims) among industrial diseases. Hence, it is hard to accept that it was the small scale and infrequency of industrial diseases that led to them being neglected for so long. To explain such neglect it is necessary to look elsewhere.

In legal theory, those who suffered ill health, or the dependents of those who died, as a result of exposure to unhealthy conditions in the workplace, could sue their employers for damages. In practice, such actions did not arise. Until 1880, for several reasons, the most important of which was the inequality of wealth between plaintiff and defendant, tort actions by injured employees against their employers were extremely uncommon. In cases of ill health, problems of diagnosis and proving a link between a specific illness and a particular employer were insuperable. After the passage of the *Employers' Liability Act, 1880,* which modified the legal barriers to successful negligence suits by employees against their employers, a few injured workers (and their dependents) did bring successful personal injury actions, but in every case, these related to accidents involving contusion, laceration, fracture, asphyxiation or burn. In 1894 the Employers' Liability Amendment Bill included a clause that would have allowed compensation to be claimed in cases of occupational ill health resulting from an employer's failure to take reasonable precautions. However, the bill foundered on the 'contracting out' question. The difficulties of establishing that sickness was contracted in a particular employment and through no fault of the plaintiff proved insurmountable throughout the nineteenth century.[19]

Only after the introduction of 'no-fault' compensation, under the terms of the *Workmen's Compensation Act, 1897*, did it become possible for victims of occupational ill health to gain financial redress from their employers. The 'no-fault' principle enabled those workers covered by the 1897 act to gain compensation without having to establish that their incapacity had been caused by the negligence of their employer. They had only to show that their injury arose 'out of and in the course of employment'. The 1897 act was limited to victims of workplace accidents, but in 1905 the House of Lords decided that a workman who contracted anthrax (one of the Home Office's 'scheduled', that is, recognised, industrial diseases) while sorting wool was entitled to benefit under the act since the entry of the anthrax bacillus into the woolsorter's body was an accident in the sense of being 'an unlooked-for mishap or an untoward event' which was not expected or designed.[20] Thus, anthrax was differentiated from other industrial diseases the development of which was gradual rather than traceable to a specific moment. Before this, as we shall see, certain china and earthenware firms in the Potteries, in an effort to deflect criticism and unwelcome regulation, had agreed to establish their own system for compensating victims of lead poisoning. Then, the *Workmen's Compensation Act, 1906* allowed claims from employees suffering from one of six specified diseases: ankylostomiasis, anthrax and lead, phosphorus, mercury and arsenic poisoning. Before long this list was extended.[21]

Until these developments in workmen's compensation in the early-twentieth century, those whose illnesses were occupationally-induced had little chance of obtaining compensation from their employers and every expectation of a future lived either as a burden on their family and friends, on public charity, or on the meagre public benefits supplied by a deterrent-led and stigmatising poor law.[22] In these circumstances, the lack of concern expressed about occupational diseases by the labour movement is surprising. After all, in a relatively low welfare and low health care society, such as Victorian Britain, nothing was of more importance to a worker than a fit and healthy body. The lack of emphasis the labour movement placed on occupational health for much of the nineteenth century reflects the fragmented and disorganised state of that movement, ignorance of the nature and extent of the hazards which existed, a preference for safeguarding employment rather than improving health and safety standards and an emphasis on achieving political change ahead of social reform.

For the reasons given above, occupational health regulation is a comparatively recent development. In Britain, in relation to any specific occupational disease, it can be traced back to the 1880s when the *Factory and Workshop Act, 1883* imposed restrictions on the manufacture of carbonate of lead, a product vital to the paint trade.[23] Although some nations, especially the Germanic, had acted to protect workers somewhat earlier than Britain, others, including the United States, were much slower to regulate the so-called 'dangerous trades'.[24] Generally speaking, the British response to the health hazards of work came long after action had been taken to deal with the problem of industrial accidents. The first significant attempt to improve safety and prevent accidents dates from the *Factory Act, 1844*, a measure that required the occupiers of textile factories to fence certain machinery and take other accident prevention measures. It was soon followed by legislation that imposed safety standards on colliery owners. In both instances government inspectors armed with powers of prosecution provided enforcement. In the second half of the nineteenth century a series of measures sought to deal with occupational safety in most manufacturing industry, mining and, to a lesser extent, transport. From about the 1860s increasing attention came to be given to the financial compensation of employees who suffered injury at work.[25] Yet even in the 1890s that indefatigable social investigator, Charles Booth, who presided over a monumental survey of life and work in London, all but ignored occupational health and safety.[26]

Why did politicians, bureaucrats and social investigators overlook occupational health at a time when questions of safety were attracting increasing attention? Although we lack hard data on industrial morbidity, it is unlikely that neglect was a reflection of the high standards of health, hygiene and sanitation in British industry. As this study will show, the surviving evidence suggests that the Victorian factory could be unhealthy as well as unsafe. The specific hazards which workers faced varied from industry to industry but dust, fume, excessive heat, poor ventilation and poisonous materials were among the perils factory hands were most likely to encounter when going about their work. The consequences of all these could be invalidity, inability to work, poverty and premature death. While the unfenced straps, cogs, cables, hoists and looms that could 'scalp' a woman, slice off a child's arm, or crush a man's bone and flesh were more obvious hazards than toxic vapours, they were not necessarily more numerous or more life threatening. On the contrary, if a recent suggestion is to be believed, for in the 1980s deaths from occupationally-induced disease were estimated to outnumber fatal accidents in a ratio as high as 10:1.[27] There is no reason to suppose that this ratio would have been much different in the 1880s.

Yet amputated, bruised and fractured limbs clearly provided more compelling reasons for state intervention than cases of nausea or colic, even if these could presage serious, sometimes fatal, illness. The policy preference for safety regulation may be explained in several ways. Accidents were visible and discrete events the immediate causes of which were often obvious and preventable; they also tended to produce the classic 'body on the floor'. In contrast, an industrial disease developed over time – sometimes a considerable period of time. In many cases its origins were unclear, even to medical science; frequently its victims had left their jobs, thereby slipping beyond the view of factory inspectors, before their conditions became critical. As a result, occupational ill health stood in more or less the same relation to an occupational accident as a single accident stood in regard to a disaster. As John Benson has observed, the contemporary and historical perception of colliery accidents and fatalities is of major disasters, caused either by roof falls or explosions, which claimed dozens, if not hundreds of lives.[28] The reality, however, is that most mining deaths involved either an individual or a handful of miners. These were men who died because of a minor roof fall, because a rock fell on a head, because a tool was dropped down the shaft or because an underground truck ran into them. Put together, however, these isolated fatalities totalled hundreds of workers each year, hence Benson's use of the phrase 'disasters by instalment'.[29] Yet it was the somewhat atypical 'single-event catastrophe' that captured newspaper attention and the public's imagination, prompted official inquiries, led to the collection of (often huge) disaster funds for the relief of victims' relatives and even, as in the case of the Hartley Colliery disaster of 1862 in which 240 miners died following the collapse of winding equipment and the consequent blockage of the only pit shaft, provoked a legislative response.[30] If the individual worker crushed by a piece of machinery was all but 'invisible' – little more than a statistic in the official tables – how much more hidden was the

Sheffield file-cutter or London compositor brought low by inhaling lead dust? Such people were not even included in the official statistics until the *Factory and Workshop Act, 1895* – fifty-one years after the collection of accident statistics had commenced – decreed that they should be.[31] In short, therefore, public opinion, the press, politicians and the law found it easier to respond to accidents than to long-term problems of occupational ill health.

Ancient and modern

Although occupational health regulation is a comparatively recent phenomenon, occupational ill health is not. Man is thought to have been mining, smelting and moulding lead, a highly toxic metal, as long ago as 7000BC. In all probability some of those involved in these ventures suffered illness as a result.[32] Later, the ancient Romans made 'prodigious' use of lead, mining it throughout their far-flung Empire. It has been suggested that occupational and non-occupational exposure in Imperial Rome were 'relatively common'. It has even been argued – though with little consensus – that lead poisoning, by lowering aristocratic birth rates and causing high child mortality, was responsible for the Empire's collapse. At most, it would seem to have been a contributory factor.[33]

Because lead was such a versatile, useful and readily obtainable metal, it remained in regular use long after its toxicity had been medically established. The Greek physician, Nikander, produced the earliest surviving description of its poisonous properties in the second century BC. Thereafter, occasional accounts of poisoning probably or possibly attributable to it were published, including by Hippocrates, but all of these focused upon non-occupational exposures. However, Hippocrates' writings do contain the earliest recorded mention of occupational disease. Among the maladies he describes are those affecting fullers (cleaners and dyers of clothes), metallurgists, tailors, farm workers and fishermen. Subsequently, a number of ancient *savants*, by no means all of whom were medical men, referred in their writings to the relationship between illness and occupation. These included such luminaries as Aristotle, Juvenal, Lucretius, Plato, Pliny the Elder and Galen. In his *Natural History* Pliny (23/4-79 AD) even referred to the use of protective bladder masks by red lead workers. Though this is thought to be the first recorded example of the practice of occupational hygiene, the efficacy such masks is open to question. Since bladders are air tight, breathing would have been possible only if gaps had existed; through such gaps dust as well as air must have inevitably passed.[34]

What do these and other references indicate about knowledge and attitudes towards occupational health in the ancient world? Opinion is divided. On the one hand, it has been suggested, the references are sufficiently numerous to suggest that the link between work and certain diseases was widely recognised. This, however, may be going to far. The brevity of the references, the long time span which separates them and the somewhat tenuous connection between some 'diseases' and occupations, for example, priests with varicose veins, might suggest the opposite conclusion. Certainly, there is no classical treatise dealing either with a specific occupation and the health hazards it posed, or with a specific disease and the occupations that might have placed an individual at particular risk of contracting it. Furthermore, as Teleky observed, allusions to protective measures are 'very scarce'.[35]

There is little extant evidence of public interest in occupational health in either the 'Dark' or Middle Ages. As Teleky says, medical science lacked the sophistication to identify the physiological damage and even if this had not been the case, neither the will nor the technology to prevent would have been available.[36] In the fifteenth century Ulrich Ellenbog (1440-1499) wrote about the diseases of miners,[37] as did the sixteenth century German physician Georg Agricola. In his twelve-volume study of the mining and metal industries, *De Re Metallica* (1556), he described the dust diseases that afflicted miners in the Carpathian Mountains. He also made suggestions for protective clothing, masks and pit ventilation in order to lessen risks. Other authors, including Paracelsus (1493-1541), described the lung ailments to which miners were prone. Paracelsus's *Von der Bergsucht und andern Krankheiten der Bergleute* (*Pthisis and Other Diseases of Miners*), published posthumously in 1567, has been described as the first comprehensive account of the diseases of any occupational group. It dealt with diseases arising from contact with metals and those that had their origins in the smelting process.[38] In the seventeenth century a number of other writers tackled the relationship between work and disease. Thus, papers on the subject appeared in the *Transactions of the Royal Society*.[39] However, the first comprehensive treatise on occupational diseases and their prevention was published by the Italian, Bernardino Ramazzini (1633-1714), in 1700. This was *De Morbis Artificum* or *The Diseases of Workers*, a book that impressed Adam Smith and, indeed, has been variously termed 'one of the most original medical works ever written' and 'the first comprehensive and systematic treatise on occupational diseases'.[40]

Inspired by observing and conversing with the cleaner who emptied his cesspit, Ramazzini made a detailed inquiry into the health conditions associated with a range of professions, trades and occupations including those of metal miner, chemist, painter, tobacco worker, laundress, midwife, athlete, corpsebearer, fisherman, wood worker, soap maker and many others. In all, he studied 53 extant and defunct occupational groups (41 in his initial study and 12 in his supplement) excluding 'learned men'. In practice these numbers were somewhat higher because three of his groups were the portmanteau categories of 'workers who stand', 'sedentary workers' and Jews. As we have seen, Ramazzini was not tilling a virgin soil, but his approach differed from all his predecessors. Whereas they had focused upon a single category of worker or a single hazard, he considered a number of risks affecting a wide variety of contrasting employments. In so doing he established a pattern which was followed, in Britain, by such distinguished investigators as Charles Thackrah, John Arlidge, Thomas Oliver and Donald Hunter, all of whom owed a considerable intellectual debt to Ramazzini. Inevitably, given the state of medical and scientific knowledge in the seventeenth century, Ramazzini was stronger on the description of diseases than on questions of causation and treatment. Nevertheless, his analysis has a relevance that goes far beyond the geographical, chronological and cultural confines in which it was made. For example, his observations that workers stuck with jobs they cursed, that they were often guilty of ignoring personal hygiene and that they neglected to take simple precautions would have struck a chord with nineteenth and twentieth century English factory inspectors and occupational health officers. By the same token, his exasperation with seventeenth century Italian farmers' neglect of their own well-being possesses a relevance to the occupational health field, which is well nigh universal:

> Now what can the medical profession do to protect these tillers of the soil whom we need so much. To suggest to our farmers in Italy any precautions of a medical sort that might safeguard them seems little short of absurd, since they seldom or never consult doctors about this and when one does make some suggestion they pay no attention.[41]

•

Medicine men

In the eighteenth and early-nineteenth centuries the literature of occupational health slowly expanded with English translations of early editions of Ramazzini's work appearing in 1705 and 1746. William Buchan made extensive use of the second of these (Robert James's) when preparing his lengthy chapter on workers' health for his popular treatise on home medicine: *Domestic Medicine or the Family Physician* (Edinburgh, 1769). The Frenchman, Philibert Patissier, also relied on Ramazzini in compiling his *Traité des Maladies des Artisans.* However, on the whole, in Britain at least, most published studies on occupational illness dealt with particular trades and/or specific ailments. They were usually written by medical practitioners whose daily duties brought them into regular contact with work-related disease. Prominent among these were military and naval medical officers. In a century of almost incessant warfare Sir John Pringle (*Observations on the Diseases of the Army in Camp and Garrison*, London, 1752 and *A Discourse upon some late Improvements of the Means for Preserving the Health of Mariners, London*, 1776), James Lind (*Essay on the Most Effectual Means of Preserving the Health of Seamen in the Royal Navy,* London, 1757) and Gilbert Blane (*Observations on the Diseases Incident to Seamen,* London, 1785 and *A Short Account of the Most Effectual Means for Preserving the Health of Seaman,* London, 1781? and *Observations on the Diseases Incident to Seamen*, London, 1785) collectively provided thoroughgoing assessments of health and disease among Britain's armed forces.[42]

Outside the armed services, Percivall Pott (in 1775) and Benjamin Bell (1794) demonstrated a link between the trade of chimney sweeping and cancer of the scrotum and testes. Pott's initial work has since come to be seen accepted as the 'first description of an occupational cancer'.[43] Meanwhile, motivated, no doubt, by the growth of manufacturing industry and the apparent link between health and work, a number of other late-eighteenth and early-nineteenth century provincial medical practitioners concerned themselves with occupational diseases. For example, James Johnstone wrote about consumption among needle pointers in Worcestershire (especially Redditch);[44] Thomas Percival about lead poisoning among miners, smelters and factory workers;[45] J. Jackson and James Kay about 'the influence of cotton manufactories on the health';[46] Arnold Knight, G.C. Holland and Charles Flavell about the lung diseases of cutlery grinders in Redditch, Sheffield and elsewhere;[47] William Allison about the respiratory problems of Edinburgh stonemasons ('I have reason to believe, that there is hardly an instance of a mason regularly employed in hewing stones in Edinburgh, living free from phthisical symptoms to the age of 50');[48] Charles Hastings about chest and other diseases among the leather dressers, glovers, needlepointers, china workers and stone cutters of his native Worcestershire.[49] In many areas of medicine the opportunity for those distant from large centres of population to contribute to medical science were strictly circumscribed. The above examples illustrate how the localised occurrence of particular diseases provided opportunities for provincial practitioners to make names for themselves by publishing papers on the relationship between health and occupation in the localities in which they resided.

By the nineteenth century occupational health had become the concern of a number of governments in continental Europe. 'In England alone', the *Lancet* observed in 1831, 'is it that the principles of popular liberty are so sagely maintained that the people are allowed... to be suffocated in the asphyxiating vapours of manufactories, without the slightest concern being manifested by the rulers of the land'.[50] The observation was made in an enthusiastic review of Charles Turner Thackrah's *The Effects of the Principal Arts, Trades and Professions and of Civic States and Habits of Living, on Health and Longevity; with a Particular Reference to the Trades and Manufactures of Leeds; with Suggestions for the Removal of Many of the Agents which Produce Disease and Shorten the Duration of Life*. Hunter has described this slim monograph, with its less than catchy title, as being 'the first treatise of any kind to be written in English on this subject, apart from translations of Ramazzini'. Judged on criteria of 'comprehensiveness, first hand clinical experience and constructive proposals for improvements', Hunter regarded it as a considerable advance on *Diseases of Workers*.[51]

Thackrah (1795-1833) was born in Yorkshire, the son of a chemist and druggist. To his mother's disappointment he declined to take holy orders, opting instead, at the age of 16, to pursue an apprenticeship with a Leeds surgeon-apothecary. In 1815 he went to Guy's Hospital in London where he came under the influence of one of the most distinguished surgeons of the period, Astley Cooper. In the following year he became a MRCS and Licentiate of the Society of Apothecaries. On returning to Leeds he began to practise medicine, including as 'town surgeon' (poor law medical officer) and, later, in partnership with the master to whom he had once been apprenticed. In 1826 he began his own School of Anatomy which, in 1831, merged with the Leeds Medical School. By this time, presumably inspired by the experience of practising medicine within a rapidly expanding industrial town, Thackrah had published the book that made his name. Written as a pro-reform contribution to the factory movement, Thackrah's 'tract' received enthusiastic reviews from the medical journals. It quickly sold out thereby encouraging its author, notwithstanding his own affliction with an advanced case of chronic tuberculosis, to produce a revised and greatly expanded version of the work. In this he discussed an additional 120 occupations, a number of which were followed only beyond the confines of Leeds. In so doing he much increased the universality of the book's appeal.

As the title of his study indicates, Thackrah appreciated the close connection between work, home and health. The starting point for his inquiry was industrialisation. While recognising that this had generated vast wealth, he questioned whether it had done so at the expense of 'the health of the millions who spend their lives in manufactories'. Did they, in short, have the same life expectancy as agricultural workers? The mere appearance of town dwellers suggested to Thackrah that they were less healthy than their rural counterparts. By studying the mortality figures for the three Ridings of Yorkshire he came to the conclusion that 'the duration of human life is considerably less in the West-Riding, the manufacturing district, than in other parts of Yorkshire'.[52] In fact he estimated that in Great Britain as a whole over 50,000 people per year died from what he called 'the effects of manufactures, civic states and the intemperance connected with these states and occupations'. Hence, Thackrah saw occupational ill health as an aspect of a larger phenomenon encompassing changed lifestyles and environments. In combination, they were responsible for high rates of urban mortality, especially among the working classes in particular occupations. But Thackrah was not merely a demographer; he believed that many of the hazards of work could be 'immediately removed or diminished' and included in his book many practical proposals for improving health and safety.

Welcomed by the medical press – the *Lancet*'s 2000 word review covered the first four pages of one issue – Thackrah's second edition was also praised by Charles Hastings, the founder of the Provincial Medical and Surgical Association (British Medical Association from 1855), of which Thackrah was one of the original members. Hastings could speak from a position of authority, having himself studied occupational illness. The factory reformer, Michael Sadler, was another admirer.[53] When Thackrah's study appeared, the *Lancet* noted, somewhat cryptically, that it 'seems to be the precursor of some public excitement on the important topic to which it relates'. If the expectation was that occupational health regulation was in the offing, it was an expectation that went unfulfilled, notwithstanding the new phase of factory legislation that was about to commence. On the other hand, if the *Lancet*'s reviewer had in mind an upsurge of medical interest in the health of workers he was closer to the mark, for while *The Effects of the Principal Arts, Trades and Professions* may have been the first major study of its kind to be published in the English language, it was not the first such work to be produced by an Englishman. Little more than a decade earlier, in 1821, John Darwall (1796-1833), who was almost an exact contemporary of Thackrah, had submitted his Edinburgh MD thesis, *Dissertatio Medica Inauguralis de Morbis Artificum, Praecipue eorum qui Birminghamiae Habitant*. Written, in line with prevailing academic custom, in Latin, it borrowed Ramazzini's title and dealt with occupational disease in Birmingham.[54]

With its focus on a particular town which, like Leeds, was at the cutting edge of industrialisation, Darwall's work, though on a far smaller scale, had much in common with Thackrah's. In it Darwall noted the close relationship between work and health and also the neglect of occupational health as a field of inquiry. His researches, which involved interviews with workers as well as visits to their homes and factories, convinced him that, regardless of the specific nature of industrial employment, there were seven basic causes of occupational ill health: long hours, over exertion, poor posture, excessive noise and light, dust, exposure to chemicals and temperature fluctuations. The object of his dissertation was to document and describe the influence of these factors. Darwall saw long hours of work as an evil mainly affecting children, particularly in terms of retarded or impaired physical development. He also regarded over exertion and poor posture in terms of injury and deformity rather than disease, though he did associate indigestion and pulmonary tuberculosis with excessive periods spent in the same position, for example at a workbench. With little to say on the subjects of light and noise and variations in temperature, Darwall's thesis comes to life only when he deals with the influence of dust and chemical inhalation. Darwall visited a number of factories in which the air was heavily loaded with dust. Personal experience alerted him to the dangers: 'I entered... a factory where gun-barrels are ground and as I went near the grindstone I was covered with dust. Carelessly I inhaled, when suddenly I was seized with coughing which remained troublesome for twenty-four hours'. Not for nothing did he regard dust as 'the most deadly cause of illnesses amongst tradesmen'.[55]

Darwall's thesis, brief and superficial as it was, compares unfavourably with the work of Ramazzini and Thackrah. As its twentieth century translator says: 'As a contribution to the literature of trade diseases, the discourse has no great merit'.[56] It is noteworthy chiefly as an early, pre-Thackrah, example of the medical interest in occupational health at a time when the profession's standard attitude was utter neglect. Taken along with his 1833 article, 'Diseases of Artisans', which Darwall contributed to the *Cyclopaedia of Practical Medicine* shortly before his death,[57] Thackrah's book and a variety of specialist papers, it provides evidence of the first stirrings of professional interest in the subject. Yet this interest developed only slowly and patchily. Although John Simon, William Guy and others (see subsequent chapters) did valuable work, it was not until the 1890s, when Thomas Arlidge published his magisterial *Hygiene, Diseases and Mortality of Occupations* (1892) that Thackrah's book was finally superseded.[58] This, as Stephen Huzzard has pointed out, speaks 'to sad neglect of the field' rather than the enduring practical relevance of Thackrah's work. All of this was in sharp contrast to the position in nineteenth century France and Germany where occupational health 'took its place in the domain of medical research', attracting what Arlidge called 'a numerous band of observers – far too numerous to designate by name'.[59]

With Thackrah's *Effects of Arts, Trades and Professions on Health and Longevity*, which it comfortably surpassed in terms of scale and scope, Arlidge's book stands as the foremost study of industrial health and medicine to be produced in nineteenth century Britain. Quite simply, it is a medical 'classic' which, because of its accessible style, concise treatment and avoidance of technicalities, received copious attention from the general medical press as well as lavish praise from specialist periodicals. Even Queen Victoria, so it is alleged, was an admirer.[60] As for the *British Medical Journal*, it considered the book to be 'the most comprehensive and important work on the subject [of occupational health] which has ever issued from the English press'.[61]

J.T. Arlidge (1822-1899) was born in Chatham, Kent. The son of a medical practitioner, he graduated MB (1846) and MD (1867) and qualified MRCP in 1847 and FRCP in 1869. Although the early years of his career were mainly devoted to the subject of mental illness, Arlidge's field of specialisation underwent an abrupt change when, in 1862, he was appointed consultant physician to the North Staffordshire Infirmary in the Potteries. Thereafter his main professional interest was in respiratory ailments. This switch of professional interest was no doubt due to the fact that the locality to which he had moved was renowned for its poor air quality. Inevitably, Arlidge's work brought him into regular contact with occupational ill health, including the dust diseases of potters, colloquially known as 'potters' phthisis' or 'potters' rot'. Indeed, as certifying surgeon of factories for three of the 'six towns' of the Potteries, Longton, Fenton and Stoke, his knowledge and experience of the diseases of pottery workers, particularly of pulmonary ailments and lead poisoning became encyclopaedic.[62] Already an accomplished author when he arrived in the Potteries – his *State of Lunacy and Legal Provision for the Insane* (London: Churchill, 1859) had been warmly reviewed in the *Lancet* – Arlidge soon began to produce a regular flow of lectures and papers on the relationship between manufacturing industry and health.[63] While most of these dealt with the diseases of potters, several tackled the health hazards of other occupations. Eventually Arlidge's reputation was such that he was invited to deliver the 1889 Milroy Lectures at the Royal College of Physicians.[64] He chose as his subject 'the hygiene and diseases of occupation'. As he later noted,

> I felt it was a subject I could best discourse upon; and that, too, it was one which possessed the charm of novelty, inasmuch as few British physicians had studied it and no treatise had been written upon it for a long series of years, although its importance could not be denied.[65]

The reception accorded his four lectures, which dealt only with dust diseases, was such that the president of the RCP encouraged Arlidge to publish them as a book. But Arlidge had other plans. To rush into print, he believed, would be to contribute 'no more than an isolated chapter of a very wide topic'. He decided instead to expand the lectures into 'a general outline of the hygiene, diseases and mortality of all the principal occupations pursued in this country. In reaching this decision Arlidge, who was no longer a young man, committed himself to what he later described as 'a task of great magnitude' involving a demanding schedule of reading and factory visits as well as the compilation of some 600 pages of text.[66] But his decision was triumphantly vindicated by a work which established him, in the few years of life left to him, as the undisputed doyen of British occupational medicine.

•

The factory question

The rise of the factory system and of a factory movement intent on reforming conditions of work, especially those experienced by children, engendered a degree of controversy about occupational health. Indeed, the fundamental justification for the factory acts, the first of which (the *Health and Morals of Apprentices Act*) was passed in 1802, was protection of the health and welfare of child workers deemed unable to safeguard themselves from the evils of excessive labour in a dangerous and unhealthy environment (prevailing ideology insisting that adult workers were fully capable of looking after themselves without state assistance). This book focuses on occupational disease in a range of manufacturing trades and processes in the Victorian and Edwardian periods. But since the starting point for subsequent chapters is around 1840, it is appropriate at this juncture to consider the degree to which health issues surfaced in the so-called factory question of the early-nineteenth century.[67]

The factory question had a number of dimensions with many reformers being particularly anxious about the moral, religious and educational consequences of child labour in textile mills. Insofar as physical damage was concerned, ill-treatment, excessive hours of labour resulting in stunted or deformed growth, the prevalence of infectious disease and, to a lesser extent, accidental injury were prime worries. Although some observers were quick to point out the unhealthiness of work within the domestic system of industry (where the workplace might consist of a cramped, low-ceilinged, damp and poorly-ventilated cellar),[68] many believed that the factory environment was, for various reasons, more or less synonymous with ill health. As the physician, Thomas Percival, wrote, even the larger, supposedly well-conducted, factories

> are generally injurious to the constitution of those employed in them, even when no particular diseases prevail, from the close confinement which is enjoined, from the debilitating effects of hot and impure air and from the want of the active exercises which nature points out as essential to childhood and youth, to invigorate the system and to fit our species for the employment and the duties of manhood.[69]

John Aikin agreed. 'The cotton trade', he observed, 'while it affords employment to all ages, has debilitated the constitutions and retarded the growth of many and made an alarming increase in the mortality'.[70] Such health hazards did not arise from exposure to invasive germs or poisons connected with the manufacturing process. Hence, when the framers of the first factory act sought to improve the hygiene of the industrial environment by requiring, in the interests of health, both the adequate ventilation of workrooms and the limewashing of internal walls, their main aim was to control the outbreaks of fever (typhus) which beset the cotton mills along with prisons, ships and other sites of huddled humanity.[71] Either because the health hazards specific to occupation were insufficiently understood, or because they seldom affected textile workers, discussion of occupational illness was not central to debates on the factory question.[72] Nevertheless, there was one aspect of textile production that a number of observers believed to pose a definite health risk arising directly out of the manufacturing process. This was dust.

Several of the early factory inquiries mentioned the dust-laden atmosphere of some textile factories and processes. In 1816 Robert Peel's Committee received a good deal of evidence about health in textile factories, much of it in relation to dust. While some witnesses minimised the dust hazard – one silk manufacturer insisting that silk was 'a perfectly clean article altogether' and not at all dusty – others emphasised that certain processes (especially the scutching and carding of cotton) were extremely dusty: As one said, 'I could scarcely see the women who worked at the engine'.[73] The best-conducted works could be well ventilated. For example, Richard Arkwright's Derbyshire mill was said to have efficient exhaust ventilation capable of clearing the air of the scutching room.[74] That such systems were not in general use was underlined when, in 1832, the Sadler Committee, appointed to consider Michael Sadler's factory bill, also highlighted the dust hazard. The Sadler Committee, was criticised at the time, as it has been since, for being 'packed' with reformers, selective in its taking of evidence and highly directive in terms of leading witnesses – in other words, biased.[75] Consequently, the evidence it took, which was published without comment, must be viewed with caution. Nevertheless, this evidence cannot simply be dismissed as unreliable, for when Edwin Chadwick's *Factories Inquiry Commission* (1833) scrutinised it, much was incapable of refutation.[76]

The Sadler Committee took evidence from a number of workers on the extent of dust in textile factories and the health consequences to which it could give rise. For example, David Brook, a Leeds cloth-dresser, said the dust (and steam) could be very bad in some premises:

> The dust from one side of the room and the steam from the other, were such, that we were under the necessity of putting a

handkerchief over our mouths at times, when we were working, for hours together. The effect produced on us was, that many men were actually obliged to be removed from the room, otherwise they would not have been able to stand the work at all.[77]

When asked whether he believed that remaining in such a room was consistent with the preservation of health, he replied: 'I am positive it is not, from experience'. Others expressed similar views. For example, Stephen Binns, who had spent thirty-seven years' in the cotton trade, described conditions in the carding department of one factory with which he was familiar. Carding was notorious for being one of the dirtiest processes in textile manufacture.[78] The dust, which was dense, got onto Binns's lungs making him fear for his life:

I was three weeks so ill that I thought I should have to give up every day, but it left such a weakness upon my lungs that I feel it now when I catch cold; but I believe that if I had stopped there I should not have lived many years; and the men who work in the old mill are all asthmatic; there is one of the name of Baxter, that was in a room under me, who said he could not run 100 yards for five guineas.[79]

Binns, who had no family history of asthma, had begun to feel the effects of the dust within an hour of starting work in the carding department. John Hannam had spent four years as an overlooker (foreman) in a carding room. He too was greatly troubled by the dust, coughing and spitting blood at the end of his day's work. Though only in his twenties, 'I might have been taken if nobody had known me, for 70 years of age'. Charles Burns also spoke of coughing up blood. The dust in the flax mills, he told the committee, (flax mills were probably the dustiest of all) could be so bad that it was difficult to see fellow workers.[80]

One of the criticisms of the evidence given to the Sadler Committee is that witnesses had not only been selected with a view to providing the worst possible picture of factories, but that they had been 'coached' in what to say by various 'short-time' committees (i.e. reform groups dedicated to the establishment of a legal ceiling to working hours). However, not all the witnesses examined were textile workers, for the committee also heard from Charles Turner Thackrah. Now while Thackrah was certainly pro-reform in outlook, he must, with his medical training and special interest in occupational health, also be regarded as an 'expert witness'. He had little to say about dust, but what he did say formed a damning indictment of occupational health standards in the textile industries:

'I may state that I do not recollect that I ever applied the stethoscope to any person who had been twenty years in a dusty mill, in whom I did not find decided marks of disease in the lungs or air tube'.[81] Yet this testimony was somewhat at odds with what Thackrah had to say in his book about the hazards of textile dust – at least in respect of one large and well-run Manchester cotton mill:

> In the first process, the *machining*, or cleaning and opening the cotton.... Much dust is necessarily produced in the process and light flakes of cotton float in the room; but the atmosphere is scarcely fouled, for a machine revolving 1200 times in a minute, produces a current of air, which, enclosed by a casing of wood, conveys the dust through a sort of chimney, quite out of the building. The children in this room made no complaint. The oldest man in it had been sixteen years at the employ. He was thin, but not sickly.[82]

In the spinning rooms there was 'little dust' even though the '[p]articles of cotton float like thistle down', while in weaving '[s]carcely any dust is produced'. Even in the carding room conditions appeared good for the 'dust is not great; the labour is light and the operatives are not crowded'.[83] Although Thackrah noted the occurrence of gastric disorders, headaches, catarrh and other ailments among operatives, he could point to few major health problems. Indeed, the only serious disease of frequent occurrence was 'intemperance'.[84]

How can these apparent discrepancies in Thackrah's opinions to be reconciled? What we cannot do is explain them in terms of the different periods in which Thackrah expressed his views, for his seemingly divergent opinions date from more or less the same time (the early-1830s). A more plausible explanation lies in the different premises to which Thackrah was referring. As observers of early-nineteenth century textile mills frequently noted, conditions varied substantially from factory to factory. In particular, working conditions in the larger, more modern premises were, in the eyes of many visitors, much pleasanter, safer and healthier than those that prevailed in small and antiquated mills. Indeed, Thackrah states in his book that in Manchester mills other than the large well-run factory he visited, 'it appears that the dust is much greater'. Furthermore, when he 'stood in Oxford Road, Manchester and observed the stream of operatives as they left the mills at twelve o'clock' he witnessed an unsettling sight:

> The children were almost universally ill-looking, small, sickly, barefoot and ill-clad. Many *appeared* to be no older than seven. The

> men, generally from 16 to 24 and none aged, were almost as pallid and thin as the children. The women were the most respectable in appearance, but I saw no fresh or fine-looking individuals among them. And in reference to all classes, I was struck with the marked contrast between this and the turn-out from a manufactory of Cloth. Here was nothing like the stout fullers, the hale slubbers, the dirty but merry rosy-faced pieceners. Here I saw, or thought I saw, a degenerate race, – human beings stunted, enfeebled and depraved, – men and women that were not to be aged, – children that were never to be healthy adults. It was a mournful spectacle.[85]

Thackrah went on to record that a mill-owner had tried to persuade him that working conditions were not responsible for the sickliness of Manchester's population. In the opinion of this industrialist, dissipation, sub-standard housing, inadequate nutrition and poor clothing were the real causes. Thackrah was not convinced however. In his opinion long hours of work, insufficient breaks for rest and meals and, above all, the employment of young children were crucial factors in explaining both the lost 'health and vigour' and the 'wretched appearance of workers'. Even so, Thackrah found little evidence of the existence either of specific occupational diseases or of heightened mortality rates. 'We had no reason', he wrote, 'to believe that either at these places [cotton mills] or at the Leeds [woollen] mill examined before, urgent diseases are often produced or the immediate mortality great'. There was some evidence of bronchitis and pulmonary maladies among adult workers, but these were 'neither prominent in feature, *as far as we have observed* nor generally prevalent' (emphasis in original).[86]

What did the Royal Commission on Factories, which reported in 1833, make of the occupational health issue? Although the Commission's reports and evidence ran to hundreds of pages and made use of three medical commissioners, it devoted comparatively little attention to health and dust. Given that the Commission's Report was a major influence upon the terms of the *Factory Act, 1833* (*3 & 4 Will.4 c.103*), this, perhaps, helps to explain why that measure ignored health questions other than in the clause (s.26), first enacted in 1802, which required the regular limewashing of internal walls. As in other factory inquiries, some witnesses played down the dust problem while others, including Robert Blincoe (he of the famous *Memoir*), did the reverse.[87] Dr Bisset Hawkins circulated a medical questionnaire in which twenty 'medical queries' were posed. This went out to twenty-eight medical practitioners based in

Lancashire, Derbyshire and Cheshire. One of the questions touched upon occupational disease: 'Have you met with many instances in which adults employed in factories have been compelled to quit their employment through diseases apparently induced by their occupations?' Twenty-seven replies were received. One merely said that he had not attended adults. Either because the respondents either did not give a direct answer to the question posed or were ambivalent in their replies, the remaining answers defy easy analysis. Some responded with an unambiguous negative, while others were equally unambiguous in reporting findings such as: 'irritation caused in the lungs by the inhalation of the fine particles of cotton floating in the atmosphere of certain rooms in the factory'.[88] The reader of these responses can do little more than record that while some of these doctors considered that employment in some areas of a cotton factory posed a clear risk to health, others believed cotton mills presented either no health hazard, nothing more than a slight risk, or no dangers that were not found in other areas of employment. The Central Commissioners also received actuarial evidence, based on comparative sickness data for East India Company labourers, government dockyard workers, children at Christ's Hospital (the City of London bluecoat school) and textile workers, that there were 'no grounds' for the belief that 'factory labour in any material degree differs in its effects on health from other labour'.[89] When the Central Commissioners, comprising Edwin Chadwick, Thomas Tooke and Thomas Southwood Smith, assessed the evidence they, like Thackrah and others before them, drew a distinction between large modern mills and small, antiquated premises noting that the latter, among their various shortcomings, had 'no contrivance for carrying off dust and other effluvia'.[90]

Discussion of the health conditions in the textile factories was not confined to official inquiries. A number of authors, medical practitioners among them, emphasised the unhealthiness of manufacturing industry. Robert Owen, for example, regarded factories as 'unfavourable to health', pointing to 'the overheated unhealthy atmosphere'.[91] In his autobiography his son recalled how, as a youth he had toured the textile factories of England and Scotland with a view to collecting evidence on the conditions of work experienced by child labour: 'and in all the cotton factories they breathed an atmosphere more or less injurious to the lungs, because of the dust and the minute cotton fibres that pervaded it'.[92] J. Jackson, who criticised the 'heat and confined air, loaded with effluvia', pointed out that cotton workers aged prematurely and that few attained the age of fifty.[93] Again, however, there was a conflict of opinion with some observers playing down the unhealthiness of factory labour. For example, John Farey stated that Derbyshire mills were not 'as unhealthy as some have represented'.[94]

Edward Baines (1800-1890), in his *History of the Cotton Manufacture of Great Britain* (first published in 1835) devoted considerable attention to the question of working conditions in cotton mills. Baines has been termed a nineteenth-century 'worthy' who was 'much troubled by the question of labour and hours and wished to rescue the cotton industry and its controllers from the bad repute into which both had fallen in the public esteem as a result of the partisan and often unscrupulous attacks of Sadler, Oastler and company'.[95] In his book he considered a variety of opinions concerning the health of the workers. He noted that some 'declamatory writers' and 'parliamentary orators' had argued that the

> high wages of the cotton spinners are earned by the entire sacrifice of health and comfort, – that the labour of the mill is so severe, incessant and prolonged, as to destroy the constitution and to exhaust the mental energies of the workmen, – that they breathe a heated and polluted atmosphere, loaded with dust and fibres of cotton, which, entering the lungs, soon produce consumption, – that the exhaustion of their bodies by labour drives them to intemperance as a relief and a stimulus, – that thus their lives are passed in an alternation of depressing drudgery and maddening excitement, without any healthy exercise of the mental faculties, or rational enjoyment.[96]

In addition, it was alleged that children were overworked and beaten, while all workers, adults included, were driven to their physical and mental limits by the pressure of keeping pace with machinery. If all such allegations were true Baines felt that factories deserved to be known as 'hells upon earth'.[97] The question to which Baines addressed himself was: were they true? Much of his analysis in this respect centred on what he termed the 'exaggerations and misstatements' of the factory movement, based on 'a few instances of deformity and injury', especially in respect of the abuse and over-exertion of child workers. Both the factory commission and the recently appointed factory inspectors had, he argued, revealed the allegations to 'contain but a small portion of truth'. While cruelty and abuse did occur, mistreatment was far from the norm. As for the health hazards of employment in a cotton factory, Baines was ready to acknowledge both that 'the labour is not so healthful as labour in husbandry' and that it was not suitable for 'delicate and infirm persons'. All occupations were in some degree hazardous but employment in a cotton factory was 'far less injurious' than a great many other occupations.[98]

For Baines the only real hazard of the cotton mill lay in the air quality:

> The only thing which makes factory labour trying even in delicate children is, that they are confined for long hours and deprived of fresh air: this makes them pale and reduces their vigour, but it rarely brings on disease. The minute fibres of cotton which float in the rooms and are called fly, are admitted, even by medical men, not to be injurious to young persons: it might have been supposed that they would have impeded respiration, or irritated the bronchial membrane, but extensive observation proves that they do so in very few cases. Workmen of more advanced years occasionally suffer from this cause: a 'spinners' phthisis' has been described by medical men and it is attributed to the irritation produced by the dust and cotton inhaled: but it is admitted that the cases are scarcely, if at all, more numerous than in other employments.[99]

Otherwise, the temperature of the mills was pleasantly warm while the air, in the absence of overcrowding, was not noisome through having been repeatedly breathed.

In Peter Gaskell's classic study of the factory system (first published in 1836), a large part of one chapter was devoted to 'the diseases to which the manufacturing population are peculiarly exposed'. Gaskell recognised that the production of cotton yarn gave rise to 'considerable quantities of dust and minute filaments' and that in certain departments in cotton factories 'much dust is diffused through the rooms'. However, he maintained not only that comparatively few workers were exposed to dust but also that in recent years there had been much improvement in terms of ventilating work rooms. Most importantly, Gaskell drew a distinction between the dangers of inhaling vegetable and mineral dusts. While he accepted the latter as being definitely injurious, he regarded cotton (as well as silk and flax) dust to be troublesome irritants only to those unused to the atmosphere of the mill. '[I]n the parties who have become accustomed to such an atmosphere it produces little or no inconvenience' beyond an aggravation of catarrhal disorders. In particular, he refuted any suggestion of a link between pulmonary disease and the inhalation of organic dusts, capping his argument by demonstrating lower mortality rates among rovers, spinners, pieceners and dressers (i.e. textile workers involved in dusty processes) than among weavers (who worked in a largely dust-free atmosphere). For Gaskell the answer to the question: 'Is the atmosphere which is breathed by the factory labourer necessarily injurious to his existence, in consequence of its being loaded with the *debris* of cotton?' was obvious: 'Public opinion says, yes; examination into the facts says no'.[100]

Notwithstanding Engels' claims to the contrary, Gaskell (along with Baines) might fairly be termed a 'champion' of the factory system.[101] Andrew Ure who, like Gaskell, was also a medical practitioner, was undoubtedly such. Ure's *Philosophy of Manufactures*, which included a chapter on the 'health of factory inmates', poured scorn on those who associated factory work with disease. Ure was particularly critical of the evidence given to the Sadler Committee. Like many others he was less concerned with specific occupational health hazards than with infectious disease, especially scrofula and deformities. However, he had much to say about the excellence of the ventilation systems installed in many mills. His judgment 'from a most extensive comparison of facts', was that 'the rustic population of England is less healthy than its factory population'.[102] Another commentator on factories, who wrote in 1841, was W. Cooke Taylor. In many respects his views were similar to those of Gaskell and Ure. He praised the healthy conditions of individual mills, believed that manufacturers understood that it was in their own self-interest to preserve the health of their operatives (after all, they comprised valuable human capital) and judged that the unhealthiness of the population of Manchester had more to do with 'the incessant tide of immigration' than with the textile trade.[103]

What is to be made of these contrasting views about the unhealthiness (or otherwise) of the early-nineteenth century textile mill? Although the health hazards of factory labour were sometimes discussed by polemicists, the factory question was not primarily concerned with occupational health. In making an evaluation it is clearly important to bear in mind that the factory system aroused strong views among both its defenders and critics. Not least because the question was so thoroughly polemicised, it is hard to determine how much of a health hazard the early nineteenth century factory represented. No doubt there was exaggeration as, also, there were differences both between factories and over time. One thing is clear, however, conditions in the pre-Victorian factory, poor though they might often have been, were merely one aspect of an unhealthy environment in which the poor, in particular, lived. Any evaluation of workplace conditions needs to take account of this fundamental fact.[104]

A historiography of occupational health

The academic disciplines of social history and medical history, not to mention the social history of medicine, have flourished in recent decades. However, while there have been many studies of workers and the workplace experience, surprisingly little attention has been paid to the history of occupational health. Instead, the major focus has been on such relationships as work and community, work and home, work and gender. Even specialist monographs such as Richard Whipp's *Patterns of Labour. Work and Social Change in the Pottery Industry* (1990), Jacqueline Sarsby's *Missuses & Mouldrunners. An Oral History of Women Pottery Workers at Work and at Home* (1988), or Burchill and Ross's *History of the Potters' Union* (1977) – to cite three works on one (notoriously unhealthy) industry and locality – deal with occupational health issues little more than in passing.[105] By the same token, this author must confess to having virtually ignored occupational health issues in his two studies of workmen's compensation in nineteenth and twentieth century Britain that were published in the 1980s.[106] Histories of medicine and labour relations have been scarcely more forthcoming. For example, Virginia Berridge's chapter on health and medicine in the period 1750-1950, written for the *Cambridge Social History of Britain*, includes only four lines on occupational health. Clegg, Fox and Thompson's studies of British trade unionism since the late-nineteenth century, perhaps reflecting the priorities of unions themselves, contains even less.[107] Until the publication of Anthony Wohl's outstanding book, *Endangered Lives,* no history of public health, surely a forum in which occupational health should have been discussed, had adequately addressed the issue, preferring to concentrate on such questions as drains, sewers, cholera outbreaks and public health acts.[108]

Rather than extend the list of historical works in which occupational health has been either ignored or insufficiently considered, much of the remainder of this chapter deals with those studies that have tackled the subject. Attention must initially be drawn to two publications in which it received considerable attention. These are Donald Hunter's *Diseases of Occupations* (1st edition, 1955), about one-third of which consisted of historical survey, and the *British Journal of Industrial Medicine* (1941-1993), which regularly included historical articles. Although academic historians, including Michael Rose and Arthur McIvor, published in the *BJIM*, both these titles were edited and, in the main, written by and for practitioners of occupational health.[109] As such, in neither was history the prime concern. Their main focus was the scientific and clinical medicine of occupational disease; history was merely background and, as such, was incidental to their main purpose. Even so it is probably fair to say that, together, these two publications dominated the history of occupational health in Britain for decades. Over the years the *BJIM* published some fine historical papers, while for some thirty years *Hunter's Diseases of Occupation* provided succinct and extremely useful historical introductions and overviews. However, what is equally true is that their approaches, for all their strengths, were far too 'Whiggish' for taste of most professional historians. In other words they tended to describe the progressive development of a sub-discipline from an unsatisfactory 'then' to a highly satisfactory, or at least, very much-improved 'now'. Moreover they often did this while ignoring the social, economic and political contexts within which occupational illness both occurred and was regulated. Instead, the emphasis was on the achievements of pioneers, 'great men' and success. Even so, at least these publications did pay attention to history. Such is no longer the case. Since the re-launch of the *BJIM* as *Occupational and Environmental Medicine* in 1994 it has shed all interest in history. As for Hunter, the most recent edition (the 9th) of this work (2000) all but excludes a historical dimension.[110] The conclusion appears to be that interest in the history of occupational health, certainly among health professionals is declining.

With the exception of the above titles, the starting point for any consideration of the recent historiography of occupational health must be Anthony Wohl's *Endangered Lives*. First published in 1983 this history of Victorian public health broke new ground by devoting a chapter to the subject of industrial disease. Although treatment of the subject is comparatively brief, this chapter provides a succinct overview of the nineteenth century history of occupational health in Britain. Soon after the appearance of Wohl's volume the history of occupational health was further elaborated in a collection of essays devoted entirely to the subject. Edited by Paul Weindling, this book grew out of a 1983 conference held by the Society for the Social History of Medicine at Portsmouth Polytechnic (as it then was) and purported to be 'the first to explore this neglected area from the perspectives of social history'.[111] Although this claim was surely a just one, the book's title suggests a comprehensiveness and coherence of a approach, which, as is so frequently the case in published conference proceedings, is not mirrored in its contents. Aside from the editor's illuminating introduction (about which, more below), those contents comprise three papers on Germany, one on Italy, regional studies on Wales and Cornwall, two papers on workmen's compensation in Britain, contributions on TNT poisoning among women munitions workers in 1914-18 Britain, factory inspection in inter-war Britain and, finally, an essay on coronary heart disease in twentieth century Britain. Valuable though these papers are, collectively they can hardly be said to constitute 'the social history of occupational medicine'. It was to be hoped that the conference and the book that resulted from it would stimulate further research and publication. By and large this has not happened. In Weindling's volume it was claimed that 'there has been virtually no published work on the social history of... work-related diseases'. Although one could not go this far today, it can hardly be said that the statement is now patently untrue. *The Social History of Occupational Health*, whatever its shortcomings, continues to dominate the field. Long after its publication it continues to be cited as the foremost British book on the history of occupational health.[112]

The one paper in Weindling's volume about which little has thus far been said is the editor's own superb overview of the field, including a review of the literature to 1982. This was so comprehensive that there is little point in trying to repeat the exercise here. The remainder of this section therefore comprises, first, a brief review of some of the British literature which has appeared since publication of *The Social History of Occupational Health* and, second, a short consideration of developments in the American history of occupational health.

The emergence of women's history as a flourishing field of research has been accompanied by an upsurge of interest in the history of women's work and health. Associated with this trend has been the appearance of a number of studies on women in the dangerous trades, especially in the late-nineteenth and early-twentieth centuries. Some of these have focused on the late-Victorian and Edwardian belief that female workers constituted a vulnerable section of the industrial workforce that was in need of the state's protection. By the end of the nineteenth century the legislative protection of women workers (on the grounds that they were incapable of looking after their own interests) already had a long history. Most notably, the *Mines Act, 1842,* had prohibited women from underground work in coal mines. Notwithstanding a lack of definite medical evidence that women workers faced greater risks than their male counterparts, controls over their freedom to work, were also imposed on health grounds. A number of historians have seen the introduction of such regulatory controls, or protective legislation, in terms of anti-feminist priorities. Thus, Carolyn Malone and others have emphasised not only the removal of women from the best paid occupations, but also the priority of confining them to the domestic sphere as wives and mothers in order to further national and imperial goals, by producing children and raising families. Robert Gray has argued that an important objective in sex-selective factory legislation was the reservation of '[j]obs involving recognised "skill", discretion and authority... as male monopolies'. In other words, it served the interests of men rather than women.[113]

Such interpretations 'correct' a more traditional view, as expressed, *inter alia,* by B.L. Hutchins and A. Harrison, that has regarded legislation which protects women from, for example, excessive hours of work in an unhealthy environment as unambiguously beneficial. Certainly, the protective principle ran counter to one strand of feminism, which held that protective legislation damaged women's interests by reducing their opportunities in the workplace. Such was the view of Jesse Boucherett and Helen Blackburn and organisations such as the Society for Promoting the Employment of Women.[114] Emma Paterson, founder of the Women's Trade Union League (WTUL), also opposed restrictions on women's working hours, on the grounds that these would circumscribe employment opportunities. Yet feminists were divided on the issue. By the 1890s, under Emilia Dilke's leadership, the WTUL supported protective legislation.[115] Finally, two studies of the women's factory inspectorate, which was set up in 1893, pay considerable attention to occupational health issues within a regulatory context. Although none of the early women factory inspectors possessed medical qualifications, they took a strong interest in the dangerous trades. Within the inspectorate, therefore, women were prominent not merely as 'victims' of occupational disease, but as 'health workers' and reformers.[116]

As is the case with the present study, the Victorian and Edwardian periods have been the main focus of recent work on women in the dangerous trades. A recent PhD thesis on potters' health covers a similar timespan.[117] Aside from Ineson and Thom (in the Weindling volume), which again highlights the particular hazards faced by women workers, only Arthur McIvor and Helen Jones have paid much attention to occupational health in the First World War.[118] Unlike Ineson and Thom, who focus on a particular disease, Jones and McIvor, in respect of both the First World War and the inter-war periods, concentrate on the problems of fatigue and overwork. During the 1914-18 war, as a result of the emphasis placed on maximising industrial production, these began to be seen as crucial aspects of workplace health.[119] Such an emphasis, McIvor and Jones argue, persisted into the twenties and thirties. Hence, in her recent survey of the history of health in the twentieth century Jones argues that:

> Most governmental activities in the 1920s and 1930s (in contrast to the pre-war years) tended to emphasise general safety, health and welfare, rather than particular diseases. The main emphasis was on light, ventilation, noise, cleanliness, accidents (particularly those associated with young people and new processes), machinery and methods and welfare facilities such as canteens.[120]

While there may be some truth in this, it should not be supposed that 'new' diseases were not emerging in this period and becoming subject to regulation. A case in point is asbestosis.

The potential health hazard of asbestos dust was first mentioned by the women's factory inspectorate in 1898. More than a quarter of a century later fibrosis of the lungs as a result of inhaling asbestos dust came to be recognised as a specific industrial disease. A factory department inquiry in the late-1920s led to the establishment of the Asbestos Regulations, 1931. In the last few years, perhaps in response to the demonisation of asbestos by the media and protracted litigation in the courts, the history of asbestos-related disease has prompted a number of historical investigations.[121] Other diseases that became the subject of concern, leading to regulation, in the inter-war period were epitheliomatous ulceration (mule spinners' cancer) and byssinosis. These too have been the subjects of historical inquiry.[122] Away from specific diseases McIvor has supplied an excellent, if brief, introduction to workplace health in the period covered by the present book. In this he argues for the ameliorative effect of legislation in terms of tackling disease in some occupations while, at the same time, emphasising the 'patchy' coverage and lax enforcement of regulations.[123] For a later period a former editor of the *British Journal of Industrial Medicine* has recently examined the place of occupational medicine during the Second World War. He has argued that the subject flourished during the war years only to return to its hitherto somewhat moribund state with the return of peace.[124] Although the author provides little in the way of an explanation for this trend, it would seem likely that government prioritised occupational health as a wartime measure in order to maximise production and sustain morale. With the end of the war and the need for retrenchment in government expenditure, these priorities ceased to exert the same attraction. Consequently, the national importance of maximising workplace health standards also ceased to be of such importance.

Turning finally to the history of occupational health in the United States. Until the 1970s this was, with the exception of George Rosen's pioneering work, at least as moribund a field as in the United Kingdom.[125] But the passing, in 1970, of the federal *Occupational Safety and Health at Work Act*, seems to have kindled historical interest in the subject. Subsequently, particularly since the early-1980s, a plethora of publications, mainly covering twentieth century developments, have appeared.[126] While it is not possible to explore the contents and findings of these volumes and other work here, it is worth noting the emphasis placed by American historians of occupational health on the distinctions between the interests of employers, employees, medical practitioners, trade unions and legislatures. Several scholars, Gersuny and Rosner and Markowitz among them, have argued that in matters of health and safety, the interests of employers and employees were diametrically opposed. With zero or minimal legislative intervention the norm in most states, standards were largely a matter of negotiation between employer and employee. Trade unions were often either excluded from this process (not least because, until 1935, there were doubts about the constitutional legitimacy of trade unionism and collective bargaining) or were unhelpful (if only because they prioritised compensation rather than prevention). As a result the negotiating process occurred within an ultra *laissez-faire* ideological framework which saw health and safety issues as somehow 'un-American' and a social context in which scientists and physicians were more or less 'in the pockets' of industry and, consequently, bent on minimising the health hazards of the workplace. Hence, the traditional view of the history of occupational health, which emphasised progress brought about by the technical and scientific advances wrought by experts, has been called into question, if not discarded, in some of the North American literature.[127]

These historiographical developments in American scholarship warrant attention in the United Kingdom given the pervasiveness of the emphasis on 'progress' in successive editions of Hunter's *Diseases of Occupations* and, until its demise, the *British Journal of Industrial Medicine*. At the same time it is arguable that significant advances in medico-scientific research and improvements workplace standards did occur in Britain, albeit unevenly, particularly in the twentieth century. In Britain, unlike the USA, occupational health has been the subject of central government regulation since at least as far back as the 1880s. Some years ago Harold Perkin argued for the emergence in late-nineteenth century Britain of a professional ideal, which also imbued bureaucracies such as the factory inspectorate. This ideal embraced selection by merit, the exercise of expertise and impartiality, not least in the pursuit of solutions to social problems.[128] One of the aims of the following chapters is to assess the extent to which, in the British context, a history of occupational health regulation which emphasises scientific and practical progress, and professional disinterestedness also stands in need of revision.

The Home Office

The department of government responsible for regulating occupational health and the dangerous trades in the Victorian and Edwardian periods (and beyond) was the Home Office.[129] This responsibility arose because the Home Office supervised the factory inspectorate and all its activities. It is appropriate, therefore, to consider the origins, general remit and administrative culture of both the Home Office and the factory inspectorate.

Although its origins can be traced to the Tudor period, if not the Middle Ages, the Home Office as a discrete department dates from 1782. For some 140 years prior to this the Crown had been served by two principal secretaries of state responsible for different areas of foreign policy. Termed the 'northern' and 'southern' departments, the former had been responsible for dealing with the protestant powers of Europe, while the latter had dealt with Roman Catholic states. In 1782 this geographical distinction ceased. Henceforth, one secretary of state handled foreign affairs, while the other took charge of domestic and colonial business. Perhaps because the first incumbent of the latter post (Lord Shelburne) was both a peer and royal favourite, whereas his foreign affairs counterpart (Charles James Fox) was a commoner and an antagonist of George III, precedence was accorded to the holder of the domestic and colonial appointment. Hence the origins of the home secretary's status, which persisted throughout the period covered by this book, as the most senior of Her Majesty's secretaries of state.[130]

Notwithstanding that the post of home secretary is usually traced to 1782 (27 March of that year, to be exact) and that the term itself came into use very soon afterwards, neither Lord Shelburne nor his immediate successors in office, were concerned purely with domestic business. Until 1794 they retained substantial responsibility for the army. Only from this date were all military obligations (with the exception of troop movements for the maintenance of internal order) jettisoned. Not until 1801 was colonial business shed. From this year, the home secretary, or secretary of state for home affairs, was responsible for all domestic matters that were not the specific concern of another minister. Although he was the recipient, throughout the nineteenth century, of a 'vast mass of statutory powers and duties' conferred by act of parliament, for some time his authority derived largely from his position as adviser to the king in the exercise of the royal prerogative powers.[131] Aside from advising on the use of these powers, especially the Royal Prerogative of Mercy, the home secretary's duties lay in two areas. First, he was the sole channel by which subjects could approach, petition or address the king, for example, for pardons or commutation of judicial sentence. Second, he was the conduit between the Crown and its officers including, lords lieutenant and magistrates. In this connection he was responsible for raising volunteers for the national defence. From the first, therefore, the Home Office was firmly linked with the maintenance of law and order and the administration of justice. Subsequent legislation consolidated and extended this connection. Thus, in the 1820s the *Prisons Act, 1823* and the *Metropolitan Police Act, 1829* conferred administrative responsibility on the home secretary. Later years saw the extension of Home Office powers for policing and punishment including, from the 1850s, into the area of juvenile crime. But the Victorian and Edwardian periods, also saw the department take on a vast ragbag of additional and seemingly unconnected jurisdictions, including for vivisection, wild birds, cremation, burial grounds, inebriates and explosives. As early as 1793 the Aliens Act gave the home secretary jurisdiction over foreigners resident in Britain. This authority over immigrants and immigration, which was extended by the *Aliens Act, 1844*, became a substantial responsibility with the influx of Russian and east European migrants to the East End of London and elsewhere from the late-nineteenth century.

As new obligations were taken on, some were dropped. Until the Poor Law Commission was abolished, in 1847, it came under Home Office supervision. The establishment of the Local Government

Board, in 1871, saw the transfer of the Home Office's local government branch to the new department. A few years later, the establishment of a Scottish Office (1885) allowed for the transfer of all Scottish business that could be separated from English affairs. Freshwater fisheries were transferred to the Board of Trade in 1886, while the establishment of a Board of Agriculture, in 1889, saw the loss of more Home Office responsibilities. Notwithstanding, these and other 'losses', the trend of nineteenth century (and subsequent) legislation was to extend Home Office jurisdictions. Beyond its core responsibilities in the areas of law and order and the administration of justice, a characteristic feature of the Home Office on which many observers have commented, has been its enormous range of duties and jurisdictions. As Sir Edward Troup, permanent under-secretary of state (1908-22) wrote in 1925:

> Generally speaking, when Parliament decides to bring any new domestic matter under government regulation, unless it is a matter coming specifically within the sphere of some other department, the Home Office, as the original department of all home affairs, is the department in which the new charge is laid and for this reason it has to deal with a great number of apparently unconnected subjects.[132]

Colourfully, Donajgrodski has termed the department 'an administrative waste-paper basket into which any new subject could be dropped'. So much was dropped in that by the 1840s the Home Office reached into 'almost every area of domestic social life'.[133] A mid-twentieth century permanent under secretary, Sir Frank Newsam, who wrote of the 'miscellany of statutory functions' acquired by the Home Office in the nineteenth century, characterised the 'unifying principle' in the Home Office's remit as 'the order, safety and well-being of the King's subjects'. As such, Newsam argued that the department was concerned with trying to hold the line between excessive and inadequate liberty of the subject.[134]

Some of the most important of the statutory powers and duties conferred on the nineteenth century Home Office were in the area of the workplace. Although the regulation of working conditions did not involve questions of public order or even, initially, industrial safety, Newsam believed it was concerned with social order insofar as it involved tackling the social consequences of the industrial revolution. Although this seems to be stretching the notion that there was some coherent theme in Home Office responsibilities, it is certainly valid to regard the factory acts as having been concerned with tackling the social costs of industrialisation. The *Factory Act, 1833*, though not the first attempt to regulate the conditions of factory labour, was the first to recognise that the state had a role to play in terms of enforcement. The act is often regarded as particularly significant by virtue of the fact that it provided for the appointment of inspectors charged with carrying its terms into effect. These inspectors may have been few in number – only four, plus a number of superintendents or sub-inspectors, were initially appointed – but they had extensive, even 'revolutionary' powers under the criminal law to enforce the legislation.[135] Until 1844 these powers included the ability to fine offenders 'on view', that is, without taking a case to court. In this respect the first inspectors could act as industrial policemen, prosecutors, juries and judges. Even after the removal (not only with the inspectors' approval but also at their behest) of the power to impose 'on-the-spot' penalties, the new officials retained substantial authority. For example, they could demand entry to any part of any factory, at any time of day or night for the purpose of enforcing the legislation. Obstruction of an inspector going about his official duties constituted a criminal offence. Furthermore, inspectors had absolute discretion over the decision of whether to prosecute.

In time, inspectors' readiness to prosecute – for reasons that historians have contested – declined. Some have seen this decline as evidence of unwillingness to penalise and stigmatise 'respectable' members of the middle-classes who did not deserve to be hauled before the courts. Others have interpreted it as a pragmatic response whereby inspectors sought to make optimal use of the resources available to them with a view to maximising compliance with the law.[136] With finite resources at their disposal, it is argued, inspectors eschewed expensive and time-consuming prosecutions involving legal uncertainty and, in many instances, victimless offences. Except in cases that they deemed serious by virtue either of the rejection of repeated advice and warnings, or, after 1844, where the actual or potential consequences were grave in terms of threatening life and limb, they tended to rely on a policy of 'negotiated compliance'.[137] With their powers of prosecution under the criminal law, the factory inspectors reflected the law and order and administration of justice culture of the Home Office.[138] However, the extension of this culture into the workplace was a novelty. As such it raised difficult questions about how inspectors should best exercise their powers, not only in terms of maximising protection for those workers covered by the legislation, but also in relation to the national interest. Industrial production was generally recognised as desirable in terms of wealth production. However, parliament also accepted that it could have undesirable consequences, including in terms of the physical abuse and exploitation of the workforce, if not in all cases, then in some. Unlike most areas of the criminal law, therefore, the factory acts and the officials who enforced them sought balance in terms of controlling evils without destroying or unreasonably hampering the industrial production. Nevertheless, any discussion of inspectors' reluctance to prosecute should take account of the fact that in the early years of their existence, they brought hundreds of prosecutions annually. At the end of the nineteenth century and indeed as late as the 1930s there were thousands of prosecutions per year (3654 in 1899 and 2586 in 1936).[139]

The Home Office possessed some minor responsibilities under pre-1833 factory legislation but these were modest and sometimes neglected.[140] Essentially, it was the 1833 act that took the department into the area of workplace regulation. This occurred simply by virtue of the fact that the factory inspectorate became one of its dependent (or semi-independent) agencies. The department had not solicited the connection. Rather, the inspectorate was imposed upon or 'tacked onto' it. Although the 1833 bill nominally originated within its walls, it was mainly drafted by Edwin Chadwick and piloted through parliament by Lord Althorp. Neither, at least in the early Victorian period, did the Home Office seek to exert any significant control over an inspectorate that it 'never… absorbed'. This was partly a matter of circumstance, partly a matter of inclination. In the first place the Home Office had little scope to assume a 'hands on' role in factory regulation given the small scale of its bureaucracy (the 22 permanent officials of 1848 had risen to a mere 36 by 1876) and the heavy, not to say 'intolerable', burden of its other responsibilities.[141] But it was not simply excessive workload and inadequate resources that ensured that Home Office control over factory inspection was minimal. Quite as important was the department's highly conservative ethos, its preference for reaction rather than pro-action and its desire to fulfil its obligations with the minimum of conflict or controversy.[142] Only slowly, comparatively late in the nineteenth century, did these departmental characteristics undergo change.

The 1833 act made no mention of the number of inspectors that were to be appointed. This decision was left to the Home Office. It is probable that the small size of the inspectorate reflected the department's lack of enthusiasm either for factory inspection as a whole or for its own administrative role in the operation. At any event, for many years the working culture of the factory inspectorate was substantially different from that of the department within which it operated. The greatest contrast was in terms of a conflict-oriented inspectorate operating within a consensus-oriented department. It is axiomatic that no inspectorate would have been created but for the recognition that there was an element of irreconcilability between public policy and entrepreneurial objectives. This is not to say that the early inspectors set out with the intention of confronting factory occupiers. On the contrary, whether out of personal preference or in response to Home Office policy, they sought to minimise friction. Thus, inspector Rickards urged his superintendents where possible to enforce the law through 'frequent personal visitation' undertaken with a 'courteous and conciliatory demeanour'. In 1838 his colleague, Leonard Horner, advised a new superintendent except in 'flagrant cases to try what admonitions would do'.[143] However, the opposition not only of many industrialists, but also of the magistrates before whom inspectors took prosecutions, made a consensual approach difficult. When inspectors clashed with manufacturers, for example over the operation of relay systems, or with magistrates over their failure to convict or to impose adequate penalties when they did convict, they received little support from Home Office. Indeed, the views of inspectors were sometimes closer to those of factory reformers such as Lord Ashley or John Fielden than they were to their bureaucratic masters. The Home Office tended to find it difficult to reign in inspectors, not least because the inspectorate could count on support in parliament. So for some years relations between inspectors and the Home Office were often distant, if not strained. Donajgrodski has summarised the relationship as follows:

> The department's stance towards the inspectors was... generally unenthusiastic. As far as it could, the Home Office seems to have withdrawn from the subject [of factory inspection] altogether. Interventions were relatively infrequent and the inspectors were left to get on with their own work. They were regarded and clearly came to regard themselves as outsiders... [144]

Where the Home Office preferred passivity, quietism and accommodation, the inspectorate favoured a more dynamic approach to its duties which embraced confrontation with industrialists and JPs, direct appeals to parliament and proposals for reform that were not necessarily welcome in Whitehall. It is well to remember that in the early Victorian period the Home Office and the factory inspectorate often did not hold identical views or speak with the same voice, either in detail or broad principal, about the regulation of the workplace. But did the culture of factory inspection in time come more closely to resemble the regulatory culture of the Home Office?

Jill Pellew, in her examination of the ten Home Office inspectorates created in the period, 1832–76, refers to the continuing independence of the dependent agencies. She observes that 'central officials below under-secretary level did not issue and rarely even proposed instructions to inspectors'. She explains this in terms of departmental recognition that inspectors possessed specialist knowledge that was not possessed by generalist officials. In addition, inspectors' social status, education and experience marked them out as the superiors of officials below the position of under-secretary. [145] Subsequently, up to 1892, 'the Home Office tended to follow a conservative policy towards factory inspection'. Pellew illustrates this point by referring to the department's distaste for reform suggestions emanating from labour organisations, but an alternative example would be its indifference to policy initiatives related to occupational health. Pellew further argues, that the permanent under-secretary, between 1885 and 1895, Godfrey Lushington, 'held a traditional view' of Home Office responsibilities and that he prioritised the law and order rather than the industrial role. Neither of the longer serving Home Secretaries of the 1880s and early-1890s, Sir William Vernon Harcourt or Henry Matthews, dissented from this view.[146] However, key changes of personnel in the 1890s, shook up both the Home Office and the factory inspectorate. Within the inspectorate, as we shall see, the retirement of the long-serving chief inspector, Alexander Redgrave (in 1891) was important in ending a period of conservatism. There followed several short-term appointments, but the arrival of B.A. Whitelegge, in 1896, meant that the inspectorate was led by a chief inspector of energy and ability. Politically, the appointment of the dynamic and visionary Herbert Asquith as home secretary (1892-5) was important. Finally, the Home Office was changed in the 1890s by civil servants of huge intellectual talent, drive and enthusiasm. Particularly significant in these respects were C.E. (Edward) Troup, who joined the Home Office as a junior clerk in 1880 under the new competitive entry arrangements and attained the position of permanent under secretary in 1908, and Malcolm Delevingne, who became a junior clerk in 1892 and was promoted to assistant under secretary in 1913. Both became closely involved with industrial business. Furthermore, both were intent on protecting and extending Home Office responsibilities rather than seeking to slough them off – which had been the attitude of an older generation of officials.[147] So, the culture of the Home Office did change in the course of the nineteenth century, but this change occurred at a relatively late stage, principally, in the last decade. Even with a change of culture, however, the factory inspectorate retained considerable autonomy. This was partly because inspectors possessed technical knowledge (usually, even at the end of the century, acquired in service rather than through academic study or experience of working in industry) that central officials lacked and could never hope to acquire. In addition, however, inspection, notwithstanding that its effectiveness was hard to gauge, had firmly established itself as 'the obvious way of enforcing certain kinds of laws'.[148]

Notes

1. Adam Smith, *The Wealth of Nations* (London: Everyman edn, 2 vols. 1970), I, 73.
2. William Cave Wright, *De Morbis Artificum. Bernardini Ramazzini. Diatriba. Diseases of Workers. The Latin Text of 1713 Revised with Translation and Notes* (Chicago: University of Chicago Press, 1940); C.T. Thackrah, *The Effect of Arts, Trades and Professions and of Civic States and Habits of Living, on Health and Longevity: with Suggestions for the Removal of Many of the Agents which Produce Disease and Shorten the Duration of Life* (London: Longman, Rees, Orme, Brown, Green and Longman, 2nd edn, 1832).
3. See John Rule, *The Experience of Labour in Eighteenth Century Industry* (London: Croom Helm, 1981), 88.
4. Though in her novel, *North and South* (1855), Elizabeth Gaskell devoted attention to the health problems of textile workers who inhaled cotton fluff (chapter 13). Industrial disease also features in Charlotte Tonna's novel, *Helen Fleetwood* (1841).
5. See Anthony S. Wohl, *Endangered Lives. Public Health in Victorian Britain* (London: Methuen, 1984), 1–2.
6. F.B. Smith, *The Retreat of Tuberculosis, 1850-1950* (Beckenham: Croom Helm, 1988), 1.
7. Rule, *op. cit.* (note 3), 76.
8. On medicine as business see Anne Digby, *Making a Medical Living. Doctors and Patients in the English Market for Medicine, 1720-1911* (Cambridge: CUP, 1994); *idem.*, *The Evolution of British General Practice, 1850-1948* (Oxford: OUP, 1999).
9. Malone's suggestion that by 1890 'an increasing number of doctors were investigating the cause and possible treatment of industrial

disease' is wide of the mark. Carolyn Malone, 'Sex in Industry: Protective Labor Legislation in England, 1891-1914', University of Rochester Ph.D. (1991), 275.

10. M.J. Cullen, *The Statistical Movement in Early Victorian Britain* (Brighton: Harvester Press, 1975); J. Eyler, *Victorian Social Medicine. The Ideas and Methods of William Farr* (Baltimore: Johns Hopkins University Press, 1979); Donald MacKenzie, *Statistics in Britain, 1865-1930: the Social Construction of Scientific Knowledge* (Edinburgh: Edinburgh University Press, 1981); Stephen M. Stigler, *The History of Statistics. The Measurement of Uncertainty before 1900* (Cambridge, Mass. and London: Belknap Press, 1986).
11. Charles Shaw, *When I Was a Child* (Firle: Caliban Books, 1980), 80.
12. Thackrah, *op. cit.* (note 2), 161.
13. Thomas Oliver (ed), *Dangerous Trades: The Historical, Social and Legal Aspects of Industrial Occupations as Affecting Health by a Number of Experts* (London: John Murray, 1902), 800–1; See also J.T. Arlidge, *Hygiene, Diseases and Mortality of Occupations* (London: Percival, 1892), 150–7.
14. *Workmen's Compensation Act, 1906 (6 Edw, 7 c.58).* Ankylostomiasis (or ancylostomiasis) involves infestation of the small intestine by a parasitic hook worm. Its spread amongst underground miners was facilitated by an absence of toilets.
15. Reports in the *Daily Telegraph* and *Independent*, 28 Sept. 1995.
16. *On the State of the Public Health. The Annual Report of the Chief Medical Officer of the Department of Health for the Year 1994* (London: HMSO, 1995), 88.
17. Allen Clarke, *The Effects of the Factory System* (Littleborough: Georges Kelsall, 1989); Wanda F. Neff, *Victorian Working Women. An Historical and Literary Study of Women in British Industries and Professions, 1832-1850* (London: Frank Cass, 1966 edn), esp. 40–7; See also Ivy Pinchbeck, *Women Workers and the Industrial Revolution, 1750-1850* (London: Frank Cass, 1969 edn). Clarke's book was originally published in 1899. Neff's first appeared in 1929, while Pinchbeck's study dates from 1930.
18. *On the State of the Public Health, op. cit.* (note 16) 88–9. See Frank Pearce and Steve Tombs, 'Ideology, Hegemony and Empiricism – Compliance Theories of Regulation', *British Journal of Criminology*, 30 (1990), 426; Theo Nichols, *The Sociology of Industrial Injury* (London: Mansell, 1997), introduction.
19. *Bill to Amend the Law Relating to the Liability of Employers for Injuries to their Workmen*, PP 1893–4 III, s.2, 61; *Employers'*

Liability Amendment Bill, PP 1894 IV, s.2, 263–72; T. Luson and R. Hyde, *The Diseases of Workmen* (London: Butterworth, 1908), 4–5; P.W.J. Bartrip and S.B. Burman, *The Wounded Soldiers of Industry. Industrial Compensation Policy, 1833-1897* (Oxford: Clarendon Press, 1983) esp. 158–65. Contracting out involved workers giving written undertakings that they would not seek compensation under the terms of the Employers' Liability Act. They might be required to contract out as a condition of employment or, more usually, induced to do so as a *quid pro quo* for their employers making a contribution to a benefit or accident relief fund.

20. Brintons Ltd. *v.* Turvey [1905] A.C. 230; See Fenton v. Thorley & Co. Ltd. [1903] A.C. 443; P.W.J. Bartrip, *Workmen's Compensation in Twentieth Century Britain* (Aldershot: Gower, 1987), 26; Karl Figlio, 'How Does Illness Mediate Social relations? Workmen's Compensation and Medico-Legal Practices, 1890-1940' in P.Wright and A. Treacher (eds), *The Problem of Medical Knowledge* (Edinburgh: Edinburgh University Press, 1982) 174–224; *idem.*, 'What is an Accident' in Paul Weindling (ed), *The Social History of Occupational Health* (London: Croom Helm, 1985), 180–206.
21. Bartrip, *op. cit.* (note 20), 53.
22. On employers' liability and workmen's compensation in the nineteenth century see Bartrip and Burman, *op. cit.* (note 19).
23. *46 & 47 Vict. c.53.*
24. The first American work devoted entirely to the subject of occupational disease appears to be Benjamin W. McCready, 'On the Influence of Trades, Professions and Occupations in the United States in the Production of Disease', *Transactions of the Medical Society of the State of New York*, 3 (1836-7), 91–150.
25. It should be recognised that since 1802 the Factory Acts had incorporated health and safety provisions. These included restrictions on the length of the working day for child workers, to prevent overstrain and physical deformity and an obligation to limewash interior walls as a means of improving hygiene and sanitation. However, the safety clauses were not concerned with accident prevention and the hygiene requirements were intended to control epidemic disease rather than health problems arising out of the work process. In the 1860s one of the Joint Chief Inspectors of factories, Alexander Redgrave, told an official inquiry that the limewashing clause had long since ceased to be enforced. *Reports of Factory Inspectors, half-year ending 31 Oct. 1864*, PP 1865 XX, 441–6, 449–51; see *Reports of Factory Inspectors, half-year ending 30*

April 1866, PP 1866 XXIV, 427–8.

26. Charles Booth, *Life and Labour of the People in London* (London: Macmillan, 10 vols, 1892–97).
27. Keith Hawkins, ' "FATCATS" and Prosecution in a Regulatory Agency: A Footnote on the Social Construction of Risk', *Law and Policy*, 11 (1989), 384.
28. See H. and B. Duckham, *Great Pit Disasters: Great Britain 1700 to the Present Day* (Newton Abbot: David & Charles, 1970). The biggest industrial disaster in nineteenth century Britain was the Oaks Colliery explosion of 1866 in which over 360 miners perished. A total of 439 miners died at Senghenydd in 1913.
29. In the fifty years between 1851, when the collection of statistics began and 1900 the annual number of coal-mining fatalities never fell below 867 (in 1864). In the worst year of this period – the year of the Oaks disaster – the figure was 1484.
30. John Benson, *British Coalminers in the Nineteenth Century: A Social History* (Dublin: Gill and Macmillan, 1980), 37–44; see the same author's 'Non-Fatal Coal Mining Accidents', *Bulletin of the Society for the Study of Labour History*, 32 (1976), 20–2; 'Colliery Disaster Funds, 1860-1897', *International Review of Labour History*, XIX (1974), 73–85 and 'English Coal-Miners' Trade Union Accident Funds, 1850-1900' *Economic History Review*, 2nd. ser 28 (1975) 401–12. The *Coal Mines Regulation Act, 1872 (35 & 36 Vict. c.76 s.20*) prohibited single shaft pits.
31. Hawkins, *op. cit.* (note 27), 384–9.
32. S. Colum Gilfillan, 'Lead poisoning and the Fall of Rome', *Journal of Occupational Medicine*, 7 (1965), 53–60; *idem.*, *Rome's Ruin by Lead Poison* (Long Beach: Wenzel Press, 1990); Jerome O. Nriagu, *Lead and Lead Poisoning in Antiquity* (New York: Wiley, 1983), 309; Christian Warren, *Brush with Death. A Social History of Lead Poisoning* (Baltimore and London: The Johns Hopkins University Press, 2000), 218.
33. Marjorie Smith, 'Lead in History', in Richard Lansdown and William Yule (eds), *The Lead Debate: The Environment, Toxicology and Child Health* (London: Croom Helm, 1986), 7–24.
34. Leonard J. Goldwater, 'From Hippocrates to Ramazzini: Early History of Industrial Medicine', *Annals of Medical History*, new ser. 8 (1936), 27–8; Henry E. Sigerist, 'Historical Background of Industrial and Occupational Diseases', *Bulletin of the New York Academy of Medicine*, 12 (1936), 597–609; Ludwig Teleky, *History of Factory and Mine Hygiene* (New York: Columbia University Press, 1948), 4.

35. Goldwater, (note 34), 27–30; Teleky, (note 34), 4.
36. Teleky, (note 34), p.4; T.M. Legge, 'Industrial Diseases in the Middle Ages', *Journal of Industrial Hygiene*, I (1919-20), 475–83.
37. For a translation see *Lancet,* 30 Jan. 1932, 270–1. See J.M. Norman (ed), *Morton's Medical Bibliography. An Annotated Check-list of Texts Illustrating the History of Medicine* (*Garrison and Morton*) (Aldershot: Scolar Press, 1991 edn), 332.
38. R.H. Major, *A History of Medicine* (Oxford: Blackwell, 2 vols. 1954), I, 387–8; see George Rosen, *The History of Miners' Diseases: a Medical and Social Interpretation* (New York: Schuman's, 1943); Norman, *op. cit.* (note 31), 332.
39. Adelaide Anderson, 'Historical Sketch of the development of Legislation for Injuries and Dangerous Industries in England', in Oliver, *op. cit.* (note 13), 26.
40. Smith, *op. cit.* (note 1), I, 73; Wright, *op. cit.* (note 2), 1, Major, *op. cit.* (note 38), I, 543; Norman, *op. cit.* (note 37), 333.
41. Wright, *op. cit.* (note 2), 343.
42. See George Rosen, 'Occupational Diseases of English Seamen during the Seventeenth and Eighteenth Centuries', *Bulletin of the History of Medicine*, 7 (1939), 751–8.
43. Percivall Pott, 'Cancer Scroti' in Sir James Earle (ed), *The Chirurgical Works of Percivall Pott FRS Surgeon to St. Bartholomew's Hospital* (London: Wood & Innes, 1808), 177–83; Norman, *op. cit.* (note 37), 333; see J.R. Brown and J.L. Thornton, 'Percivall Pott and Chimney Sweepers' Cancer of the Scrotum', *British Journal of Industrial Medicine,* 14 (1957), 63–70; H.A. Waldron, 'A Brief History of Scrotal Cancer', *British Journal of Industrial Medicine*, 40 (1983), 390–401; Alan Fowler and T.J. Wyke (eds), *The Barefoot Aristocrats: A History of the Amalgamated Association of Operative Cotton Spinners* (Littleborough: George Kelsall, 1987), chapter 10.
44. James Johnstone, 'Some Account of a Species of Pthisis Pulmonalis, peculiar to Persons Employed in Pointing Needles in the Needle Manufacture', *Memoirs of the Medical Society of London*, V (1799), 89–93.
45. Thomas Percival, *Observations and Experiments on the Poison of Lead* (London: Johnson, 1774), 21–5, 36–7.
46. J. Jackson, 'On the Influence of the Cotton Manufactories on the Health', *London Medical and Physical Journal*, xxxix (1818), 464–6; James Phillips Kay, 'Observations and Experiments Concerning Molecular Irritation of the Lungs as One Source of Tubercular Consumption and on Spinners' Pthisis', *North of England Medical*

and Surgical Journal, 1 (1830-1), 348–63; *idem.*, *The Moral and Physical Condition of the Working Classes Employed in the Cotton Manufacture in Manchester* (London: Ridgway, 1832).

47. Arnold Knight, 'On the Grinders' Asthma', *North of England Medical and Surgical Journal*, 1 (1830-1), 85–91 and 167–79; G.C. Holland, *Diseases of the Lungs from Mechanical Causes; and Inquiries into the Condiotion of Artisans Exposed to the Inhalation of Dust* (London: John Churchill, 1843); Charles Fox Flavell, 'On Grinders Asthma', *Transactions of the Provincial Medical and Surgical Association*, new ser. vol.2 (1846), 143–84; M.P. Johnson, 'Grinders' Asthma in Sheffield', *Bulletin of the Society for the Social History of Medicine*, 16 (1975), 7–8.
48. W. P. Allison, 'Observations on the Pathology of Scrofulous Diseases with a View to their Prevention', *Transactions of the Medico-Chirurgical Society of Edinburgh*, I (1824), 373. See also D. Noble, 'On the Influence of the Factory System in the Development of Pulmonary Consumption', *Journal of the Statistical Society of London*, V, 1832.
49. Charles Hastings, *Illustrations of the Natural History of Worcestershire* (London & Worcester: Sherwood, Gilbert & Piper, 1834); Charles Hastings, *A Treatise on the Inflammation of the Mucous Membrane of the Lungs* (London: Thomas & George Underwood, 1820), 335–45; William H. McMenemy, *The Life and Times of Sir Charles Hastings. Founder of the British Medical Association* (Edinburgh and London: Livingstone, 1959), 109.
50. *Lancet*, 9 July 1831, 450.
51. P. A. B. Raffle, W. R. Lee, R. I. McCallum, R. Murray (eds), *Hunter's Diseases of Occupations* (London: Hodder and Stoughton, 1987), 125.
52. Thackrah, *op. cit.* (note 2), 3–4.
53. On Thackrah see A. Meiklejohn, *The Life Work and Times of Charles Turner Thackrah, Surgeon and Apothecary of Leeds (1795-1833* (Edinburgh and London: E&P Livingstone, 1957), 1–43; J. Cleeland and S. Burt, 'Charles Turner Thackrah: a Pioneer in the Field of Occupational Health', *Occupational Medicine*, 45 (1995), 285–97.
54. See A. Meiklejohn, 'John Darwall, MD (1796-1833) and Diseases of Artisans', *British Journal of Industrial Medicine*, 13 (1956), 142–51; John Conolly, 'Biographical Memoir of the Late John Darwall of Birmingham', *Transactions of the Provincial Medical and Surgical, Association*, 2 (1834), 489–546.
55. Meiklejohn, *op. cit.* (note 53), 146–7.

56. *Ibid.*, 142.
57. J. Forbes, A. Tweedie and J. Conolly, *Cyclopaedia of Practical Medicine* (London: Sherwood, Gilbert and Piper and Baldwin and Cradock, 1833), I, 149–60.
58. In the 1860s and 1870s papers on aspects of occupational health were regularly read at meetings of the National Association for the Promotion of Social Science. These included contributions on the health of merchant seamen, military and naval personnel, London postmen and mill workers as well as more general questions, for example: 'On the Influence of Occupation on Health and Life'. See *Papers and Discussions on Public Health: Being the Transactions of the Fourth Department of the National Association for the Promotion of Social Science* (London: Emily Faithful, 1862) and *Transactions of the National Association for the Promotion of Social Science.*
59. Arlidge, *op. cit.* (note 13), 7–9; Stephen Huzzard, 'The Role of the Certifying Surgeon in the State Regulation of Child Labour and Industrial Health, 1833-1973', Manchester University, M.A. thesis (1976), 124.
60. Elliot Isaacson, *The Forgotten Physician* (no publishing details), 9–10.
61. *BMJ*, 4 Nov. 1899, 1325; see G.H. Brown (comp.), *Munk's Roll. Lives of the Fellows of the Royal College of Physicians of London, 1826-1925* (London: RCP, 1955), IV, 167–8.
62. On Arlidge see Isaacson, *op. cit.* (note 60); E. Posner, 'Thomas Arlidge (1822-1899) and the Potteries', *British Journal of Industrial Medicine*, xxx (1973), 266–70; Clare Holdsworth, 'Potters' Rot and Plumbism: Occupational Health in the North Staffordshire Pottery Industry', Liverpool University, Ph.D. thesis (1995); *idem.*, 'Dr John Thomas Arlidge and Victorian Occupational Medicine', *Medical History*, 42 (1998), 458–75.
63. *Lancet*, 20 Aug. 1859, 189.
64. The Milroy endowment, which had been set up under the terms of Gavin Milroy's will in 1886 consisted of a bequest of £2000 to fund an annual series of lectures on a public health or sanitation theme. On Milroy (1805-86) see *Lancet*, 27 Feb. 1886, 425; Brown, *op. cit.* (note 61), 71–2.
65. Arlidge, *op. cit.* (note 13), vii.
66. *Ibid.*, 7–8.
67. For discussion of the relationship between health, medical practitioners and the factory (though not specifically in terms of occupational health) see Robert Gray, *The Factory Question and*

Industrial England, 1830-1860 (Cambridge, CUP, 1996), chapter 3, esp. 72–85 and the same author's 'Medical Men, Industrial Labour and the State in Britain, 1830-1850', *Social History*, 16 (1991), 19–43. There is, of course, a large literature on the factory question more generally.

68. See for example, *Minutes of Evidence Taken before the Select Committee on the State of the Children Employed in the Manufactories of the United Kingdom*, PP 1816 III, 288, 385, 492–3.
69. Quoted in Alfred (Samuel H.G. Kydd), *The History of the Factory Movement from the Year 1802, to the Enactment of the Ten Hours' Bill in 1847* (London: Simpkin, Marshall and Co., 1857), 177.
70. John Aikin, *A Description of the Country from Thirty to Forty Miles Round Manchester* (London: John Stockdale, 1795), 456.
71. See A. Meiklejohn, 'Outbreak of Fever in Cotton Mills at Radcliffe', *British Journal of Industrial Medicine*, 16 (1959), 68–9; Charles Webster, 'Two-Hundredth Anniversary of the 1784 Report on Fever at Radcliffe Mill', *Bulletin of the Society for the Social History of Medicine*, 36 (1985), 65–70; Charles Webster and Jonathan Barry, 'The Manchester Medical Revolution' in Barbara Smith (ed), *Truth, Liberty and Religion. Essays Celebrating Two Hundred Years of Manchester College* (Oxford: Manchester College, 1986), 169.
72. Two witnesses (Ashley Cooper, the surgeon and Josiah Wedgwood, the pottery manufacturer) gave oral evidence to Peel's Committee about the occupational health hazards of lead and arsenic. See *Minutes of Evidence Taken before the Select Committee on the State of the Children*... PP 1816 III, 267, 294.
73. *Ibid.*, 532. Scutching was the process by which seeds and other impurities were separated from the cotton fibre. The term had a slightly different meaning when applied to the preparation of other textile materials (e.g. flax, silk or hemp). Carding involved the combing of fibres (cotton, wool, flax etc).
74. *Minutes of Evidence Taken before the Select Committee on the State of the Children*... PP 1816 III, 544–5.
75. See e.g. U.R.Q. Henriques, *Before the Welfare State. Social Administration in Early Industrial Britain* (London: Longman, 1979), 74–83; Eric Hopkins, *Childhood Transformed. Working Class Children in Nineteenth Century England* (Manchester: Manchester University Press, 1994), 78–9.
76. Bartrip and Burman, *op. cit.* (note 19), 16. See Frederick Engels, *The Condition of the Working Class in England* (London: Panther,

1969 edn), 198, where the Sadler Committee is described as 'emphatically partisan'. Witnesses spoke 'the truth, but truth in a perverted form'. Engels has much to say about the unhealthiness of factory work.

77. *Report from the Select Committee on the 'Bill to Regulate the Labour of Children in the Mills and Factories of the United Kingdom'; with the Minutes of Evidence, Appendix and Index*, PP XV 1831-2, 60.
78. Neff, *op. cit.* (note 17), 44–5.
79. *Report from the Select Committee on the 'Bill to Regulate the Labour of Children...'* PP XV 1831-2, 178.
80. *Ibid.*, 166 and 286. See also the evidence of James Kirk, 16; Joshua Drake, 38–9 and 40; Alonzo Hargreaves, 85; Eliza Marshall, 148; Mark Best, 172–74; Elizabeth Bentley, 196; and Charles Aberdeen, 440–1.
81. *Ibid.*, 513–14. The medical evidence presented to the early factory inquiries is reviewed in W.H. Hutt, 'The Factory System in the Early Nineteenth Century' in F.A. Hayek (ed), *Capitalism and the Historians* (London: Routledge and Kegan Paul, 1954), esp. 166–71.
82. Thackrah, *op. cit.* (note 2), 144.
83. *Ibid.*
84. *Ibid.*, 145.
85. *Ibid.*, 145–6. Slubbers, sometimes called "rovers" looked after slubbing (or roving) machines. These machines elongated fibres following carding and before spinning. Slubbers were assisted by pieceners. They were normally children or young persons. Their job was to carry "cardings" from the carding to the slubbing (or roving) machines and to join threads when they broke. Pieceners were employed and paid by rovers or slubbers. See Oxford English Dictionary on-line (2nd edn, 1989).
86. Thackrah, *op. cit.* (note 2), 147.
87. John Brown, *A Memoir of Robert Blincoe, an Orphan Boy; Sent from the Workhouse of St. Pancras, London, at Seven years of Age, to Endure the Cotton-Mill, through His Infancy and Youth, with a Minute Detail of his Sufferings, being the First Memoir of the Kind Published* (Firle: Caliban Books, 1977). The *Memoir*, first published in 1828, is one of the classic accounts of the early nineteenth century factory.
88. *Supplementary Report of the Central Board of His Majesty's Commissioners for Inquiry into the Employment of Children in Factories; with Minutes of Evidence and Reports by Medical Commissioners. Dr Bisset Hawkins's Reports on Lancashire, Derbyshire*

and Cheshire, D3, PP 1834 XIX, esp. 542–3.

89. *Second Report of the Central Board of His Majesty's Commissioners for Inquiry into the Employment of Children in Factories; with Minutes of Evidence and Reports by Medical Commissioners. Dr James Mitchell's Report*, PP 1833 XXI, 305–19.
90. *Irish University Press Reprints of British Parliamentary Papers (Industrial Revolution Children's Employment 3). First Report of the Central Board of His Majesty's Commissioners for Inquiring into the Employment of Children in Factories*, 16.
91. See R. Owen, 'On the Employment of Children in Manufactories' (1818) in Robert Owen, *A New View of Society and Other Writings* (London: Everyman, 1927), 131, 135.
92. Robert Dale Owen, *Threading My Way. Twenty Seven Years of Autobiography* (London: Trubner, 1874), 101.
93. Jackson, *op. cit.* (note 39),464–6.
94. E. Baines, *General View of the Agriculture and Minerals of Derbyshire* (London: Board of Agriculture, 3 vols, 1811-17), quoted in Stanley D. Chapman, *The Early Factory Masters* (Newton Abbot: David & Charles, 1967), 205.
95. W.H. Chaloner, 'Bibliographical Introduction' to Edward Baines, *History of the Cotton Manufacture of Great Britain* (London: Frank Cass, 1966 edn), 12–13. Richard Oastler, a leading light in the factory movement, was author of the renowned exposé of child labour in factories, published under the heading 'Yorkshire Slavery' in the *Leeds Mercury*, 16 Oct. 1830.
96. Baines, *op. cit.* (note 95), 451.
97. *Ibid.*, 452.
98. *Ibid.*, 452–7.
99. *Ibid.*, 457.
100. P. Gaskell, *Artisans and Machinery: the Moral and Physical Condition of the Manufacturing Population considered with Reference to Mechanical Substitutes for Human Labour* (London: Frank Cass, 1968), chapter 9 esp. 221–7.
101. Engels, *op. cit.* (note 76), 98; see Gray *op. cit.* (note 66), 85.
102. Andrew Ure, *the Philosophy of Manufactures: or, an Exposition of the Social, Moral and Commercial Economy of the Factory System of Great Britain* (London: Charles Knight, 1835), 374–84.
103. W. C. Taylor, *Notes of a Tour in the Manufacturing Districts of Lancashire* (London: Frank Cass, 1968), 26, 114–15, 260–69,
104. See Malcolm I. Thomis, *The Town Labourer and the Industrial Revolution* (London: Batsford, 1974), chapter 6 and the same author's *Responses to Industrialisation. The British Experience, 1780-*

1850 (Newton Abbot: David & Charles, 1976), 145–56.

105. Frank Burchill and Richard Ross, *A History of the Potters' Union* (Stoke-on-Trent: CATU, 1977). Burchill and Ross note that 'Potteries were unhealthy places in which to work and they looked it' (232) but they devote only a very small proportion of their study to health issues. Whipp notes that ill health was not an issue for mobilising workers, many of whom opposed state intervention because they associated it with unemployment and loss of autonomy. Richard Whipp, *Patterns of Labour. Work and Social Change in the Pottery Industry* (London: Routledge, 1990), 190, 209–10

106. Bartrip and Burman, *op. cit.* (note 19); Bartrip, *op. cit.* (note 20).

107. F.M.L. Thompson (ed), *The Cambridge Social History of Britain, 1750-1950. vol.3 Social Agencies and Institutions* (Cambridge: CUP, 1990), 171–242; H.A. Clegg, Alan Fox and A.F. Thompson, *A History of British Trade Unions since 1889* (Oxford: Clarendon Press, 3 vols. 1964-94). Volumes 2 and 3 are by Clegg alone.

108. Chapter 10 deals with 'the canker of industrial diseases'.

109. Michael Rose, 'The Doctor in the Industrial Revolution', *British Journal of Industrial Medicine*, 28 (1971), 22–6; A.J. McIvor, 'Employers, the Government and Industrial Fatigue in Britain, 1890-1918' *British Journal of Industrial Medicine*, 44 (1987), 724–32.

110. On Hunter as a historian see Paul Weindling, 'Linking Self Help and Medical Science: the Social History of Occupational Health' in Weindling, *op. cit.* (note 20), 3. Since Hunter's death in 1978 *Diseases of Occupation* has been updated by editors and re-issued as *Hunter's Diseases of Occupation*.

111. Weindling, *op. cit.* (note 20), dustwrapper 'blurb'.

112. See, for example, Arthur F. McEvoy, 'Working Environments: An Ecological Approach to Industrial Health and Safety', *Technology and Culture Supplement*, 36 (1995), S145–72.

113. Malone, *op. cit.* (note 9); *idem.*, 'The Gendering of Dangerous Trades: Government Regulation of Women's Work in the White Lead Trade in England, 1892-1918', *Journal of Women's History*, 8 (1996), 15–35; *idem.*, 'Gendered Discourses and the Making of Protective Labor Legislation in England, 1830-1914', *Journal of British Studies*, 37 (1998), 166–91; Robert Gray, 'Factory Legislation and the Gendering of Jobs in the North of England, 1830-1860', *Gender & History*, 5 (1993), 56–80.

114. J. Boucherett and Helen Blackburn, *The Condition of Working Women and the Factory Acts* (London: Elliot Stock, 1896).

115. There is now a very large historical literature on these themes. Aside from works cited in note 113 see B.L.Hutchins and A. Harrison, *A History of Factory Legislation* (London: P.S. King, 1926 edn), chapter 9; A. Davin, 'Imperialism and Motherhood', *History Workshop* 5 (1978), 9–66; C. Dyhouse, 'Working Class Mothers and Infant Mortality, 1895-1914', *Journal of Social History*, 12 (1978), 248–67; Elizabeth Roberts, *Women's Work, 1840-1940* (Basingstoke: Macmillan, 1995); J. Lewis, *The Politics of Motherhood. Child and Maternal Welfare in England, 1900-1939* (London: Croom Helm, 1980); R. Feurer, 'The Meaning of "Sisterhood": The British Women's Movement and Protective Labor Legislation', 1870-1900', *Victorian Studies*, 31 (1988) 233–60; Holdsworth, *op. cit.* thesis, (note 62), 18–25; *idem.*,'Women's Work and Family Health: Evidence from the Staffordshire Potteries, 1890-1920', *Continuity and Change*, 12 (1997), 103–28; S. Walby, *Patriarchy at Work. Patriarchal and Capitalist Relations in Employment* (Cambridge: Polity, 1986); Sonya Rose, 'Gender Antagonism and Class Conflict: Exclusionary Strategies of Male Trade Unionists in Nineteenth Century Britain', *Social History* 13 (1988), 191–208; *idem.*, '"From behind the Women's Petticoats": Factory Act Reform and the Politics of Motherhood in Britain, 1870-1878', *Journal of Historical Sociology*, 4 (1991), 32–51; *idem., Limited Livelihoods. Gender and Class in Nineteenth Century England* (Berkeley: University of California Press, 1992); Barbara Harrison, '"Some of Them gets Lead Poisoned": Occupational Health Exposure in Women, 1880-1914', *Social History of Medicine*, 2 (1989), 171–95; *idem.*, 'Suffer the Working Day. Women in the "Dangerous Trades", 1880-1914', *Women's Studies International Forum*, 13 (1990), 79–90; B. Harrison and H. Mockett, 'Women in the Factory: The State and Factory Legislation in Nineteenth Century Britain' in L. Jamieson and H. Corr (eds), *State, Private Life and Political Change* (London: Macmillan, 1990), 137–62; B. Harrison, 'Women's Health or Social Control? The Role of the Medical Profession in Relation to Factory Legislation in Late Nineteenth-Century Britain', *Sociology of Health and Illness*, 13 (1991), 469–91; *idem.*, 'Feminism and Health Consequences of Work in Late Nineteenth and Early Twentieth Century Britain' in S. Platt *et al.* (eds), *Locating Health. Sociological and Historical Explorations* (Aldershot: Avebury, 1993), 75-96; *idem., Not Only the 'Dangerous Trades'. Women's Work and Health in Britain, 1880-1914* (London: Taylor & Francis, 1996); J Lewis and C. Davies, 'Protective Legislation in Britain, 1870-1900:

Equality, Difference and their Implications for Women', *Policy and Politics*, 1 (1991), 13–25; P.W.J. Bartrip, ' "Petticoat Pestering": the Women's Trade Union League and Lead Poisoning in the Staffordshire Potteries, 1890-1914', *Historical Studies in Industrial Relations*, 2 (1996), 3–26.

116. Mary Drake McFeely, *Lady Inspectors. The Campaign for a Better Workplace, 1893-1921* (Oxford: Blackwell, 1988); Helen Jones, 'Women Health Workers. The Case of the First Women Factory Inspectors in Britain', *Social History of Medicine*, 1 (1988), 165–82.

117. Holdsworth, *op. cit.* thesis, (note 62); other useful theses not mentioned in Weindling's review include Huzzard, *op. cit.* (note 59); Rhoda H. Bledington, 'The Growth in Awareness of Health and Safety at Work, 1780-1900', University of Aston M.Phil. (1983); Helen Jones, 'The Home Office and Working Conditions, 1914-1940', University of London Ph.D. 1983.

118. Antonia Ineson and Deborah Thom, 'T.N.T. Poisoning and the Employment of Women Workers in the First World War' in Weindling, *op. cit.* (note 20), 89–107; A. J. McIvor, 'Manual Work, Technology and Industrial Health, 1918-39', *Medical History*, 31 (1987), 160–89. See also A. Watterson, 'Occupational Health Education in the United Kingdom Workplace: Looking backwards and Going Forwards? The Industrial Health Education Society at Work, 1922-40', *British Journal of Industrial Medicine*, 47 (1990), 366–71.

119. This is evident in Jones, *op. cit.* (note 116) and also in McIvor, *op. cit.* (note 109).

120. Helen Jones, *Health and Society in Twentieth Century Britain* (London: Longman, 1994), 71.

121. These include N.J. Wikeley, 'The Asbestos Regulations 1931: A Licence to Kill?', *Journal of Law and Society*, 19 (1992), 365–78; *idem.*, *Compensation for Industrial Disease* (Aldershot: Dartmouth, 1993); *idem.*, 'Turner & Newall: Early Organizational Responses to Litigation Risk', *Journal of Law and Society*, 24 (1997), 252–75; Morris Greenberg, 'Knowledge of the Health Hazard of Asbestos Prior to the Merewether and Price Report of 1930', *Social History of Medicine*, 7 (1994), 493–516; David J. Jeremy, 'Corporate Responses to the Emergent Recognition of a Health Hazard in the UK Asbestos Industry: The Case of Turner & Newall, 1920-1960', *Business and Economic History*, 24 (1995), 254–65; P.W.J. Bartrip, 'Too Little Too Late? The Home Office and the Asbestos Industry Regulations, 1931', *Medical History*, 42 (1998), 421–38; *idem.*, *The Way from Dusty Death. Turner & Newall and the*

Regulation of Asbestos-Related Disease in Britain, 1890s-1970s (London: Athlone Press, 2001); Geoffrey Tweedale and Philip Hansen, 'Protecting the Workers: the Medical Board and the Asbestos Industry, 1930s-1960s', *Medical History*, 42 (1998) 439–57; Geoffrey Tweedale, *From Magic Mineral to Killer Dust. Turner & Newall and the Asbestos Hazard* (Oxford: OUP, 2000).

122. Fowler and Wyke, *op. cit.* (note 43), 184–96; Peter Neild, *Byssinosis – 'The Lancashire Disease'* (London: Chartered Insurance Insurance Institute, 1982).
123. Arthur McIvor, 'Work and Health, 1880-1914. A Note on a Neglected Interaction', *Scottish Labour History Society Journal*, 24 (1989), 47–67; *idem.*, *A History of Work in Britain*, 1880-1950 (Basingstoke: Palgrave, 2001), 113–30.
124. H.A. Waldron, 'Occupational Health during the Second World War: Hope Deferred or Hope Abandoned?', *Medical History*, 41 (1997), 197–212.
125. *The History of Miners' Diseases, op. cit.* (note 38).
126. Joseph A. Page and Mary-Win O'Brien, *Bitter Wages: Ralph Nader's Study Group Report on Disease and Injury on the Job* (New York: Grossman, 1973); Nicholas Askounes Ashford, *Crisis in the Workplace: Occupational Diseases and Injury* (Cambridge, Mass.: MIT Press, 1976); Daniel Berman, *Death on the Job. Occupational Health and Safety Struggles in the United States* (New York: Monthly Review Press, 1979); Carl Gersuny, *Work Hazards and Industrial Conflict* (Hanover NH: University Press of New England, 1981); Bennett M. Judkins, *We Offer Ourselves. Towards Workers' Control of Occupational Health* (Westport: Greenwood Press, 1986); David Rosner and Gerald Markowitz (eds.), *Dying for Work. Workers' Safety and Health in Twentieth-Century America* (Bloomington: Indiana University Press, 1987); Barbara Ellen Smith, *Digging our Own Graves: Coal Miners and the Struggle over Black Lung Disease* (Philadelphia: Temple University Press, 1987); Ronald Bayer (ed), *The Health and Safety of Workers. Case Studies in the Politicsd of Professional Responsibility* (New York: OUP, 1988); Alan Derickson *Workers' Health, Workers' Democracy. The Western Miners' Struggle for Health and Safety, 1891-1925* (Ithaca: Cornell University Press, 1988); *idem.*, *Black Lung. Anatomy of a Public Health Disaster* (Ithaca and London: Cornell University Press, 1998); Jaqueline Karnell Corn, *Response to Occupational Health Hazards. A Historical Perspective* (New York: Van Nostrand Reinhold, 1992); David Rosner and Gerald Markowitz, *Deadly Dust: Silicosis and the Politics of Occupational Disease in Twentieth Century America*

(Princeton: Princeton University Press, 1991); Christopher C. Sellers, *Hazards of the Job. From Industrial Disease to Environmental Health Science* (Chapel Hill and London: University of North Carolina Press, 1997); Warren, *op. cit.* (note 32).

127. See Christopher Sellers, 'Working Disease In: Silicosis, Science and the Social History of Medicine. An Essay Review', *Journal of the History of Medicine and Allied Sciences*, 48 (1993), 98–109; P.W.J. Bartrip, 'Accidents and Ill-Health: The Hidden Wages of the Workplace', *Social History of Medicine*, 3 (1990), 291–6.

128. Harold Perkin, *The Origins of Modern English Society, 1780-1880* (London: Routledge & Kegan Paul, 1969), 268–70, 319–26, 338, 428–9, 451.

129. This responsibility remained until 1940 when the factory inspectorate was transferred, initially on a temporary basis, to the Ministry of Labour and National Service (MLNS). In 1946 this transfer was made 'permanent'. The MLNS reverted to its (pre-September 1939) title of Ministry of Labour in 1959. In 1968 the factory inspectorate became the responsibility of the Department of Employment and Productivity (Department of Employment from 1970). In 1974, following the *Health and Safety at Work Act (22&23 Eliz. 2 c 37)* factory inspection was brought under the control of the Health and Safety Executive.

130. On the origins of the Home Secretary and the Home Office see C.E. Troup, *The Home Office* (London and New York: G.P. Putnam's Sons Ltd., 1925) and Sir Frank Newsam, *The Home Office* (London: George Allen & Unwin, 1954).

131. Troup, *op. cit.* (note 130), 19.

132. *Ibid.*, 24.

133. Antony Peter Donajgrodski, 'The Home Office, 1822-48', University of Oxford. D.Phil. thesis (1974), 4 and 23.

134. Newsam, *op. cit.* (note 130), 26.

135. Troup, *op. cit.* (note 130), Preface.

136. See W.G. Carson, 'The Conventionalization of Early Factory Crime', *International Journal of the Sociology of Law*, 7 (1979), 37–60; P.W.J. Bartrip and P.T. Fenn, 'The Conventionalization of Factory Crime – a Re-assessment' Crime', *International Journal of the Sociology of Law*, 8 (1980), 175–86; P.W.J. Bartrip and P.T. Fenn, 'The Evolution of Regulatory Style in the Nineteenth Century British Factory Inspectorate', *Journal of Law and Society*, 10 (1983), 201–22.

137. Before the passing of the *Factory Act, 1844* (*7 & 8 Vict. c.15*), factory legislation did not mention industrial safety or accident

prevention.

138. Pellew divides the Home Office inspectorates – of which there were ten by 1876 – into three groups: industrial, law and order and medical. In so doing she excludes the factory inspectorate (along with the mines and explosives inspectors) from the law and order category, notwithstanding the policing and enforcing responsibilities of all three. Her distinction is based on the subject matter of inspection rather than differences in inspectors' policies, practices and powers. See Jill Pellew, *The Home Office, 1848-1914. From Clerks to Bureaucrats* (London: Heinemann Educational Books, 1982), 122–3.
139. *Annual Report of HM Chief Inspector of Factories and Workshops,* (1898) PP 1899 XII, 40–1; *Annual Report of HM Chief Inspector of Factories and Workshops,* (1936) *PP 1936–7 X*, 477.
140. Donajgrodski, *op. cit.* (note 133), 69.
141. *Ibid.*, 70–1, 149; Pellew, *op. cit.* (note 138), 30–1.
142. On the conservatism of the Home Office see Donajgrodski, *op. cit.* (note 133), 6; Pellew, *op. cit.* (note 138), 5, 8 and 179.
143. *Report of Inspector Rickards, PP 1835 XL*, 697–8; *Report of Inspector Horner*, PP 1837-8 XLV, 57.
144. Donajgrodski, *op. cit.* (note 133), 469.
145. Pellew, *op. cit.* (note 138), 148–9, 179.
146. Harcourt was Home Secretary in Gladstone's second ministry (1880-85). Matthews held the post from 1886-1892.
147. See my articles on Troup and Delevingne in the *New Dictionary of National Biography* (Oxford: OUP, forthcoming).
148. Pellew, *op. cit.* (note 138), 179–82.

2

Lead: The Road to Regulation

Introduction

Lead poisoning was, both statistically and politically, one of the most significant occupational diseases of the Victorian factory. Its symptoms include colic, constipation, anaemia, sterility, paralysis, blindness and encephalopathy. In its severest form it can be fatal. In women it can produce gynaecological problems. Indeed, in Victorian Britain it was deliberately used by women in some localities as an abortifaceant.[1] Reasonably safe in its metallic state, because in such a form it cannot normally enter the human body, lead becomes dangerous when converted into a dust or vapour that can be easily inhaled or ingested and thus absorbed into the bloodstream.

In the nineteenth century lead poisoning was not, any more than at other times, restricted to the industrial workforce. Obviously the Victorian era was free from problems associated with the use of lead additives to petroleum, but there were numerous other ways in which lead could impair the health of the general population. Notwithstanding well-established knowledge of its toxicity, lead was everywhere. It was a constituent of paint, textile dyes, food and drink containers, pottery and earthenware glazes, shotgun cartridges, water pipes, cosmetics and many other products. Ironically, the provision of piped water, usually considered to be one of the most crucial factors in the improvement of Victorian public health, also facilitated the spread of a metallic poison in the nation's drinking water. In the early-Victorian period lead, in its non-metallic form, was even a common ingredient of medicines. Thus in 1840 the *Provincial Medical Journal* noted that 'profuse perspiration' was treatable with sugar of lead, adding only that 'in some cases this remedy has produced serious inconvenience'. Acetate of lead was used to treat cholera victims in the late-1840s.[2] While the extent of low-level lead poisoning is unknown, it is reasonable to assume that it was more widespread than has usually been appreciated. Intriguingly, Gore Vidal has argued that many of the characters in Charles Dickens' fiction, far from being the gross caricatures that they sometimes appear, were actually realistic pen portraits drawn from a population among whom chronic lead poisoning, with attendant personality disorders, was widespread.[3]

Within the workplace lead poisoning was not associated with the textile trades and since factory regulation was confined, until 1864, to textile manufacture, the problem attracted little official recognition before this date. This is not to say that the health hazards of lead were unknown; as we have seen, these had been recognised in the ancient world and reasonably well understood, at least by some men of science, since the seventeenth century. Liquid lead glaze dates from the 1740s and Charles Turner Thackrah indicates that lead poisoning affected potters in the pre-Victorian period.[4] In 1793 the Society of Arts offered a prize of either a gold medal or £20 to anyone who could produce a viable leadless glaze for use on earthenware. Although prizes were awarded in 1820 and again in 1822, the glazes concerned were rejected as unsuitable by pottery manufacturers. As a result the Society renewed its offer in the 1850s.[5] In 1818 Samuel Taylor Coleridge inquired of the lawyer and diarist, Henry Crabb Robinson, 'whether there is not some law prohibiting, or limiting, or regulating the employment of children or adults, or of both, in the White Lead Manufactory'. He went on to say that when the surgeon, Astley Cooper, had appeared as a witness before a select committee of the House of Commons, he had expressed his belief that there was such a law. Coleridge's idea was that if his recollection was correct, the existence of protective legislation could be used to counter the *laissez-faire* argument that there was no precedent for laws to safeguard child workers.[6] Coleridge was clearly referring not to Astley Cooper, but to Ashley Cooper who had appeared before the 1816 Select Committee on the State of the Children Employed in the Manufactories of the United Kingdom. Cooper had said that, with the exception of arsenical colour production, the most dangerous occupation involved manufacture of sugar of lead. He had also 'seen many children suffer most severely from white lead manufactories'. When asked whether he knew of any law 'to restrain children from going to such manufactories', he had replied: 'Yes, I think there is a law'.[7] In fact, Cooper was misinformed. Hazardous as the processing of lead might have been, in 1816 and, indeed, for long afterwards, there was no legislation to protect the workforce.

Aside from these references, there is little evidence of sustained public interest in occupational lead poisoning until much later in the nineteenth century. However, the Children's Employment Commission did broach the subject in the 1840s. This Commission, established in 1842 at the behest of Lord Ashley (later the Seventh

Earl of Shaftesbury) to investigate conditions of child labour in mines and industries not covered by existing legislation, did uncover a problem of lead poisoning in the Staffordshire Potteries. The Commission comprised a central board, consisting of two factory inspectors, Leonard Horner and Robert Saunders, plus Thomas Tooke and Thomas Southwood Smith, both of whom had served on the 1833 Royal Commission on Factories.[8] Like that earlier inquiry the Children's Employment Commission also employed sub-commissioners for the purpose of collecting information from the regions. The Commission's first report, which dealt with coal mining and led to the passing of the *Mines Act, 1842*, is its best known. This is largely because, with its emphasis on the exploitation of (often semi-naked) women and children, it was also the most sensational; indeed, few official publications have ever surpassed it in terms of public impact. But it is the second report, which covered many hitherto unregulated manufacturing industries, including metalware, earthenware, glass, lace, hosiery, calico printing and paper making, that concerns us here. This report 'did not make the impression on the public which that on Mines had done' and Ashley 'made no immediate move to act upon it'.[9] It was in this that the existence of lead poisoning in earthenware was documented, albeit at no great length.

Samuel Scriven and the Children's Employment Commission

The British pottery industry has been centred in North Staffordshire since the seventeenth century. Its initial location there owed much to the plentiful availability of the three main raw materials of production: coal, clay and lead. Subsequently, the presence of a skilled workforce encouraged the concentration of the industry in the area. Major expansion took place in the second half of the eighteenth century as consumer demand and technical innovation brought about huge growth in the number of potbanks (pottery factories). In 1841 the workforce comprised nearly 25,000 workers; these were distributed among some 150 potbanks. Every subsequent census throughout the rest of the nineteenth century showed further growth in both the number of workers and of potbanks. By 1891 some 90% of pottery workers and 80% of national production were to be found in the Staffordshire Potteries. In 1901 about 46,500 workers, employed in 400 potbanks, were turning out goods to the value of £3m pa.[10]

The report of the Children's Employment Commission on the Staffordshire Potteries was based on the investigations of one of its sub-commissioners, Samuel Scriven. It drew attention to the 'most pernicious and destructive' effects of the processes of dipping, scouring and throwing and of plate, saucer and dishmaking. Scriven was particularly concerned about lead poisoning among dippers (those who immersed the 'biscuit' ware in the glazing liquid), noting that for coarse goods a 'large proportion' of carbonate of lead was used in the glaze.[11] Workers' constant handling of such rough ware led to smoothing of fingers, loss of cuticle and, occasionally, bleeding. Scriven believed these conditions facilitated the absorption of lead into the system – though later medical opinion minimised the importance of cutaneous absorption as against ingestion via the gastro-intestinal tract or pulmonary inhalation.[12]

Although dipping was an occupation of adult males, newly-glazed ware was passed on to boys for shelving and drying. Some of the children employed in these tasks were as young as five, while hundreds were between the ages of six and eight. Both the adult dippers and their juvenile assistants, Scriven noticed, had 'their hands and clothes almost always saturated' with glazing liquid. Furthermore, 'reckless of the danger they... seldom or ever change, or use precautionary measures, frequently taking their meals in the same room, sufficiently satisfied to wipe their hands on their aprons'.[13] It is instructive to note Scriven's observation that wages for dipping-house workers were relatively high – about 30s (£1.50) per week for men and 5s (25p) for boys. Indeed, he explained such rates in terms of danger money: 'This pay', he believed, 'is a strong temptation to the thoughtless and improvident parent, who, regardless of consequences to their offspring, permit them, so long as they reap the advantages of their labour, to continue in this pest-house'.[14]

In response to Scriven's report and the evidence he produced, the Central Commissioners reached a number of conclusions. These were that in the great majority of workplaces healthy conditions were absent and that even where harmful materials were in use there were no facilities for workers to change their clothes or to wash before meal breaks. While the work required of children and young persons was seldom oppressive, laborious, or injurious, there were 'some lamentable exceptions', including within earthenware manufacture. What the Commissioners did not do, on the grounds that their terms of reference did not permit it, was propose any solutions. In terms of recommendations they went no further than to suggest that the moral and physical condition of the working classes called for the serious consideration of parliament and government.[15]

Dippers had informed Scriven that poisoning was less prevalent in 1842 than it had been formerly when higher concentrations of lead were present in the glaze. Their anecdotal evidence may be compared with the recollections of Charles Shaw who, recalling the pottery industry of the 1840s from an Edwardian perspective, wrote:

> I don't think lead was such a deadly factor in those days as now, except among 'the dippers,' who were always using it. The same processes were not carried on then as now, such as have been required by modern developments. Earthenware then was a very different thing from what it is to-day, with its dirty, brownish-looking glaze, whereas to-day it has to look brilliant and white as china ware.[16]

When assessing Shaw's value as a witness it should be remembered not only that he was looking back over many decades but also that he was writing at a time of fierce public controversy about lead poisoning in the pottery trade. It may be, therefore, that Shaw, contrasting the prevailing furore with the relative lack of concern some sixty years earlier, concluded that the poison itself, rather than the disquiet, was the new phenomenon. In the 1890s some observers were of the opinion that lead poisoning in pottery and earthenware had been more prevalent in earlier decades.[17] Certainly, the historian, Neil McKendrick, has dubbed Shaw a polemicist and questioned his reliability as a witness. Even so, McKendrick does suggest that Shaw could 'speak with some authority of conditions of work'.[18] In the absence of statistical or other compelling evidence, there is no way of determining whether lead poisoning among pottery and earthenware workers became more or less prevalent in the course of the nineteenth century. Shaw acknowledges that serious dangers existed in the 1840s. On the other hand, the autobiography downplays lead poisoning as having been a major health hazard for potters in that decade.

Lord Shaftesbury (as he became in 1851) attributed the *Print Works Act, 1845*, which he had introduced in parliament, and the *Bleaching Works Act, 1860*, to the second report of the Children's Employment Commission.[19] He explained the lack of additional legislation in the following terms:

> ...although the Report of that Commission disclosed some terrible facts as regards the health and morals of the children, the country was not then ripe for propositions such as these and the consequence was that I was very much obstructed in my endeavours to carry into effect many of the recommendations of that Commission.[20]

Although historians might quibble over the vagueness of the term 'ripeness', dismissing it as a *post hoc* rationalisation for inaction, many would agree that *laissez-faire* sentiment was a significant factor in forestalling major reform of working conditions outside the established areas of textile factories and coal mines, where the emotional impact of the first report of the Children's Employment Commission made legislative action almost inevitable. Elsewhere, it was not until the passing of the *Factory Acts Extension Act, 1864* that the regulation of labour in non-textile employment was introduced. This act, which represented a first tentative step towards limiting workers' exposure to lead, followed the deliberations of another Children's Employment Commission and a report by the Medical Officer of the Privy Council, Sir John Simon, on the health risks faced by lead workers. We may now look at what the findings of these two inquiries, undertaken more or less simultaneously, reveal about occupational lead poisoning in the 1860s, that is, shortly before the beginning of statutory regulation. First, the Privy Council report.

Whitley's report

In the late-1850s and early-1860s Sir John Simon, as head of the Privy Council's medical department, undertook a systematic inquiry into the outstanding health problems of the day. Assisted by an expert staff, his investigations centred upon occupational health and hygiene, a subject that greatly interested him. As Simon's biographer states, 'between 1860 and 1863, he directed a series of major investigations into the health circumstances and consequences of manufacture: [this was] the most meticulous and comprehensive survey of the sanitary condition of labour so far undertaken directly by English government'.[21] In 1862 three occupational health inquiries were undertaken; one of these, conducted by Dr George Whitley, medical registrar at Guy's Hospital, investigated the health risks encountered by workers in trades in which lead and mercury were used.[22] Whitley's report is important for two reasons. First, it covered eleven trades in which lead was used. This was unusual since most observers, until the last years of the century, looked at individual lead processes in isolation. Second, Whitley attempted, though with little success, to analyse such issues as the extent and severity of poisoning, the reasons for increasing or decreasing rates of incidence and the value of the remedial measures hitherto employed.

Whitley found that lead smelters were little exposed to a risk of lead poisoning owing to the measures adopted to prevent the wasteful loss of lead during the smelting process. Neither was his report notably pessimistic about the dangers of employment in the manufacture of lead preparations such as white lead, red lead, or sugar of lead. Although he was refused permission to visit one of the large white lead works in London, he was allowed to inspect two Newcastle-upon-Tyne factories in which white and red lead and shot were produced. These inspections led him to conclude that while white lead manufacture was one of the most hazardous branches of the lead industry, 'even here it appears that if they [the workers] would strictly observe the precautions suggested the ill effects would be comparatively slight'.[23] Despite the fact that medical practitioners were attached to both the factories he visited, Whitley succeeded in obtaining little precise information about the extent and severity of poisoning. He was merely informed that the incidence had declined in recent years owing to a combination of improved sanitation and modified manufacturing techniques. However, the one doctor prepared to speak to him expressed the opinion that no precautions could ever obviate the dangers of two processes, namely, the removal of white lead from the 'stacks' in which it was produced, or the packing of it into casks. As for the dangers of red lead or sugar of lead manufacture Whitley was able to uncover little evidence. Either the processes appeared to be relatively safe (as in the former case) or, as in the latter case, production was on a small scale.

Whitley also minimised the risks of lead poisoning in pottery manufacture. Although considerable amounts of white lead were used in glazes, and although dippers tended to remain in their jobs for long periods, Whitley judged that few were exposed to serious health hazards. He received evidence that poisoning had diminished in recent years owing to the adoption of the practice of 'fritting' lead before use (that is, converting it to a powderless, crystallised form), the abandonment of arsenic as an ingredient of glaze and a reduction in the lead content of glazes. Whitley's investigation of other trades, namely, painting, plumbing, printing, type-founding, shot-making, enamelling, floor-cloth manufacture and glass-making yielded similar results. For none of these occupations could he find evidence of serious health hazards; indeed, the indications were that where lead poisoning had been more-or-less prevalent, sanitary and technical improvements had done much to eradicate it. Whitley summed up his findings by stating that whereas a 'very considerable' number of people were employed in the lead industries, in 'a very few only of these occupations does the amount of danger from lead-poisoning appear to be at all serious, while in the others very little inconvenience is felt'.[24] Even in the riskier occupations precautionary measures that could render dangers 'very insignificant' were available. Whitley specified a number of general precautions, including temperance, use of overalls, general cleanliness, ventilation, use of respirators and occasional doses of aperient medicine, all of which could do much to safeguard lead workers. For white lead manufacture, he suggested that where dry grinding was unavoidable, the machinery should be housed in enclosed and properly-ventilated chambers. Otherwise grinding, pulverising and packing should be undertaken only in wet conditions. Finally, Whitley considered the prospects for legislative interference with the lead industries. He was, in fact, strongly opposed to any such interference:

> While it appears almost certain that the full adoption of the above precautions would reduce the amount of lead-poisoning amongst persons employed in the various branches of lead industry [sic] to a minimum, it is only just to the principals generally to state that the neglect of those precautions lies almost exclusively with the workpeople themselves. Since, therefore, except in cases where the neglect of the precautions prescribed endangers the lives of others, as in the case of coal-miners, the work-people cannot well be actually compelled to adopt them, there appears to be no call for legislative interference in reference to any of the branches of the lead industry.[25]

In a very brief reference to Whitley's report Royston Lambert suggests that it revealed the 'serious and common dangers' faced by lead workers. In fact as the above summary indicates, Whitley's intention was to demonstrate that in general danger was neither serious nor common. Equally puzzlingly Bledington suggests that Whitley's report showed the existence of a large-scale health problem and consequently was a factor in turning industrial lead poisoning into a topic of public interest, persuading the government to include potbanks in the *Factory Acts Extension Act, 1864*.[26] In reality, Whitley upheld *laissez-faire* dogma and in so doing repudiated any notion that adults, whether they be employers or workers, should be treated by the state as anything other than free agents in a free labour market.

Although Simon evidently accepted the general tenor of Whitley's report, he was impressed by the fact that his colleague had failed to obtain statistics indicating the full extent of the disease among those engaged in the most dangerous occupations. He also suspected that Whitley had inspected premises that were 'very favourable specimens'.[27] Presumably for these reasons Simon was much less sanguine than Whitley about prevailing conditions in some of the lead trades. He concluded his brief report by observing that 'in my opinion it deserves more particular consideration than it has yet received, whether the processes which diffuse lead dust and which occasion the chief danger of his industry, are not processes which ought to be discontinued or modified'. Such a conclusion was far closer in mood to the views of Francis Longe who, more-or-less contemporaneously with Whitley, investigated lead poisoning in the Staffordshire Potteries for the Children' s Employment Commission. It would therefore appear reasonable to conclude, especially in the light of subsequent findings, that Whitley's assessments were somewhat complacent.

Francis Longe and the Children's Employment Commission

The Children's Employment Commission (CEC) was established in February 1862, for the purpose of examining the employment of children and young persons in trades and manufactures not already regulated by law.[28] Its main concern, in common with most of the early factory inquiries, was with the education and hours of labour of juveniles. As we have seen, it was not the first such commission. In the early-1840s a CEC had also examined the case for extending the legal protections of the Factory Acts to a variety of industries. Though this led directly to the passing of the (Coal) *Mines Act, 1842,* which prohibited women and children (below the age of 10) from working underground, it had no such payoff in other areas of employment even though conditions of labour in the so-called 'free industries' were 'much more melancholy than anything that had been reported with reference to the great factories'.[29]

The 1862 appointment appears to have been made partly because Lord Shaftesbury's Commons appeal (of 15 August 1861) for an inquiry into unregulated trades met with support, including from some employers. As the debates on the *Factory Acts Extension Act, 1864* showed, opposition to the regulation of child labour was much less entrenched than it had been in preceding decades. This opened the way to an extension of the factory acts beyond the few occupations, and those not necessarily the most dangerous, unsanitary or arduous, to which they had applied for decades. During the late-1850s and early-1860s John Simon and Edward Greenhow began to show not only the relationship between occupation and mortality, but also that existing legislation largely ignored matters of health and hygiene.[30] '[No] existing law', wrote Simon in 1861, 'is more than very imperfectly applicable to procure the mitigation of unwholesome industrial conditions'.[31] By this time factory safety regulations compelling, *inter alia*, the fencing of machinery, dated back some seventeen years but, Simon observed, 'deaths from unboxed machinery would probably count as nothing in comparison with those which the unventilatedness of factories occasions'.[32]

The Children's Employment Commissioners were Hugh Seymour Tremenheere, who in 1842 had become the first mines inspector, Edward Carleton Tufnell, an inspector of Poor Law schools and Richard Dugard Grainger, an anatomist and physiologist who served on a number of official inquiries. Faced as they were with a vast array of unregulated industries, the commissioners had to select both the trades that were to be investigated and the manner in which their investigations should be conducted. They decided that three classes of industry warranted examination: those in which the masters, workers, or both had called for intervention; those which had grown in importance since the 1840-2 inquiry, some of which came into the category of 'noxious trades'; and those identified by the previous commission as being in need of regulation but which remained unregulated. They proposed, in the first instance, to look at enterprises that came within the first two of these categories. As for the method of investigation, they opted for a strategy 'tried and tested' by earlier commissions, namely the appointment of assistant commissioners responsible for investigating particular trades. The assistants appointed were: Francis Davy Longe, John Edward White and Henry William Lord, all of whom were barristers.[33]

The commissioners' first report was signed on 15 June 1863. It dealt with eight trades, one of which, pottery, particularly concerns us here. The report on potteries was based largely upon inquiries carried out in the Staffordshire Potteries by Francis Longe in 1862. The Potteries was selected for investigation partly because the commission received a memorial from twenty-six employers, representing most of the principal works, calling for legislative protection of the young and partly because of the dominant position of Staffordshire in relation to the rest of the trade.[34] It is noteworthy that the manufacturers' memorial made no mention of dangers to health from toxic substances, but dwelt upon the evils of employing the very young, particularly since this meant they they could not acquire any education.

Longe took evidence from a variety of sources including manufacturers, workers, medical men, clergymen and schoolmasters. One of the doctors with whom he corresponded was Thomas Arlidge, who, since May 1862, had been senior physician at the

North Staffordshire Infirmary. Three decades later, as we have seen, Arlidge established himself, following publication of his book, *The Hygiene, Diseases and Mortality of Occupations* (1892), as the leading authority on industrial health. His opinions, which were based on regular visits to potbanks and frequent contact with pottery workers are, therefore, of great interest. Arlidge told Longe that:

> The potters as a class, both men and women, but more especially the former, represent a much degenerated population, both physically and mentally. They are, as a rule, stunted in growth, ill-shaped and frequently deformed in the chest; they become prematurely old and are certainly short-lived; they are phlegmatic and bloodless and exhibit their debility of constitution by obstinate attacks of dyspepsia and disorders of the liver and kidneys and by rheumatism.[35]

One of the factors responsible for this sorry tale of ill health was, according to Arlidge, the use of lead in glazes.

Longe's report indicated that there had been little improvement in the physical condition of the Potteries workforce since Scriven's inquiry twenty years earlier. It is clear from the report, however, that lead poisoning was not the sole, or even the main, reason for high mortality and morbidity rates among pottery workers; the dust-laden atmosphere was probably more significant. Longe's references to lead poisoning concentrated on the dippers; here too his findings were similar to Scriven's. He found boys of a 'very young age' engaged in the 'specially injurious employment' of carrying the ware to the dipper and thereby spending much time in a 'poisoned atmosphere':

> The injurious effects of the dipping tub are well known. Few dippers continue many years at their work without suffering from painter's colic or paralysis; many becoming crippled at an early age. Boys of about 14 or 15 years of age are employed to 'gather' the ware from the dipper; they are brought more in contact with the glaze than the other boys. Women are also employed in the dipping house to brush the ware. Nearly all the boys whom I found engaged in this work had felt its effects more or less; some had suffered very seriously. There seems to be ground for supposing that some constitutions are more affected by the lead poison than others.[36]

Longe, in common with Whitley, went on to suggest that some health improvements in the dipping room had been achieved by the withdrawal of arsenic as a glazing ingredient. He also held out hope that in the future lead too might be dispensed with without making the glaze more expensive to produce or less efficient in operation.

The commissioners, who suggested that pottery manufacture should be brought under the factory acts, proposed a number of remedies for safeguarding the health of children and young persons. These included improved ventilation, abolition of overtime, regular mealtimes and 'specific regulations' for the protection of health in particular departments. One novel proposal, which was not taken up, was for the temporary appointment of a medical inspector. In fact, it was not until 1898 that such an official was appointed. The main way in which the commissioners proposed to extend protective measures to the young people employed in potteries owed as much to the precedent of the mines acts as to the factory acts. The *Mines Acts, 1855* and *1860* (*18 & 19 Vict. c.108* and *23 & 24 Vict. c.151*) had provided for the establishment of general health and safety rules applicable to all coal mines, plus 'special rules', which took account of local conditions, applicable to individual collieries. These special rules were compiled by mine owners and submitted to the Home Office for approval. If the Home Office registered no objection within a period of forty days, the rules were established. However, subject to an arbitration procedure, it was also open to the secretary of state to propose additions or alterations. The Children's Employment Commissioners recommended the use of special rules to regulate occupational health in potteries.[37]

Factory Acts extension

Under pressure from Lord Shaftesbury and others, the government's Factory Acts Extension Bill, received a first reading in March 1864.[38] After speedily passing through all its parliamentary stages, it received the Royal Assent on 25 July 1864. The act brought five trades: pottery and earthenware, lucifer matchmaking, percussion cap making, paper staining and fustian cutting under regulation, applying the provisions of the existing factory acts, to all of them. In addition the newly regulated trades were to be subject to sanitary provisions relating to cleanliness and ventilation, so 'as to render harmless so far as is practicable any Gases, Dust, or other impurities generated in the Process of Manufacture that may be injurious to Health'. Occupiers who failed to comply with sanitary measures would be liable to fines of between £3 and £10. The act also provided for the establishment of special rules, to be drawn up by employers and approved by the Home Office, relating to the conduct of workers. This was 'to prevent the requirements of this act as to

Cleanliness and Ventilation in a Factory being infringed by the wilful Misconduct or wilful Negligence of the workmen'. Workers convicted of breaching special rules would be liable to fines of up to £1. In the last third of the nineteenth century and beyond, the regulation of unsanitary conditions and unhealthy processes by means of special rules specifying workers' and employers' duties, came to characterise the regulation of the dangerous trades. This, however, was for the future.[39]

The 1864 act also made specific provision for limiting operatives' exposure to the lead hazard. Although it included no reference to lead, it provided that 'at no time after the passing of this Act shall any Child, Young Person, or Woman be allowed to take her or his Meals, or to remain during any time allowed for Meals, in the Dipping Houses, Dippers' Drying Rooms, or China-scouring rooms'. The potential effect of this clause was to offer some protection to certain workers against deleterious dusts and other harmful substances, including lead. The extent to which it represented a significant attack on lead poisoning is questionable. Indeed, the extent to which such protection as the act offered ever became a shop-floor reality is unknown. Mess suggests that rules compiled and enforced by employers under the terms of the 1864 act 'did not amount to much'. In any case, they 'fell into disuse between 1878 and 1891' when they were re-enacted in the *Factory and Workshop Act, 1891*.[40] This author's research on factory legislation and inspection in this period supports the notion that the impact of the 1864 act was very limited.[41] The *Factory Acts Extension Act, 1867*, which followed further reports of the Children's Employment Commission, was significant from an occupational health viewpoint, in that it included the first prohibitions from work on dangerous processes (*30 & 31 Vict. c.46*). Some of the restrictions introduced under the terms of the act promised to limit exposure to lead poisoning. But the act did not, any more than earlier legislation, represent an assault on the problem. Indeed, the onset of regulation was delayed until the factory inspectorate, more than a decade later, began to refer to dangers posed by white lead works.

If we ask why lead poisoning gained little significant official attention till the mid-1870s, we are faced with the difficult historical problem of explaining a negative. Attention is directed to Chapter 1 of this volume where various reasons for the 'delayed' regulation of occupational health are discussed. Beyond, this, it is important to avoid reliance upon hindsight, the use of which might convey the erroneous conclusion that inaction stemmed from a wilful determination to ignore the problem. It is more fruitful to consider how the Victorian Home Office obtained information about the existence of social problems and was prompted to propose remedies. Classically, this would occur either as the result of an MP raising and pursuing a question in the House, through press campaigns – to which the Home Office could be very sensitive – or through individuals or groups lobbying by letter, memorial, or deputation ('moral entrepreneurs' as they have been called).[42] Whatever extra-parliamentary strategies were employed though, the question would inevitably have to come before parliament if legislation were to be passed. Moreover, for a successful outcome to be achieved, parliamentary 'champions', of Lord Shaftesbury's ilk, would be needed. For much of the nineteenth century there was little popular demand for occupational health reform for the benefit of lead workers. One reason for this is that employees in the lead industries were not very numerous. Of course, the pottery industry, which employed about 63,000 people in 1907, was large but more then half of these were deemed by the factory inspectorate to be engaged in safe processes. Fewer than 11% worked with lead. Those who suffered from lead poisoning appear often to have suffered their fates with resignation. As the factory inspector, J.H.Walmsley, commented in 1898, some workers considered lead poisoning 'a necessary consequence of their work and when unable to withstand the poison had dropped out from the ranks and been forgotten'. As for employers, they 'have apparently been unable to realise, *individually*, the pernicious effect which lead has had upon the operatives. Not being aware of such cases having occurred on their works, they evidently concluded that their neighbours were likewise exempt'.[43] These observations raise several questions. How, for example, can such a rationalisation explain the behaviour of those employers on whose premises poisoning actually occurred? How could employers ignore the poisoning statistics that were published by the factory inspectorate from 1896? More fundamental is the possibility that Walmsley's comment indicates the condescension of a middle-class bureaucrat towards working class misery and death. How much less painful for those with the power to ameliorate conditions or to reduce poisoning rates if suffering could be viewed in terms of acceptance and inevitability?

Certainly, some historians would contest Walmsley's opinions, particularly insofar as they seek to explain employer behaviour, preferring an explanation that emphasises the exploitation of the workforce.[44] Employers' opposition to remedial measures and their reluctance to deal with well-known dangers lends support to the notion of exploitation. On the other hand, employers had no interest in crippling their employees and the pathology of lead poisoning was imperfectly understood in the nineteenth century. Moreover, widespread use of lead and lead-based products in middle-class homes indicates that outside the workplace, at least, neither contact with lead, nor the occurrence of lead poisoning were restricted by social class. When, from the 1890s, the extent of lead poisoning was more fully appreciated, significant improvements, if the official statistics are to be believed, occurred fairly rapidly. Hence, in the case of industrial lead poisoning, it is going too far to see occupational ill health exclusively in terms of class oppression or indifference. Manufacturers were keen to protect their economic interests which, no doubt, they felt were shared by workers who were dependent upon them for their livelihood, against what they saw as meddlesome regulations that threatened the viability of their businesses. As we shall see, most employers were willing to adopt, without protest, measures aimed at improving occupational health. Truly recalcitrant employers probably constituted an atypical minority that attracted disproportionate press and political attention.

To revert to our examination of how and why the lead poisoning question came to attract public attention when it did. Parliamentary and extra-parliamentary pressure was necessary to prompt government interest and action. Such pressure might almost be termed a necessary precondition of government intervention, for governments, of whatever political persuasion were almost always reactive rather than pro-active on social questions. Given that departments of state, in the Victorian period, had limited facilities for information-gathering, had relatively small bureaucracies for assessing incoming information, were required by the Treasury to place a high priority on economy and fiscal discipline and were likely to be ideologically averse to investigation and legislation, intervention generally needed some strong external stimulus.[45] In the case of social welfare questions associated with manufacturing industry, Lord Shaftesbury was clearly a dominant figure; the factory inspectorate also played a prominent part. But neither Shaftesbury, who, in the 1830s and 1840s had interested himself in the subject of factory safety, nor anyone else, took up the question of industrial lead poisoning before the inspectorate did so in the mid-1870s. Up to this point none of the pre-conditions for government intervention had been met, for although several reports of the Children's Employment

Commission and other inquiries had referred to lead poisoning in industry,[46] the matter had never been brought before the Houses of Parliament. However, within a very few years of the inspectorate raising the issue, all the pre-conditions had been met and governments – Conservative and Liberal – became committed to action.

The first government to show concern was Disraeli's Conservative administration of 1874-80, a government which has been highly regarded, perhaps excessively so, in terms of its social reform record.[47] But Gladstone's governments of 1880–5 and 1892–4, which are generally regarded as having been somewhat inert in social reform terms, were equally active. This is probably because continuity of staffing at the Home Office meant that, in this context, electoral change was of little significance. The question that remains, however, is why the factory inspectorate did not raise the question of lead poisoning until the mid-seventies at which point, as we have seen, the issue was not new, even within the official consciousness. To answer this, account needs to be taken of the leadership of the factory department. Alexander Redgrave, who was born in 1818 and was, therefore, 58 (and, hence, in Victorian terms, comparatively old) when he became chief inspector of factories, was far from being an adventurous innovator. Indeed, he was a cautious man who was loath to antagonise employers and stressed the advantages of a conciliatory approach when dealing with factory occupiers. Before his appointment as chief inspector Redgrave had been, with Robert Baker, joint chief inspector of factories. Because Baker and Redgrave were, literally, not on speaking terms, the scope for joint policy initiation was limited.[48] In any case Baker, notwithstanding that he was the first medically-trained inspector of factories, never showed much interest in occupational health.[49] Aside from such personal influences upon policy, it is also important to stress the legislative context. The nineteenth century factory acts were primarily concerned with restricting the hours of labour and ensuring the education of children; they were far less concerned with promoting health and safety. Safety regulations, it is true, dated from 1844, but their enforcement constituted only a relatively small part of inspectors' responsibilities. The most satisfactory, though less than ideal way of demonstrating this is to plot the incidence of safety prosecutions relative to prosecutions arising from non-safety breaches of the acts. By doing this we find that, in 1879-80, for example, fewer than 5% of all prosecutions were for breach of safety regulations.[50] As for protecting the general health of factory operatives, little legislation was concerned with this till the 1880s. The sanitary provisions established by the *Factory Acts Extension Acts, 1864* and *1867*, which represented only minor incursions into the field, affected relatively few workers. Thus, it is reasonable to conclude that the factory inspectorate failed to raise the lead question because their normal duties did not bring them directly into contact with the problem. Given that the inspectorate's resources, relative to workload, were always stretched, it is also understandable that they tended to avoid raising controversial issues not strictly within their terms of reference. Why, though, did this position change in the mid-seventies? The explanation lies partly in the terms of the two extension acts, the *Workshop Regulation Act, 1867* and the *Factory and Workshop Act, 1871* which together extended the provisions of the factory acts to all manufacturing employment, large or small; and partly in the growth of the 'new journalism' which viewed health 'scares' in terms of good copy and high sales. As a result inspectors' attention was drawn to the question of industrial lead poisoning, initially among white lead workers.

Notes

1. P. Knight, 'Women and Abortion in Victorian and Edwardian England', *History Workshop*, 4 (1977), 57–69.
2. *Provincial Medical Journal*, 31 Oct. 1840, 88; *Provincial Medical and Surgical Journal*, 30 May 1849, 297.
3. 'Bookshelf', BBC Radio 4, 20 Oct. 1985.
4. Lorna Weatherill, *The Pottery Trade and North Staffordshire, 1660-1760* (Manchester: Manchester University Press, 1971), 28–30; C.T. Thackrah, *The Effect of Arts, Trades and Professions and of Civic States and Habits of Living, on Health and Longevity: with Suggestions for the Removal of Many of the Agents which Produce Disease and Shorten the Duration of Life* (London: Longman, Rees, Orme, Brown, Green and Longman, 2nd edn, 1832), 120–21; Clare Holdsworth, 'Potters' Rot and Plumbism: Occupational Health in the North Staffordshire Pottery Industry', Liverpool University, Ph.D. thesis (1995), 42.
5. Rhoda Helena Bledington, 'The Growth and Awareness of Health and Safety at Work, 1780-1900', Aston University M.Litt. thesis (1983), 78; *Transactions of the Society of Arts* (1793) xi; (1820), xxxviii; (1822) xl, 44–6; *Journal of the Society of Arts* 31 Dec. 1852, 65; *Report of the Departmental Committee Appointed to inquire into the Dangers attendant on the Use of Lead and the Danger or Injury to Health arising from Dust and other Causes in the Manufacture of Earthenware and China and in the Processes incidental thereto*

including the Making of Lithographic Transfers, PP 1910 XXIX,105.

6. Thomas Sadler (ed), *Diary, Reminiscences and Correspondence of Henry Crabb Robinson, Barrister-at-Law* (London: Macmillan, 3 vols. 1869), II, 93–5; see B.L. Hutchins and A. Harrison, *A History of Factory Legislation* (London: P.S. King, 1926 edn), 29.
7. *Select Committee on the State of the Children Employed in the Manufactories of the United Kingdom*, PP 1816 III, 267.
8. *His Majesty's Commission of Inquiry into the Employment of Children in Factories*, PP 1833 XX & XXI.
9. G.B.A.M. Finlayson, *The Seventh Earl of Shaftesbury, 1801-1885* (London: Eyre Methuen, 1981), 190.
10. R. Whipp, *Patterns of Labour. Work and Social Change in the Pottery Industry* (London: Routledge, 1990), 11,15–24.
11. Biscuit ware is pottery or earthenware that has undergone its first firing prior to glazing, painting or other embellishment. Throwing was the process whereby clay was fashioned into ware. Scouring involved the cleaning of the ware. See Oxford English Dictionary on-line (2nd edn, 1989).
12. *Appendix to the Second Report of the Children's Employment Commission. Trades and Manufactures, part 1. Reports and Evidence from the Sub-Commissioners, Reports by Samuel Scriven*, PP 1843 XV, 216.
13. *Ibid.*, 216–17.
14. *Ibid.*, 217
15. *Irish University Press Reprints of British Parliamentary Papers (Industrial Revolution Children's Employment 9). Second Report of the Commissioners on Trades and Manufactures*, 195–204.
16. Charles Shaw, *When I was a Child* (Firle: Caliban, 1977 edn), 80.
17. *Report on the Conditions of Labour in Potteries, the Injurious Effects upon the Health of the Workpeople and the Proposed Remedies*, PP 1893-4 XVII, 46–7.
18. Neil McKendrick, 'The Victorian View of Midland History: a Historiographical Study of the Potteries', *Midland History*, I (1971), 39.
19. 3 *Hansard*, 172 (24 July 1863), 1337.
20. Quoted in Finlayson, *op. cit.* (note 9), 227.
21. R. J. Lambert, *Sir John Simon and English Social Administration* (London: MacGibbon & Key, 1963), 331.
22. On Whitley see C. Fraser Brockington, *Public Health in the Nineteenth Century* (Edinburgh & London: E.S. Livingstone, 1965), 244–46.
23. *Sixth Report of the Medical Officer of the Privy Council. Appendix by*

George Whitley, PP 1864 XXVIII, 354–55.

24. *Ibid.*, 360.
25. *Ibid.*, 361. This outlook reflected the common law notion that in entering an employment a workers voluntarily accepted all the risks posed by their occupation. See P.W.J. Bartrip and S.B. Burman, *The Wounded Soldiers of Industry. Industrial Compensation Policy, 1830-1897* (Oxford: Clarendon Press, 1983).
26. Lambert, *op. cit.* (note 21), 334; Bledington, (note 3), *op. cit.* 69.
27. *Sixth Report of the Medical Officer of the Privy Council*, PP 1864 XXVIII, 21.
28. In 1862 the Factory Acts applied only to the textile trades. In no other branch of *manufacturing* industry were there any restrictions on, for example, the age at which children could begin work, or the length of their working day. The *Factory Act, 1844* (*7 & 8 Vict. c.15*) defined a child as someone below the age of 13 and a young person as anyone between the ages of 13 and 18.
29. Edwin Hodder, *The Life and Work of the Seventh Earl of Shaftesbury K.G.* (London: Cassell, 1893), 242.
30. Edward Greenhow (1814–88) was a London-based physician who carried out a number of investigations on epidemics and public health on behalf of the Privy Council and the Board of Health. See *Dictionary of National Biography* (London: Smith, Elder, 1908), VIII, 524.
31. *Fourth Report of the Medical Officer of the Privy Council*, PP 1862 XXII, 493.
32. *Ibid.*, 495.
33. *First Report of the Children's Employment Commission*, PP 1863 XVIII, 7.
34. *Ibid.*, 8 and Appendix: Memorials of Employers in the Potteries, 322; Marguerite W. Dupree, *Family Structure in the Staffordshire Potteries* (Oxford: Clarendon Press, 1995), 218, 220, 238.
35. *First Report of the Children's Employment Commission*, PP 1863 XVIII, Appendix: Reports and Evidence of Assistant Commissioners, J.T. Arledge (sic) to F.D. Longe, 31 Oct. 1862, 120; See Thomas Arlidge, *On the Mortality of Stoke-upon-Trent and its Causes, with Especial Reference to Children and Potters*, (Newcastle-under-Lyme: np, 1864), 1–23.
36. *First Report of the Children's Employment Commission. Appendix: Reports and Evidence of Assistant Commissioners*, PP 1863 XVIII, 101.
37. *First Report of the Children's Employment Commission*, PP 1863 XVIII, 8–48.

38. 3 *Hansard*, 172 (16 July 1863), 870; (24 July 1863), 1331–8; Finlayson, *op. cit.* (note 9), 407–08.
39. *27 & 28 Vict. c.48, s.4.*The regulation of industry only to the extent that it was 'practicable' (or, later, 'reasonably practicable') which subsequently became a legislative commonplace, dates from the 1864 Act.
40. H.A. Mess, *Factory Legislation and its Administration, 1891-1924* (London: P.S. King, 1926), 51–2.
41. P.W.J. Bartrip, 'State Intervention in mid-Nineteenth Century Britain: Fact or Fiction?', *Journal of British Studies*, xxxiii (1983), 63–83.
42. R.M. Hartwell, 'Entrepreneurship and Public Inquiry: the Growth of Government in Nineteenth Century Britain', in F.M.L. Thompson, (ed), *Landowners, Capitalists and Entrepreneurs* (Oxford: Clarendon Press, 1994); P.W.J. Bartrip and R.M. Hartwell, 'Profit and Virtue. Economic Theory and the Regulation of Occupational Health in Nineteenth and Twentieth Century Britain', in Keith Hawkins (ed), *The Human Face of Law. Essays in Honour of Donald Harris* (Oxford: Clarendon Press, 1997), 47.
43. *Annual Report of the Chief Inspector of Factories and Workshops,* (1899) PP 1900 XI, 118.
44. Pat Kinnersly, *The Hazards of Work. How to Fight Them* (London: Pluto Press, 1973); Carl Gersuny, *Work Hazards and Industrial Conflict* (Hanover N.H. and London: New England University Press for University of Rhode Island, 1981).
45. M. Wright, *Treasury Control of the Civil Service, 1854-1874* (Oxford: Clarendon Press, 1969); Jill Pellew, *The Home Office, 1848-1914. From Clerks to Bureaucrats* (London: Heinemann Educational, 1982), 24; P.W.J. Bartrip, 'British Government Inspection, 1832-1875. Some Observations', *Historical Journal*, 25 (1982), 605–26. See R. Davidson and R. Lowe, 'Bureaucracy and Innovation in British Welfare Policy, 1870-1945' in W.J. Mommsen (ed), *The Emergence of the Welfare State in Britain and Germany, 1850-1950* (London: Croom Helm, 1981), 264–5 where a different line is taken with regard to the Board of Trade.
46. Aside from those already mentioned, attention is drawn to the *Fifth Report of the Children's Employment Commission*, which contained information on Bristol white lead works where a few children were employed. PP 1866 XXIV, 10.
47. Paul Smith, *Disraelian Conservatism and Social Reform.* (London: Routledge & Kegan Paul, 1967).
48. See Public Record Office (hereafter PRO) HO45/OS8002 for

correspondence on differences between Baker and Redgrave; also, this author's entry on Redgrave for the *New Dictionary of National Biography* (Oxford: OUP, forthcoming).

49. On Baker see W.R. Lee, 'Robert Baker: the First Doctor in the Factory Department', *British Journal of Industrial Medicine*, 21 (1964), 85–93, 167–79.
50. *Annual Report of the Chief Inspector of Factories and Workshops,* (1880) PP 1881 XXIII.

3

The White Lead Trade[1]

Dickens and Tressell

White lead was the popular name for lead carbonate, a white powder used, among other things, as a basic ingredient of paint (along with linseed oil and turpentine).[2] Although most white lead was used in paint manufacture, it was also widely employed in pottery glazes and, to a lesser extent, by plumbers, as a sealant. The dangers of white lead derived from its toxicity combined with the facility with which the body could absorb it.[3] In the nineteenth century most white lead was manufactured by the 'Old Dutch' method (the alternative being the chamber process). In this, thin perforated sheets of the purest possible metallic lead were placed in a corroding house, otherwise known as 'stacks' or blue beds. The floor of the house was covered with a 2-3 inch layer of tan upon which, in earthenware pots, stood dilute acetic acid. The lead sheets were placed over the pots and covered with boards. Tan, pots, lead and boards made up the first layer of the stack upon which further layers, usually between 12 and 15, were placed. The average dimension of a completed stack was some 20 feet (in height), by 16 feet, by 13 feet. Once the stack was constructed the door of the corroding house was closed for a period of 10 to 15 weeks. During this time the tan would warm up and give off carbonic acid. The chemical reaction between the lead, the carbonic and acetic acids converted the metallic lead into a carbonate. When the process was believed to be complete the stack was opened and the thick white incrustation stripped from what was left of the lead strips. This was then rolled, crushed, washed, dried and packed. It was in the dismantling of stacks and these subsequent processes that workers, many of whom were casual women workers from the poorest classes, were placed at most risk as the lead dust covered them and was absorbed in various ways.[4] Thomas Oliver, writing at the beginning of the twentieth century, stated that 'No industry, unless, perhaps it be that of pottery manufacture, has caused so much plumbism [lead poisoning] as the manufacture of white lead'.[5] In *The Ragged Trousered Philanthropists* Robert Tressell, a housepainter himself, vividly depicted the dangers of handling white lead:

> One of the worst jobs that he [Bert, the apprentice painter] had to do was when a new stock of white lead came in. This stuff came in wooden barrels containing two hundredweight and he used to have to dig it out of these barrels with a trowel and put it into a metal tank, where it was kept covered with water and the empty barrels were returned to the makers.
>
> When he was doing this work he usually managed to get himself smeared all over with the white lead and this circumstance and the fact that he was always handling paint or some poisonous material or other was doubtless the cause of the terrible pains [presumably colic] that sometimes caused him to throw himself down and roll on the ground in agony.[6]

In 1869 the problem of poisoning in white lead works was discussed in an article published in Charles Dickens' *All the Year Round*,[7] and in 1875 the question came to the attention of the factory inspectorate, at least partly, it would seem, because of the Dickens connection. Alexander Redgrave, then one of the joint chief inspectors of factories, requested his metropolitan sub-inspectors 'to make special inquiries into the subject, so that we might if possible arrive at some definite conclusions as to the actual prevalence of danger and surest means of averting it'.[8] On the basis of their reports Redgrave included a substantial section on the white lead trade in his next half-yearly report to the secretary of state. In this he suggested that while progress had been made in tackling the causes of occupational ill health, 'much suffering' and 'considerable danger' remained. Redgrave, rather uncharacteristically, distanced himself from the extreme *laissez-faire* views that were often to be heard when the subject of regulating the conditions of adult labour was discussed:

> I do not think it is sufficient for an employer to say that the operatives who come to him accept the work with its consequences. Is he justified in placing men and women in jeopardy without providing and insisting upon the adoption of some sufficient precautions? The people employed in these works are all adults; the women especially are of the very poorest class and loss of employment through sickness means deprivation of sustenance to a whole family, which has then to be supplied by the relieving officer.[9]

In order to effect further improvement Redgrave proposed the introduction of five rules. In essence these involved the provision of respirators and protective clothing, an obligation on workers to wash and change their clothes before leaving their places of work and authorising manufacturers to make special rules 'which should render any of his workpeople amenable to law for disregarding them'.[10] It appears that these suggestions, through the proselytising efforts of factory inspectors did exert some influence on manufacturing practice. But it is noteworthy that while Redgrave anticipated a role for the state in occupational health regulation, his specific reform proposals envisaged the imposition of obligations almost entirely upon workers. Under threat of prosecution they were to be compelled to modify their habits and practices; the main obligation to be placed upon the employer was that of disciplining the neglectful worker. Such an approach, which was by no means out of character for Redgrave, set an enduring example for the regulation of the dangerous trades whereby the onus for protecting employees from occupational health hazards was placed on the employees themselves.

Nothing came of Redgrave's proposals. Neither did occupational health figure as a matter of central importance in the Royal Commission on Factories and Workshops, which reported in 1876. In his evidence to it Redgrave pointed out that some employments, including white lead manufacture, carried health risks. He also repeated his suggestion for regulations to uphold cleanliness. The commission's report accepted that white lead manufacture was 'absolutely destructive of the health of those employed, unless careful precautions as to the washing and changing of clothes, etc. are taken'. However, its recommendations followed the well-worn path of proposing the exclusion of children from the trade while leaving those deemed capable of making rational decisions in the market place (that is, adults, regardless of gender) to fend for themselves. The *Factory and Workshop Act, 1878*, which was based on the report of the Royal Commission, reflected this approach by banning the employment of children in the white lead industry.[11] As a result, the freedom of action of the white lead manufacturer was impeded only in relation to pre-production hiring policy. Since all white lead workers were adults anyway, they were completely unaffected by the regulation. *Laissez-faire* principles therefore remained inviolate.

In 1880 the home secretary, on Redgrave's advice, issued an order prohibiting the consumption of food in white lead factories except in rooms used solely for meal taking. As has often been acknowledged, there is a substantial difference between the making of rules and their observance or enforcement. Redgrave maintained that there was compliance with the order in all white lead works. But even if this were so, it was still the case that the freedom of white lead producers, regarding the maintenance of healthy conditions on their premises, remained virtually unfettered. The provision of healthy working conditions remained a matter of employer choice. In the early 1880s pressure from backbench MPs, Poor Law authorities and journalists encouraged the government to press Redgrave to make a further inquiry. This led to the passing of the *Factory and Workshop Act, 1883*, the first part of which regulated the white lead industry.

The *Factory and Workshop Act, 1883*

The regulatory process began in April 1882 when Thomas Burt and Henry Broadhurst, two newly-elected working-class Liberal MPs, prompted by a newspaper report in the *Daily News*, asked the home secretary, Sir William Vernon Harcourt, if his attention had been drawn to the case of Hannah McCarthy, who had died of lead poisoning at Shoreditch Infirmary on the previous Thursday. Burt referred to the inquest evidence of Mr Forbes, the medical officer of the Shoreditch workhouse, in which Forbes stated that lead poisoning was of frequent occurrence and that little was done to protect workers. Burt went on to inquire whether the home secretary had the power to compel factory occupiers to adopt preventive measures against what the coroner's jury had termed 'the wholesale poisoning by lead' which was occurring in white lead factories. If he did not, Burt went on, would he apply to parliament for such powers? The prospect of preventive measures inevitably raised questions about how to regulate an industry in the interests of the health of its workers without destroying its commercial viability. Redgrave was asked to investigate and produce a special report on the subject. Meanwhile, Burt received two letters that indicated the occurrence of lead poisoning outside of the East End of London. The first, from the Rector of Gateshead, referred to the 'terrible murders (for they are nothing else) that are being daily committed in our white lead factories'. It suggested that female employment should be permitted only on a six months on, six months off basis. The second letter was from J.O. Caris, a member of the Gateshead Board of Guardians. This too suggested that there was a widespread problem of industrial lead poisoning, the solution to which was the substitution of mechanical for female labour in the dismantling of stacks and packing of white lead. Caris made no mention of whether such machinery was available and, in fact, one of Redgrave's recent reports had suggested that it was not.[12]

When forwarding these two letters to the Home Office Burt stated his belief that lead poisoning was as prevalent on Tyneside as in London and also his hope for the relief of the problem. These letters and the parliamentary questions to which they led are of interest not least in terms of what they indicate about the formation of social policy. They show how some rather flimsy, anecdotal evidence, based on little more than two proven fatalities and no precise indication of the dimensions of the problem, could be transformed, almost by sleight of hand, into evidence of a major hazard in two large cities that justified public concern and government action. Indeed, that action, in the form of Redgrave's inquiry, was initiated simply in response to the questions of Burt and Broadhurst. As such, the episode exemplifies the influence of backbench working-class MPs on the formulation of government policy.

Redgrave's five page report on 'precautions which can be enforced under the Factory Act and...the need for further powers for the protection of persons employed in white-lead works' was completed by the end of April 1882. It argued that while the *prevention* of poisoning was impossible, 'mitigation of the evil lies in excessive and enforced cleanliness and with the use of special clothing and appliances when at work'. He rejected a ban on female employment, arguing that although white lead work was both hard and hazardous, it did offer an employment opportunity. As for the attainment of appropriate standards of hygiene, he maintained that it was the responsibility of employers, rather than the state, to adopt and enforce preventive measures, if necessary by the dismissal of uncooperative workers.[13] His reluctance to recommend anything other than self regulation stemmed from the belief that it would be unfair to penalise employers for the neglect of their workers, particularly as the victim of irresponsible behaviour was the careless worker himself and nobody else.[14] However, such an argument was based on a misconception about the way in which lead entered the bodies of workers. As later became clear, most absorption came about through inhalation and only the employer was in a position to improve the quality of a factory's atmosphere. Redgrave can hardly be criticised for this misconception. However, he was more at fault in failing to consider the possibility that there might be employers who would show little interest in making and enforcing rules, not least because there would be an obvious competitive advantage for those who did nothing. Neither did he consider banning white lead even though possible alternatives were becoming available.[15]

In a memorandum written in 1882, following receipt of Redgrave's report, Godfrey Lushington, under secretary of state at the

Home Office, summarised the government's objectives and the options available for achieving them. The 'main object', he wrote, was to procure a substitute for white lead, for no preventive measures could ever be totally effective and, even if they were, the poisoning problem would remain for others such as painters. But Lushington doubted whether the government could ever obtain the power to prohibit white lead manufacture and compel the use of a substitute. Furthermore, apparently disregarding the precedent of the *Mines Act, 1842*, he felt it was impossible for the 'Government [to] take upon itself to prohibit the employment of adult women', one of the groups deemed to be most at risk from lead. The perceived impossibility of these options led Lushington to recommend three courses of action: first, legislation empowering inspectors to require manufacturers to provide preventive appliances such as respirators, the installation of machinery wherever it could be substituted for human labour and the provision of medical examinations; second, statutory authority for employers to frame penal rules against employees who failed to make use of 'prophylactic appliances'; third, more frequent inspection of the most dangerous premises.[16]

In response to Lushington's suggestions Redgrave was requested to report upon what regulations could be adopted to reduce health risks. In preparing his report Redgrave visited most of the UK's white lead works. In the course of his tour he became impressed by the 'serious unhealthiness' of the industry and decided that 'it is necessary that those manufacturers who have neglected that which is a moral duty, should be compelled to place their works in at least as good a condition as those of most of their competitors in the trade'. He proposed six rules, relating to the provision of clean working conditions, that manufacturers would have to observe if they were to obtain a Home Office certificate allowing them to remain in production.[17] These were for the provision of overalls and other protective clothes for the most exposed workers, plus the general provision of dining and washing facilities, acidulated drinks (which were believed to neutralise absorbed lead) and adequately ventilated stacks and stoves. Redgrave personally favoured the regular (and free) medical examination of employees but stopped short of recommending this on the grounds that:

> It would be carrying legislative regulations to too extreme a point..., especially as it has been urged upon me in the strongest terms that English firms have already to strain their utmost to contend with foreign competition, and that great care must be taken not to burden

> manufacturers with restrictions which would still further hamper the trade.[18]

Notwithstanding this reservation, Redgrave's report differed significantly from that of April 1882, for whereas on that previous occasion he had recommended little more than vigilance on the part of manufacturers, by November of the same year he was recommending compulsion and, if necessary, that the non-compliant should be made to cease trading. The explanation for this change of heart would seem to lie in Redgrave's factory visits and his personal observation of working conditions in white lead works. Implicit in this change of heart was an acknowledgement that *laissez-faire*, market forces and collective bargaining could not be relied upon to solve the problem of lead poisoning; instead, state intervention, enforced by an inspectorate and, where appropriate, the courts, would be required.

In response to Redgrave's report Lushington observed that white lead manufacture 'is a dreadful trade and ought to be put under stringent regulation'. His one reservation was that employers should be required to provide the services of a doctor 'who should weekly examine the women employed and attend to the case of any man who required it'.[19] On 1 January 1883 the home secretary, Harcourt, sanctioned the immediate preparation of a bill to give effect to Redgrave's recommendations. In June a bill, which Redgrave had helped to draft, was introduced in the House of Lords. The first part, which dealt with the white lead industry, was closely modelled on Redgrave's report (there being no requirement for medical examinations). In committee Lord Wemyss, who had extensive industrial interests in Scotland, launched a vigorous attack on the bill. Wemyss, as founder of the ultra *laissez-faire* Property and Liberty Defence League, particularly objected to the six regulations listed in the bill's 'schedule' (i.e. those specifying the employer's obligation to provide such things as protective clothing and washing facilities). He scoffed that 'they might as well introduce a provision requiring that every day or every second, one of the workmen should take a dose of Epsom salts'. Although Wemyss professed his willingness to support any legislation that would alleviate the harshness of working-class lives, he opposed what he termed 'grandmotherly legislation' and, in particular, interference between adult male workers and their employers.[20] Although, these opinions received some support, the bill emerged from the Lords unscathed.[21] After quickly progressing through the Commons, it received the Royal Assent in August. The act specified that all operational white lead factories had to be certificated and that all certificated factories were obliged to operate in compliance not only with the act and its scheduled conditions on hygiene, but also with approved special rules for the guidance of employees, the object of these rules being 'to prevent injury to health in the course of...employment'. The penalty for non-possession of a certificate was a fine of up to £2 per day; the penalty for breaching special rules was a fine of up to £2 with employers subject to fines of up to £5 unless they could demonstrate that they had done everything possible to prevent the contravention. Failure to comply with the act could lead to the withdrawal of certification and, thereby, the right to trade.[22]

A fool's paradise?

The 1883 act was significant as a first attempt to suppress, by means of legislation, a specific industrial disease. Furthermore, the chosen method of doing this, by means of 'special rules' that specified precise precautions to be undertaken and obligations to be observed, set a pattern which was to be followed in the regulation of the dangerous trades from the 1890s onwards (on the origins of special rules see above 70). Assessment of the act's impact is difficult, for there are no statistics that allow a comparison of pre- and post – 1883 positions. It was surely an omission on the part of the act's drafters that they made no provision for the collection of statistics. But once the idea of regular medical inspection had been jettisoned, there was an absence of the appropriate diagnostic and monitoring facilities. As inspector Richmond noted in 1891, it was difficult to trace poisonings because '[n]ot being "accidents" within the meaning of the Act no reports have been made: whilst [until recently] no inquests have been held on men certified as having died from lead poisoning'.[23] In the absence of statistics, judgments about the act's effectiveness must rest upon flimsier ground. In 1890 Redgrave, in his final full report as chief inspector, claimed that except for 'a lack of sufficient supervision and a repugnance to the use of the bath' the regulations were 'in most cases well observed'.[24] However, Redgrave's successor as H.M chief inspector of factories, Frederick Whymper, spoke of 'widespread' disregard of white lead rules and of the need for more to be done 'to check a mortality which has been far from entirely suppressed by the measures already taken'. The rules, he suggested, 'had hardly been enforced' in the past.[25] In 1892 the *Daily Chronicle* stated that 'people who flatter themselves that the white lead trade has been rendered harmless by the White Lead Act of 1883 [i.e. *Factory and Workshop Act*, 1883] are living in a fool's paradise'.[26]

The perceived inadequacies of the 1883 act led to a policy shift within the Home Office in favour of stricter regulations more stringently enforced. Self-regulation had been tried and found wanting. Thus, an unsigned Home Office memorandum of 1891 emphasised that 'too great pains cannot be spent in ascertaining what are the most effectual and practicable precautions and the use of them should be rigorously enforced... . No indulgence should be shown and the excuse should not be accepted that it is of no use to provide the things [i.e. protective items], because, if provided the men would not use them'.[27] This was certainly not the kind of language that Redgrave had been accustomed to using. In practice, however, the only significant change introduced in Whymper's 1892 special rules was the introduction of medical examinations. This is not to say that Whymper was opposed to the tougher approach signalled by the Home Office memorandum. However, the most important factor affecting the reform of the dangerous trades was not internal civil service memoranda, but the legislative framework. Regulation had to be accomplished within the terms of the *Factory and Workshop Act, 1891*. This measure, which a *Daily Chronicle* leader later termed 'cruelly inadequate', allowed the home secretary to certify factories and workshops as dangerous or injurious to health and either to propose special rules or to require the adoption of such special measures as appear to the chief inspector of factories 'to be reasonably practicable and to meet the necessities of the case'.[28] But as well as discontinuing the procedure in the 1883 act whereby workers could play a role in the rule-making process via a power of objection, the 1891 act gave employers power to object to special rules which they opposed. Moreover, they could push these objections to the point of insisting upon independent and binding arbitration. This meant that between 1891 and 1901 (when the employer's right to insist upon arbitration was removed) manufacturers possessed considerable scope to block proposals to which they objected. As a result the Home Office was obliged to moderate proposals in order to avoid employer opposition.

The impact of Whymper's rules upon conditions in white lead factories was vigorously criticised in articles published in the *Daily Chronicle* towards the end of 1892 as part of its long-running campaign against occupational disease. The newspaper attacked the 'absolute sway of the Amateur at Whitehall', the uselessness of medical examinations paid for by manufacturers rather than out of public funds and, more generally, a regulatory approach which focused upon effects rather than causes. Briefed by the occupational health authority, Thomas Oliver, it pressed for an inquiry into the practicability of producing a harmless white lead. Further criticism of white lead works (in the *Pall Mall Gazette*, *Fortnightly Review* and *Whitehall Review*), questions in parliament and claims by the White Lead Company that it could manufacture a harmless and practicable product, encouraged the recently-elected Liberal government, in which Asquith was home secretary, to set up a departmental committee of inquiry.[29]

The Lead Committee and Labour Commission

This committee (hereafter the Lead Committee), which had scientific expertise at its disposal, had far wider terms of reference than had originally been anticipated, but the largest part of its report dealt with white lead and its potential substitutes. The committee believed lead sulphate to be relatively safe, both in its manufacture and application, but regarded it as inferior to lead carbonate for paint manufacturing purposes. Other alternatives, including zinc oxide, were dismissed out of hand. The committee recognised the danger of making recommendations that could damage indigenous industries and therefore confined itself to proposals that would safeguard workers without unduly burdening employers. One set of recommendations focused upon eligibility for employment. These included the medical examination and certification of all female employees both before employment and before return to work following illness. All female employees, it was proposed, should be required to furnish a certificate from a works medical superintendent specifying that they were at least twenty years of age and physically fit for work. In order to avoid the possibility of women moving from one employer to another under assumed names, it was suggested that they be required to furnish birth or baptismal certificates to prospective employers. A second category of recommendations specified tasks and locations from which female labour should be banned. Accordingly, it was proposed that no woman of any age should be employed on white beds, rollers, washbecks, stoves, or in packing white lead. The committee realised that this would represent a 'drastic' change, notwithstanding that they had visited four works where no women were employed in white beds, stoves or packing, consequently, they felt its implementation should be delayed till 1 January 1896. Further proposals dealt with respirators, protective clothing and work practices.[30]

The emphasis in these proposals on introducing restrictions on women's employment continued a trend that went back to the early decades of the nineteenth century. The ostensible agenda was the removal of women, as a vulnerable group of workers, from occupations that placed them at particular risk. Yet the medical evidence that women were particularly susceptible to attack was, at best, debatable. As we have seen, some historians have argued that the enactment of 'protective legislation' or introduction of 'gender-specific restrictions' in the workplace (and not merely in relation to specific occupational diseases) reflected a social and political agenda which went beyond a simple desire to safeguard vulnerable and defenceless women.[31]

At around the same time that the Departmental Committee on Various Lead Industries' inquiry was proceeding, industrial lead poisoning was also receiving attention from the Royal Commission on Labour. This commission was set up in 1891 to inquire into industrial relations in a period of labour unrest. As part of its investigations an inquiry into the employment of women was undertaken by four 'lady assistant commissioners': Eliza Orme, Clara Collet, May Abraham and Margaret Irwin. Collet, who reported upon working conditions in Birmingham, Walsall, Dudley and the Staffordshire Potteries, investigated several trades, notably china and earthenware manufacture, in which lead poisoning was a problem. As for the white lead trade, this was investigated by Abraham, who later became one of the first lady inspectors of factories. In 1892 she visited nine white lead factories; in addition she met lead poisoning victims and medical experts. Her report gave case histories of workers and details of the conditions she encountered in each factory she visited. It also included such statistical data as it was possible to acquire. But the most valuable part of the report was Abraham's review of compliance with special rules under section 8 of the 1891 act. Here she wrote of insufficient bathroom accommodation, insufficient use of baths, dirty baths, inadequate supplies of towels, overalls and respirators, unsatisfactory medical inspection, insufficient supplies of drinks, failures to ensure that workers leaving factories were free of lead and little attention to ventilation. While it was true that compliance with some rules was generally good and that not all firms were unsatisfactory in all respects, Abraham's report indicated both lax observance of the rules and the continuing occurrence of poisoning.[32]

As a result of the departmental committee's findings and May Abrahams's report on the employment of women in white lead works, new special rules were drawn up by the factory inspectorate and issued in April 1894. Although these differed little from the previous rules and did not prohibit female labour from any part of white lead works, they did go into greater detail about the enforcement of cleanliness. The most notable innovation was in the requirement that employers should report every case of lead poisoning to the factory inspectorate and certifying surgeon. This gave promise that some statistics would, for the first time ever, be available to inspectors and the Home Office. In the event, the *Factory and Workshop Act, 1895* required that medical practitioners who diagnosed industrial lead poisoning, as well as certain other diseases, should notify the chief inspector of factories. Such reporting was to be encouraged by the payment of a fee (2s. 6d.) for each notification and a penalty imposed (fines not exceeding £2) for failure to report.[33] The statistics generated by these regulations are presented and discussed in the next chapter. Otherwise, the most significant change in the 1894 rules was to make it an offence to seek work under an assumed name or 'any false pretence'.

Although the 1894 rules did not ban female employment in the white lead industry, section 28 of the 1895 act, building on section 8 of the 1891 act, facilitated the exclusion of women by empowering the secretary of state to prohibit or restrict employment in the dangerous trades of any person subject, in the case of adults, to parliamentary scrutiny. Almost as soon as the act came into operation the Home Office began to consider the case for making a rule to exclude women. The women inspectors of factories, May Abraham and Mary Paterson, had collected data from five Newcastle white lead works that appeared to lend support to the notion that women were more susceptible to poisoning than men (see Table 3.1). Putting aside the important question of how illness was defined, the value of the figures is compromised by a lack of information on the nature of the employment undertaken. Yet the evidence is that female workers in the white lead trade were from the poorest backgrounds, were often malnourished and therefore susceptible to disease and that they were employed on the most menial and dangerous tasks, such as stripping the white beds following 'corrosion' of the metallic lead. What the Abraham/Paterson data indicated was merely that the most vulnerable workers were also the most afflicted workers. Lead is an abortifaceant and foetotoxic. As such it poses reproductive hazards, but it is not inherently more hazardous to women than to men.[34] Consequently, substitution of male for female workers promised no net reduction in levels of poisoning except in so far as men might

TABLE 3.1:
Lead Poisoning and Employment in Five Newcastle-upon-Tyne Factories

	1894		1895	
	Average Number Employed	Number Ill	Average Number Employed	Number Ill
Men	**409**	**34**	**409**	**39**
Women	**385**	**234**	**385**	**268**

prove better able to persuade employers to improve standards of care, or employers felt impelled to adopt protective measures in order to safeguard workers who represented a greater investment in human capital, or men's superior nutritional status rendered them less likely to attack.[35] Nevertheless, the factory inspectorate supported the exclusion of women from certain tasks in white lead works.[36]

In March 1896 chief inspector Sprague Oram drew up a rule to this effect. Several firms, as well as some women workers fearful of losing their livelihoods, objected to the exclusion proposal, but their arguments were weakened by the fact that some manufacturers had already dispensed with female labour either *in toto* or in certain processes. There was, therefore, a competitive aspect to the rule-making in that such firms had an interest in seeing the regulations which they voluntarily observed, along with their associated costs, imposed upon their competitors. Hence, Cooksons, the Tyneside firm, not only accepted the rule but were prepared to support it before the arbitrator. This lack of solidarity among the manufacturers enabled the Home Office to secure agreement on the new rule without recourse to arbitration, subject to the concession of delaying its introduction for one year. C.E. Troup, who in 1896 was appointed head of the department's new parliamentary and industrial department, deemed this a 'very satisfactory result'.[37]

Liberating the white slaves

Even after its success in excluding women from the most dangerous production processes, the Home Office continued to maintain the pressure on the white lead producers. This was partly because the lead poisoning statistics, collated since 1896, revealed a disturbing incidence of disease. An additional factor may have been the continuing press publicity given to the issue by R.H. Sherard. In 1897 the journalist, Sherard, following the lead of the *Daily Chronicle*, published a series of articles in *Pearson's Magazine* on conditions of work in British factories. The attention these attracted led him to publish them in book form under the emotive title: *The White Slaves of England*.[38] The articles, based on materials gathered in Spring 1896 from six districts in the English Midlands and North, focused on the alkali workers of Widnes and St Helens, nailmakers of Bromsgrove, slipper makers and tailors of Leeds and white lead workers of Newcastle. They were largely concerned with such issues as 'sweated labour', heavy work and poor wages rather than specific occupational diseases, but the chapter on white lead, much of the material for which was supplied by Thomas Oliver, devoted considerable attention to the issue of lead poisoning. The subject was treated in a more or less sensationalised way, with poverty-stricken women nobly opting for low-wage and high risk employment in the white lead works rather than taking to prostitution ('we prefer anything to dishonour'). At the same time Sherard took the authorities to task for their relative inactivity in tackling iniquities.[39]

Whether in response to Sherard or to factory inspectorate returns which showed 370 cases of poisoning in white lead works for 1897 (as against 239 for 1896), in 1898 a Home Office issued a circular calling for information on numbers employed, number of poisoning notifications over a given period and current methods of production. B.A. (Arthur) Whitelegge, who had been appointed chief inspector of factories in 1896, in succession to Sprague Oram, was called upon to analyse the twenty-three replies received.[40] Overall, he found the position 'by no means unsatisfactory'. Employers, he felt, generally admitted the need for improved methods. Some firms had discarded traditional technologies, while others had introduced mechanical drying and packaging; some limited the time spent by workers on the more hazardous tasks. Whitelegge directed Thomas Legge, the newly appointed (in 1898) medical inspector of factories, to visit and report upon those firms that had failed to respond to the circular. At the same time he proposed a conference between manufacturers and Home Office officials. Legge's report showed the need for structural changes to white lead works, along with modifications in the packing, handling and storing of the product, plus decasualisation and avoidance of long-term exposure to dangers.[41] A Home Office memorandum noted that manufacturers deserved credit for their observance of the existing rules and their co-operation with officials.

But it also referred to the 'heavy incidence' of poisoning in the industry as a whole and in some firms in particular, and of the necessity for action to abate this. Whitelegge's idea for a conference was considered by Troup who was struck by the high incidence of poisoning in a few firms, with the worst offender located on Tyneside. He approved of the conference provided its object 'is to insist on something being done and done speedily in all works where the proportion of cases is large'. The conference was held at the Home Office on 2 February 1899 under the chairmanship of Kenelm Digby, permanent under secretary.

In addressing the manufacturers Digby emphasised the dangers of the white lead trade and the need to strengthen existing rules so as to improve standards in the minority of firms with a poor record. Proposed new rules, drawn up by Legge, were placed before the conference where it was decided, in line with the decision reached by the manufacturers at their own private meeting on the previous day, that the employers would nominate some of their number to consult with officials over the draft rules. Two meetings held in February resulted in a substantial measure of agreement.[42] The manufacturers' delegates then sought approval of the rules from all white lead manufacturers. In May 1899 Troup noted that the 'matter is progressing satisfactorily. It has been possible to meet the objections of the manufacturers in nearly every point without materially impairing the efficiency of the new rules'. Kenelm Digby observed that the episode 'shows what can be done by negotiations with the employers'.[43]

The new rules were placed before parliament on 1 June 1899. They imposed tough new controls upon producers. From as early as 1 July 1899 any new or structurally altered white lead factory had to have its construction plans approved by the chief inspector of factories. From 1901 any existing factories would have to comply with certain structural and ventilating requirements. Women were banned from undertaking any work that might expose them to white lead dust. These represented the major rule changes adopted in 1899. So dramatic was the subsequent decline in official statistics of poisoning, that the 1899 rules remained in force until 1921, at which time a new code, containing few significant additions, was compiled. An analysis of the relationship between regulation and the reduction in poisoning statistics is presented in the next chapter.

Notes

1. On this see P.W.J. Bartrip, 'Expertise and the Dangerous Trades, 1875-1900' in R.M. MacLeod (ed), *Government and Expertise. Specialist, Administrators and Professionals, 1860-1919* (Cambridge: Cambridge University Press, 1988), 89–109; Barbara Harrison, '"Some of the Gets Lead Poisoned": Occupational Health Exposure in Women, 1880-1914', *Social History of Medicine*, 2 (1989), 171–95; D.J. Rowe, *Lead Manufacturing in Great Britain. A History* (Beckenham: Croom Helm, 1983); Carolyn Malone, 'The Gendering of Dangerous Trades: Government Regulation of Women's Work in the White Lead Trade in England, 1892-1898', *Journal of Women's History*, 8 (1996), 15–35; *idem.*, 'Sex in Industry: Protective Labor Legislation in Engand, 1891-1914', University of Rochester Ph.D. (1991).
2. In the Victorian period paint was usually mixed from the basic ingredients by the painters themselves.
3. On the question of absorption see *Royal Commission on Labour. The Employment of Women. Report of May Abraham on the White Lead Trade*, PP 1893-4 XXXVII, 700 where equal weight is attached to respiratory, digestive and cutaneous absorption. See also A.R.L. Clark, 'Industrial Plumbism. A Study of Theories and Attitudes which Inhibited its Control in the Nineteenth Century', (unpublished essay presented for the *Diploma in the History of Medicine of the Society of Apothecaries*, 1984).
4. See R.H. Sherard, *The White Slaves of England. Being True Pictures of Certain Social Conditions in the Kingdom of England in the Year 1897* (London: James Bowden, 1897), 173–203. On the characteristics of the workforce see *Annual Report of HM Inspector of Factories*, (1878-9) PP 1880 XIV, 138; *Communications Addressed to the Secretary of State on the Subject of White Lead Poisoning, with Report by the Chief Inspector of Factories upon the Same Subject*, PP 1883 XVIII, 929–41.
5. Thomas Oliver (ed), *Dangerous Trades. The Historical, Social and Legal Aspect of Industrial Occupations as Affecting Health by a Number of Experts* (London: John Murray, 1902).
6. Robert Tressell, *The Ragged Trousered Philanthropists* (London: Lawrence & Wishart, 1955 edn), 453.
7. 27 Feb. 1869, 302–3, reprinted in *The Uncommercial Traveller* (London: Everyman edn, 1911), 343–6; see Harrison, *op. cit.* (note 1), 171–95.
8. *Report of Inspector Redgrave for the Half-Year Ending 31 October*

1875, PP 1876 XVI, 27.

9. *Ibid.*, 34–5; see *Report upon the Precautions which can be Enforced under the Factory Act and as to the need of further powers for the Protection of Persons employed in White Lead Works*, PP 1882 XVIII, 960.
10. *Report of Inspector Redgrave for the Half-Year Ending 31 October 1875*, PP 1876 XVI, 27–37.
11. *Report of the Commissioners Appointed to Inquire into the Working of the Factory and Workshops Acts with a View to their Consolidation and Amendment*, PP 1876 XXIX, lxxxv; *Factory and Workshop Act, 1878 (41 Vict. c.16)* s.38 and first schedule.
12. 3 *Hansard*, 268 (4 April 1882), 666–7; *Daily News*, 3 April 1882; Public Record Office (PRO) HO45/A15330, W. Moore Eden to Thomas Burt, 5 April 1882; J.O. Caris to Thomas Burt (undated); *Report of HM Chief Inspector of Factories and Workshops*, PP 1880 XIV, 138.
13. *Report upon the Precautions which can be Enforced under the Factory Act and as to the Need of Further Powers for the Protection of Persons Employed in White Lead Works*, PP 1882 XVIII, 957–61.
14. *Ibid.* Note that Whitley had rejected legal intervention on the same grounds some twenty years earlier. See above 66.
15. Discussions regarding such alternatives are covered in Bartrip, *op. cit.* (note 1), 96–7.
16. PRO HO45/A15330, Lushington's memorandum, 10 May 1882.
17. *Communications Addressed to the Secretary of State on the Subject of White Lead Poisoning, with Report by the Chief Inspector of Factories upon the Same Subject*, PP 1883 XVIII, 929–41.
18. *Ibid.*, 941.
19. PRO HO 45/A15330, Lushington's note, 18 July 1882.
20. Gertrude Tuckwell who, as we shall see, was a leading figure in campaigns against the dangerous trades, referred to Wemyss as 'that famous die-hard of the Individualist school'. She noted that any attempt to protect the 'under-dog' was likely to be termed 'Grandmotherly' and that 'among my own particular circle of friend of the progressive school I had been dubbed "Grannie"'. See TUC Library Collections. North London University Library. Gertrude Tuckwell Papers. Unpublished Reminiscences of Gertrude Tuckwell, 104 and 182.
21. 3 *Hansard*, 281 (19 July 1883), 1865-67; 282 (23 July 1883), 121–5.
22. *Factory and Workshop Act, 1883* (*46 & 47 Vict. c.53*). Special rules were framed by the employer, but they had to be approved by the

secretary of state. The act allowed employees to object to special rules prior to their establishment. On procedures for establishing these rules see ss.7–10.

23. *Annual Report of HM Chief Inspector of Factories and Workshops,* (1890-91) PP 1892 XX, 468–9.
24. *Annual Report of HM Chief Inspector of Factories and Workshops,* (1889-90) PP 1890-1 XIX, 477.
25. *Annual Report of HM Chief Inspector of Factories and Workshops,* (1890-91) PP 1892 XX, 499.
26. *Daily Chronicle*, 15 and 21 Dec. 1892.
27. PRO HO 45/A15330. Incomplete note possibly dated 16 Sept. 1991.
28. 54 & 55 Vict. c.75; *Daily Chronicle*, 24 Nov. 1892. See also TUC Library Collections. North London University Library. Gertrude Tuckwell Papers. Unpublished Reminiscences of Gertrude Tuckwell. Unpublished Reminiscences of Gertrude Tuckwell, 100, 105–06.
29. *Daily Chronicle*, 15, 21 Dec. 1892; PRO HO 45/A15330, Superintending Inspector Henderson to Chief Inspector Sprague Oram, 29 Dec. 1892; HO 45/9848, J. Foster to A.J. Mundella and H.H. Asquith, 21 Dec. 1892; Sprague Oram to Lushington, 9 Feb. 1893; minute of 15 Feb. 1893; 4 *Hansard*, 8 (17 Feb. 1893), 1704.
30. *Report from the Departmental Committee on the Various Lead Industries*, PP 1893-4 XVII, 723–41.
31. A. Davin, 'Imperialism and Motherhood', *History Workshop*, 5 (1978), 9–66; C. Dyhouse, 'Working Class Mothers and Infant Mortality, 1895-1914', *Journal of Social History*, 12 (1978), 248–67; Elizabeth Roberts, Elizabeth Roberts, *Women's Work, 1840-1940* (Basingstoke: Macmillan, 1995); J. Lewis, *The Politics of Motherhood. Child and Maternal Welfare in England, 1900-1939* (London: Croom Helm, 1980); R. Feurer, 'The Meaning of "Sisterhood ": The British Women's Movement and Protective Labor Legislation', 1870-1900', *Victorian Studies*, 31 (1988), 233–60; Robert Gray, 'Factory Legislation and the Gendering of Jobs in the North of England, 1830-1860', *Gender & History*, 5 (1993), 56–80; Clare Holdsworth, 'Potters' Rot and Plumbism: Occupational Health in the North Staffordshire Pottery Industry', Liverpool University Ph.D. thesis (1995); *idem.*,'Women's Work and Family Health: Evidence from the Staffordshire Potteries, 1890-1920', *Continuity and Change*, 12 (1997), 103–28; S. Walby, *Patriarchy at Work. Patriarchal and Capitalist Relations in Employment* (Cambridge: Polity, 1986); Sonya Rose, 'Gender Antagonism and Class Conflict: Exclusionary Strategies of Male Trade Unionists in Nineteenth Century Britain',

Social History, 13 (1988), 191–208; *idem*., '"From behind the Women's Petticoats": Factory Act Reform and the Politics of Motherhood in Britain, 1870-1878', *Journal of Historical Sociology*, 4 (1991), 32–51; *idem., Limited Livelihoods. Gender and Class in Nineteenth Century England* (Berkeley: University of California Press, 1992).

32. *Royal Commission on Labour. The Employment of Women. Report of May Abraham on the White Lead Trade*, PP 1893-4 XXXVII, 699–703.
33. *58 & 59 Vict. c.37* s.29.
34. Kathleen Irwin, 'Reproductive Hazards in the Victorian Lead Trades: Blessing or Curse' (unpublished paper dated 18 March 1983). I am indebted to Dr Elliot Isaacson, late of the North Staffordshire Infirmary, Stoke-on-Trent for a copy of this paper.
35. PRO HO 45/B12393AC, undated (1896) Report of May Abraham and Mary Paterson. See M. Pember Reeves, *Round About a Pound a Week* (London: Virago, 1979 edn) – first published in 1913 – for evidence of the custom of feeding male breadwinners in preference to other members of the family.
36. PRO HO 45/9856/B12393AC, H.P. Smith to Sprague Oram, Feb. 1896; J. Vaughan to Sprague Oram, 15 Feb. 1896; to Sprague Oram, 20 Feb. 1896; R. Johnson to R.W. Cooke Taylor, 21 Feb. 1896; E. Gould to Sprague Oram, 25 Feb. 1896.
37. PRO HO 45/B12393AC, Troup's minutes of 30 April 1896 and 23 June 1897; S. Tudor & Co to Sprague Oram, 8 April 1896.
38. This title self-consciously echoed Richard Oastler's famous 'Yorkshire Slavery' letter to the *Leeds Mercury* in 1830 while, at the same time, contrasting Britain's imperial, civilising mission with a continued state of barbarism at home. There were also echoes of W.T. Stead's 1885 *Pall Mall Gazette* articles about female 'white slavery', in which it was alleged that British women and girls were being kidnapped and sold overseas as prostitutes. See General William Booth, *In Darkest England and the Way Out* (London: Charles Knight, 1970 edn); Cecil Driver, *Tory Radical. The Life of Richard Oastler* (New York: OUP, 1946); E.J. Bristow, *Vice and Vigilance. Purity Movements in Britain Since 1900* (Dublin: Gill & Macmillan, 1977), 106–14.
39. R.H. Sherard, *The White Slaves of England. Being True Pictures of Certain Social Conditions in the Kingdom of England in the Year 1897* (London: James Bowden, 1897), 17, 20–5, 39–41, 158–9, 182–200.
40. Tuckwell described ['d]ear old' Sprague Oram as a 'kind old man' and Whitelegge as 'wise and humane'. TUC Library Collections. North London University Library. Gertrude Tuckwell Papers.

Unpublished Reminiscences of Gertrude Tuckwell. Unpublished Reminiscences of Gertrude Tuckwell 108 and 163.

41. PRO HO45/9939/B27900, Legge's Report, 11 Nov. 1898; Whitelegge to Kenelm Digby, 15 Nov. 1898.
42. PRO HO45/9939/B27900, Undated and unsigned memorandum on the white lead conference of 1899.
43. PRO HO45/B27900, Troup's minute, 12 May 1899.

4

Pottery and Earthenware

First moves

As we have seen (Chapter 2) the adverse effects of lead on pottery workers were documented by Samuel Scriven for the Children's Employment Commission in 1842. But as Dupree has pointed out, although the link between pottery work and ill health was recognised in 1842, there were few suggestions of the need for legislative intervention until the early-1860s.[1] Following further official inquiries the *Factory Act Extension Act, 1864* introduced some regulations aimed at improving health in pottery manufacture. As previously stated, it is doubtful whether these had much impact at shop-floor level.[2] For more than twenty years after 1864 the hazards of lead poisoning in pottery and earthenware manufacture largely fell into abeyance as a matter of public concern. One of the few who remained interested in the question in these years was the physician, Thomas Arlidge.[3] In 1871 he read a paper on lead poisoning in the Potteries to the Social Science Congress in Leeds. Arlidge's survey of 800 hospital out-patients over the age of ten indicated that 8% of men and 5% of women pottery workers suffered from lead poisoning. This made it the fifth commonest ailment for male potters and the sixth for women.[4] Although Arlidge pointed out that non-potters were not entirely immune, referring in particular to the occurrence of the disease among house painters, his 'control group' of 100 other artisans yielded no other case of lead poisoning. He believed that 'probably no members of a craft suffer in so large a proportion from it as do potters, except it be the men engaged in the manufacture of white lead'. Among potters Arlidge found that it was dippers, dippers' helpers and 'glost placers' (the operatives who applied the 'glost' or glaze) who were most affected. The extent to which any individual suffered depended, in Arlidge's view, partly on personal proclivity, but also on the individual care and cleanliness exercised. Even so, he regarded the disease as 'absolutely and relatively a preventable one'. It was for working potters to exercise caution, but also for chemists, in tandem with pottery manufacturers, 'to discover another mode of glazing pottery'.[5]

Although Arlidge continued to take an interest in the diseases of pottery workers, including lead poisoning (he read a paper on the subject at the BMA's 1876 annual meeting), few shared his concern.[6] The Royal Commission on Factories and Workshops, which reported in 1876, took some evidence about industrial lead poisoning (among Sheffield file-cutters) and heard from the manager of a Hanley pot bank that dipping was 'at the best...a very unhealthy business', but it produced no recommendations for further regulation of occupational health in china and earthenware manufacture.[7] The *Factory and Workshop Act, 1878* contained general provisions relating to sanitary conditions in factories and workshops; it also included special provisions applicable to particular premises. In addition, the act's first schedule introduced restrictions on the employment of children and young persons in certain industrial processes.[8] As we have seen, it was under this schedule that minors were excluded from white lead factories. However, the schedule did not apply to china and earthenware production. Consequently, no restriction was placed on the use of lead in pottery manufacture. Occupational health in potbanks was safeguarded only by the general requirement in the act (s.3) for ventilating works 'in such a manner as to render harmless... all the gases, vapours, dust, or other impurities generated in the course of the manufacturing process'. But the obligation to provide such ventilation was qualified by the phrase, 'so far as is practicable'. In the absence of intrusive factory inspection, or of specialists in medicine and engineering within the inspectorate, manufacturers had considerable freedom to reject any system that threatened to interfere with the manufacturing process. Consequently occupational health remained largely a matter for employers to take seriously or ignore as they saw fit. Since the installation of ventilating equipment imposed costs on individual employers which could be avoided by competitors, there was a financial disincentive to invest. So, at the beginning of the 1890s the problem of lead poisoning in potteries was virtually untouched by regulation. As a leading article in the *Daily Chronicle* noted, the factory acts more or less ignored 'the evil' of 'the poison death'.[9]

Special rules[10]

The regulatory process really got underway only with the passage of the *Factory and Workshop Act, 1891*, a measure that, as we have seen, empowered the secretary of state, to certify factories and workshops as dangerous or injurious to health. As in the white lead industry, a home secretary who did this could then propose special rules or require the adoption of such special measures as appeared to the chief inspector of factories to be 'reasonably practicable and to meet the necessities of the case'.[11] However, the minister had no power of imposition. Employers had a statutory right to object to the establishment of such rules or measures. This right was particularly important in the pottery industry, for it was freely used by prosperous and well-organised manufacturers to impede the Home Office's regulatory objectives. If an employer objected to the proposed regulations he could attempt to persuade the Home Office to change its proposals. If he was unable to do this he could insist upon arbitration. H.J. (Jack) Tennant, chairman of the Dangerous Trades Committee, which sat between 1895 and 1899, described what might happen in event of arbitration:

> the matter in dispute is referred to two arbitrators. In the event of their disagreement they may appoint an umpire whose decision is final. Thus matters which ought to be settled by the Secretary of State with the guidance and control of Parliament, are taken out of his hands and placed either in the hands of the prejudiced or of an irresponsible power.[12]

The Women's Trade Union League, with which Tennant was associated, pressed for these arrangements to be changed and for 'the establishment of special rules for *Dangerous Trades* based on the recommendation of the Home Office experts without submission to arbitration or any other system of reference'.[13] Under the terms of the *Factory and Workshop Act, 1901* the power of objection was extended to 'persons affected', including workers, as well as employers. In addition, the employer's right to insist upon arbitration was removed. As a result of these developments occupational health regulation came to be a process of negotiation between the Home Office, employers and trade unions, rather than a matter over which employers exercised effective control.[14]

Following the passing of the 1891 act, the appearance of four publications prompted the home secretary, in December 1892, to declare pottery manufacture a process dangerous to health. The first was Thomas Arlidge's book, *The Hygiene, Diseases and Mortality of Occupations* (1892), a volume that was extremely influential in encouraging the regulation of occupational disease in late-Victorian and Edwardian Britain.[15] The second was the published evidence of the Labour Commission on the harmful effects of dust and lead in potteries.[16] The third was a report on china and earthenware manufacture by William Dawkins Cramp, one of HM superintending inspectors of factories (for the Midlands division). Cramp, who had read Arlidge's book and interviewed its author, was ordered to undertake his inquiry in consequence of the Labour Commission's reports. In making his investigations he came across 'numerous cases of sickness and death' and concluded, on the basis of in-patient numbers at the North Staffordshire Infirmary, that recent years had seen but little improvement in the problem. Cramp, who carried out his inquiry in 1892, produced a report in which he proposed a number of rules aimed at making pottery and earthenware manufacture safer. [17] The fourth was the *Daily Chronicle*'s exposée of lead poisoning in the Staffordshire Potteries, coupled with the same newspaper's editorial calling upon Asquith to act.[18]

Once Asquith had certified earthenware manufacture as a dangerous trade (on Christmas Eve, 1892), it was possible to draw up special rules for its regulation.[19] In order to avoid a confrontation that could lead to objections from employers and arbitration, the Home Office and factory inspectorate sought to persuade employers to agree the rules in advance of their promulgation. At the same time, although they were not legally required to do so, officials also consulted with the trade unions in order to ascertain workers' views about the proposals and in so doing maintain their position of neutrality between employers and employees. These discussions revealed fundamental disagreements between manufacturers and workers. Whereas the latter wished to see raw lead banned and the use of leadless or 'fritted' (i.e. dustless) glazes made compulsory, employers were outraged that their industry should even be certified as dangerous. As for the factory inspectorate, there were doubts about the extent to which there should be interference in what were essentially matters of business. Cramp, who compiled the special rules, believed that a ban on lead glazes or even specification of the type of glaze to be used was carrying legislative intervention too far. Reluctant to take far-reaching decisions without the sanction of experts, in March 1893 Sprague Oram and his four superintending inspectors decided unanimously that the special rules question ought to be evaluated by an official committee (hereafter referred to as the Pottery Committee).[20]

The Pottery Committee and the Women's Trade Union League

The Pottery Committee, appointed on 21 April 1893, comprised three factory inspectors (Samuel May, who occupied the chair,

William Dawkins Cramp and J. H. Walmsley) plus J.T. Arlidge, A.P. Laurie, a Cambridge University chemist, and W.D. Spanton, a surgeon who was a colleague of Arlidge at the North Staffordshire Infirmary. They were required to look 'into the conditions under which the manufacture of pottery is carried on, with the object of diminishing any proved ill effects in the health of the workpeople engaged therein'. Their eleven-page report was submitted to the secretary of state in July 1893. The bulk of this comprised a sub-report by Arlidge and Spanton on medical issues. They pointed out that 'the potter's occupation is one fraught with injury to health and life'. However, the statistics available to them confirmed their personal suspicions that 'there is less prevalence of plumbism among the pottery population than in past times and this, notwithstanding a growing number of factories and workers'. They had little to suggest in terms of remedial measures, confining themselves to the recommendation that it should be 'a subject for serious consideration whether a periodical examination should not be insisted upon in the instance of all workers with lead, to be made by the certifying surgeon visiting the factories'. Laurie's laboratory experiments indicated that it would be premature to interfere with manufacturers' glazing recipes and techniques. On the other hand 'everything should be done to encourage the manufacturers to continue their experiments in fritted lead'.[21]

The main reason for the Committee's appointment was to consider and amend the draft special rules drawn up for the pottery industry. The Committee decided that the secretary of state had been justified in scheduling potting as dangerous. Of the thirteen rules it considered, four were unchanged and seven altered only slightly. Neither the new rule the Committee proposed, nor the one significantly altered, related to lead. The Committee therefore supported bans on both the employment in any lead process of anyone below the age of fourteen and on the preparation and consumption of meals in rooms where lead was present. In addition they recommended that employers should provide protective clothing (overalls and hoods) and personal washing facilities for those who worked with lead. Responsibility for washing and storing protective clothing would rest with the employer. In terms of maintaining a hygienic and healthy working environment, the Committee proposed that in dusty processes employers should install ventilation by mechanical fans or other means; that employers should supply brooms, brushes and such other cleaning equipment as was necessary for work benches, workroom floors, stairs and stoves to which workers had access to be kept clean; and that workplace temperatures should be kept within reasonable bounds. As for employees, they would be obliged to wear the protective clothing supplied, to wash both before meals and before leaving their places of work, to participate in cleaning and not impede the ventilation. The Committee expressed the hope that manufacturers and workers would accept the special rules 'and cheerfully obey them with a view of taking away from one of the most beautiful, interesting and useful of our manufactures, the reproach of being also one of the most unhealthy'. But more important than such hopes was likely to be both the extent to which employers and employees deemed it to be in their interests to comply and the degree to which the factory inspectorate could achieve compliance.[22]

Effective enforcement of regulation depends to a large extent on the availability of adequate resources; in 1892 these were in limited supply, with only 57 inspectors in post.[23] In a note written in December 1893, by which time he had already raised the number of inspectors to 86, Asquith argued for further expansion on the grounds that 'both the staff and the expenditure [£36 300 in 1893-4] are still upon an extremely modest scale'.[24] Numbers were increased to 99 in 1894; further significant expansions occurred in 1896 and 1899. On the eve of the First World War the number in post stood at 206. In so expanding the factory department Asquith and his successors at the Home Office, created conditions in which the factory acts might be more effectively enforced. Even so, in 1901, at which time there were 107 inspectors in post, Gertrude Tuckwell recognised their numerical inadequacy in relation to the scale of the tasks that faced them (i.e. inspecting 'the hundred thousand workplaces, thronged with workers, throughout the country'). She also recognised that effective enforcement depended upon the attitudes of the regulated, that is, co-operative employers and vigilant workers who understood the law and were willing to notify the authorities about infractions. In the pottery and earthenware industry such conditions were by no means universal.[25]

In December 1893 the Home Office issued draft rules that were almost identical to those approved by the Pottery Committee. The main change involved the jettisoning of the rule that excluded young workers from lead processes. Notwithstanding this concession, pottery manufacturers, bitterly critical of the way in which the Pottery Committee had conducted its business, opposed several of the proposed rules, including the one that required them to provide, wash and store protective clothing. Following negotiations with two superintending inspectors of factories (Cramp and May) and a conference at Stoke in April 1894, the industry secured several amendments.[26] It was agreed, for example, that employers would have to supply protective clothing only for women workers. It was also agreed that employers would not have to wash these clothes, merely have them delivered to a laundry or washhouse of the worker's choice. The temperature clause was retained but modified to the effect that anything up to 90°F was acceptable. Such modifications amounted to significant dilutions but equally as significant, perhaps, was the fact that employers' hostility to regulation did not bode well for voluntary compliance.

The special rules for pottery and earthenware were established in 1894. At first there was considerable optimism that they would be effective in tackling the lead poisoning problem. Thus, in 1895 Inspector J.H. Walmsley reported the view of local doctors in the Potteries that a reduction in the frequency and severity of cases was occurring. In 1897 the *Women's Trade Union Review* (*WTUR*) expressed the belief that, notwithstanding the 'clumsy machinery' of the special rules and the 'difficulty of getting them to work', they had effected 'a considerable amount of good'.[27] However, the number of in-patients admitted to North Staffordshire Infirmary with lead poisoning symptoms showed no immediate sign of declining and before long Walmsley was expressing the view that the rules had made little difference to standards of employer and employee care. Many manufacturers continued to take the view that lead poisoning was the result of workers' carelessness and their disinclination to make use of soap and water. They consequently argued that education, rather than statutory intervention, offered the best prospect of improving workers' health. At the same time some sought either to evade the law or wrest further concessions from inspectors. Evasion was facilitated by drafting deficiencies in the rules. Thus, Inspector Walmsley, whose area included the North Staffordshire Potteries, noted in 1898: 'we were much disappointed to find that when the rules came to be enforced we had not been sufficiently careful to specify exactly what we required.'[28] In contrast with this view, which saw the shortcomings of the 1894 rules in terms of misfortune, Mess, writing in the 1920s, blamed the 'weakness' of the Home Office and its willingness to make concessions 'freely' in the face of pressure from manufacturers.[29] As for workers, Walmsley felt that they were 'suspicious of the rules' as 'a hardship forced upon them by the Factory Department, to which the masters had been privy'. He found little evidence of compliance on the part of operatives: 'the high wages of lead workers', he reported, 'induces them to run all risks'.[30] So, while Mess's judgment is harsh, particularly because it overlooks the limitations placed on bureaucratic power by the 1891 act, it does appear that the 1894 rules, 'largely failed' in terms of controlling hazards. As the *Daily Chronicle* went on to point out, the real problem for those who sought to create special rules to safeguard worker health was that the 1891 Act allowed employers too much influence in their compilation. As a result:

> They [the 1894 special rules] were based on the impossible principle that questions of safety were susceptible to arbitration. To avoid arbitration the new standard of protection was pitched too low. the poison was diluted, just a trifle watered down, but not enough to bring the employer to his right mind, not enough to stop the monumental waste of life which stands recorded in the death registers of the Potteries.

Asquith agreed. In his opinion the rules 'turned out in practice to be entirely inoperative'.[31]

Initially, there were no statistics of lead poisoning cases, for the requirement to collect such data commenced only with the *Factory and Workshop Act, 1895*. When the first figures for lead poisoning (for 1896) were published, in 1897, they appeared to confirm that lead poisoning among pottery workers remained a serious hazard. It emerged that of the 432 reported cases, about 42% had occurred in pottery and earthenware manufacture, most of them in North Staffordshire. The factory inspectorate and the Home Office recognised that official figures represented 'but a very small proportion of the total number suffering'. [32] Nevertheless the statistics provided a basis for further regulation, for even if they were incomplete, they still indicated the existence of a significant problem. They were also helpful in enabling inspectors to investigate individual poisoning cases on a more systematic basis than had previously been possible. Thus, in 1897 two of the recently appointed women inspectors, Mary Paterson and Lucy Deane, undertook a special investigation of the leading china and earthenware works in the UK. In the course of this they interviewed lead poisoning victims, analysed 404 cases of lead poisoning reported from North Staffordshire in the period April 1896-March 1897, and reviewed the annual statistics of local hospital admissions since 1889. Paterson and Deane's report, depicting, as it did, cases of blindness, miscarriage, paralysis and death attributable to industrial lead poisoning painted a grim picture of conditions in the Potteries some three years after the establishment of the special rules. It recorded the 'general opinion' in North Staffordshire that in spite of recent legislation and increased activity on the part of factory inspectors, the incidence of poisoning had not declined. The inspectors attributed 'this unsatisfactory result' to both the superficiality of existing regulations and the difficulty of enforcing them. They recommended the exclusion from lead processes of women, children and those whose 'personal idiosyncrasy' as revealed by periodic medical examination, rendered them liable to attack.[33]

The official poisoning statistics for 1898 seemed to confirm the shortcomings of the existing regulations for they showed an increase of 14 in the number of reported cases. Expressed as a percentage of all lead poisoning notifications, china and earthenware showed some slight improvement on the previous year, but the industry was still supplying almost 40% of all reported cases. Against this background criticism of the 1894 rules became intense and numerous demands for further reform arose. For a while and for the only occasion in the nineteenth century, perhaps the only occasion ever in the UK, it might be said that there was popular demand for government action on occupational health. This reform campaign has been explored in my article: '"Petticoat Pestering": the Women's Trade Union League and Lead Poisoning in the Staffordshire Potteries, 1890-1914' and will, therefore, be examined here only briefly.[34] The campaign, which got underway in 1897, mainly involved members of the Women's Trade Union League (WTUL), the Christian Social Union, the Labour Church movement, sections of the press, especially the *Daily Chronicle* (the 'sworn enemy of the pottery manufacturers', as it has been called), sympathetic MPs, particularly Sir Charles Dilke, and prominent public figures such as the Duchess of Sutherland and George Bernard Shaw.[35] Together these institutions and individuals formed a powerful, if informal, reform network capable of exerting considerable influence upon government and countering the voice of the manufacturers. The leading organisation within this network was the WTUL.

Founded as the Women's Protective and Provident League (WPPL) by Emma Paterson in 1874 (Women's Provident League from 1889), the WTUL, as it became known in 1890, was not itself a trade union, but an 'umbrella' organisation that sought to foster trade unionism among working women. At the time of Paterson's death, in 1886, there were still only some 3000 members of WPPL-affiliated unions. From 1886 till 1904 the league was led, with considerable dynamism, by Emilia Dilke (assisted for much of the period by her niece, Gertrude Tuckwell). In the later-1890s the number of women trade unionists affiliated to the league grew dramatically – to about 70,000 – as the result of a scheme whereby any union admitting women as members could become affiliated at a cost of $^1/_2$d p.a. per female member.[36] WTUL activity on behalf of lead-poisoned pottery workers had two main aspects: the medical and financial relief of individual victims and the introduction of voluntary and legal restrictions on the use of lead. It pursued its aims in four ways: by encouraging (though with little success) trade unionism among women pottery workers; by organising a public appeal for funds to finance the education, maintenance and medical treatment for the sick, on whom it maintained detailed personal records; by seeking a consumer boycott of lead-glazed ware; and by campaigning for further a statutory controls. The controls it sought included regular medical examinations, compulsory use of leadless or fritted glazes, appointment of a specialist (preferably, woman) factory inspector for the Potteries, exclusion of women and children from dangerous processes and extension of workmen's compensation to cover lead poisoning victims.[37]

The need for further reform was receiving endorsement from a number of other quarters, including from within the factory inspectorate. In February 1898 William Dawkins Cramp informed Whitelegge that the large number of poisoning cases indicated the inadequacy of the special rules. Although he described the *Daily Chronicle*'s accounts of conditions in the Potteries as highly-coloured, he favoured the use of fritted lead, prohibition of glazes with a high lead content, additional protections for young workers and more forceful enforcement. Following a personal tour of inspection Whitelegge recommended changes including medical inspection and further restrictions on the employment of young workers. In parliament Charles Dilke, husband of the WTUL's president, addressed MPs about the need to appoint a specialist woman inspector for the Potteries and to exclude young persons from working on dangerous processes. He was supported by Tennant whose wife, the first woman factory inspector, was a staunch supporter of the WTUL. He particularly stressed the need for another committee of inquiry to be appointed and for the regular medical examination of those who worked with lead. The home secretary, Sir Matthew White Ridley agreed that pottery and earthenware manufacture posed considerable health risks, especially for women and children and that existing rules were inadequate.[38]

In May 1898 the factory inspectorate completed the draft of a new set of (seventeen) special rules. At about the same time the home secretary, on Whitelegge's recommendation, appointed two scientific experts, Professors Thomas Oliver and Edward Thorpe to examine the extent to which allegedly harmless substitutes to glazes incorporating raw lead were in fact danger free and to advise manufacturers.[39] Meanwhile government inquiries were being made on the continent in order to establish what steps (if any) had been undertaken to tackle the question of lead glazes. In June, a month that saw further revelations involving fatalities in the pottery industry, the draft rules were served on 576 known pottery manufacturers.[40] The most significant innovations in these were for a minimum age limit of fourteen for anyone who worked with lead (to be raised to fifteen on 1 August 1899); monthly medical examinations for women and young persons below the age of twenty-one – with mandatory suspension from work for anybody found to be suffering from lead poisoning; and the keeping of a health register in which would be recorded the visits of the certifying surgeon and the results of his examinations. The prospects for a rapid settlement of the new rules faded when, following a meeting of the North Staffordshire Chamber of Commerce on 15 June, the Home Office began to receive objections from the employers. This meant that unless the employers could be persuaded to change their minds, the question would have to be settled by arbitration under the terms of the *Factory and Workshop Act, 1891*. Although many firms (ultimately, 476 of the 576 involved) either accepted the rules or were induced to drop their objections, the rest refused to compromise, thereby making arbitration necessary. This took place in October 1898 at the North Stafford Hotel in Stoke with Chester Jones (for the Home Office) and A.P. Llewellyn representing the manufacturers) acting as arbitrators, and J.S. Dugdale serving as the independent 'umpire'. Although this arbitration resulted in the modification of seven of the Home Office's seventeen regulations, it is fair to say that the changes were comparatively minor.[41]

Notwithstanding the relatively slight differences between the two sets of rules issued in 1898 (the May and October codes), the position on the ground had become considerably more complicated. This was because the rules settled by arbitration applied to 100 firms, whereas the original rules, accepted without arbitration, applied to the other 476. Thus when the rules came into effect the pottery industry became subject to two different codes. As a result two adjacent manufacturers engaged in producing identical ware and possibly sharing some common workers might find themselves subject to different regulations. This state of affairs posed obvious administrative problems for the factory inspectorate. It also produced an unfair situation ('farcical' in the view of the *WTUR*) whereby the more co-operative employers were penalised relative to other firms by having to adhere to a stricter code of practice.[42] However, even while the 1898 special rules for pottery were being settled, the codes they established were being rendered obsolete by the work of Oliver and Thorpe, for their researches threatened to change the regulatory debate into one concerned about the contents of the glazing tub.

The two professors

Thorpe and Oliver presented their report to the home secretary in February 1899. When embarking on their inquiry they accepted that lead poisoning had 'prevailed extensively' in the early-1890s and had set out to determine what improvements had been effected in the course of the decade. Their conclusion was that 'very little of an effective character had been attempted'.[43] They found that

> Certain manufacturers have substituted 'fritted' lead for 'raw' lead in compounding their glazes, and a few persons have made more or less successful efforts to produce, or to re-introduce, leadless glazes, but no concerted action had been taken by the trade. Beyond what may have been effected by the operation of the Special Rules issued by the Home Office in 1894, there had been little or no improvement during this period of five years.[44]

By taking the number of persons 'working in the lead' (in July 1898) and dividing by the number of 'lead cases' for 1898 Thorpe and Oliver found that 12.4% of at-risk females and 4.9% of at-risk males went down with lead poisoning. For specific processes attack rates were much higher; among colour and litho-dusters – the most extreme case – as many as 62.5% of males and 20.8% of females were found to be suffering from lead poisoning.[45]

As we have seen, the main purpose of the Thorpe-Oliver inquiry was to ascertain how lead poisoning could be diminished by means of safer glazing without damaging the pottery trade in the process. The report was unequivocal on this point: '*We have no doubt whatever that leadless glazes, of sufficient brilliancy, covering power and durability and adapted to all kinds of table ware, are now within the reach of the manufacturer*' (italicised in original).[46] They therefore recommended an absolute prohibition on the use of lead as an ingredient for glazes and colours. Because they accepted that such a ban could not be introduced overnight without crippling the industry, they also proposed a number of interim measures. These included the use only of fritted lead of low solubility in acids, the exclusion of women and children from dipping houses and the laying down of concrete floors that could be hosed clean. But if all else failed they favoured legal powers to shut down factories that could not be made fit for occupation.[47]

The main significance of the Thorpe-Oliver Report was the scientific credence it gave to the reformers' case. It endorsed the view that little progress had been made in cutting lead poisoning rates, but in supporting the use of leadless glazes, it went further than most campaigners. As such it changed the nature of the regulatory debate for, subsequently, argument centred upon the abolition of raw lead and compulsory use of leadless glazes. The WTUL welcomed the report as a complete endorsement of its policies. Many manufacturers, on the other hand, were aghast at the prospect of having to use leadless glaze, contending that no such glazes were commercially viable. In fact, even a local doctor who was active in his support of regulations on behalf of pottery workers who handled lead, Dowling Prendergast, expressed doubts as to the practicality of dispensing with the material that caused the problem.[48]

For its part, the Home Office dithered. Although senior officials had prior knowledge of the report's contents, when the final version arrived in their hands it still caused consternation. One described it as 'most drastic' and expressed grave misgivings about several findings and recommendations. Another thought that Thorpe and Oliver had exceeded their brief: 'and instead of confining their report to chemical and biological questions which they...understand...[they] have endeavoured to embrace the whole industrial and economic problem without hearing the case for the employers and workmen'.[49] For his part Whitelegge considered that the report 'threw much new light on the question' and that, overall, its findings were 'most important'. At the same time he harboured a number of doubts, especially about some of the medical judgments. He accepted that there was a need for further regulation but advocated caution in order to avoid alienating employers. On his recommendation the report was distributed to all employers, but with a covering circular indicating that while tougher rules were under consideration, the Thorpe-Oliver Report did not constitute a full and final expression of official policy. The WTUL took a jaundiced view of these developments. 'Is it possible [inquired the *WTUR*] that the circular issued to the Potteries employers by the Home Office is to be the only outcome of the experts' investigations and recommendations'.[50]

The Home Office's resort to tact and diplomacy in its dealings with the manufacturers cut little ice with the industry. Indeed, the pottery manufacturers rejected the case for leadless glazes out of hand. Although they were willing to use fritted lead, they felt that reasonable time for experimentation should be allowed before the adoption of 'frits' became compulsory. They also opposed any idea of an upper limit on lead content. They were prepared to meet Home Office officials to discuss the questions raised by the Thorpe-Oliver report. But when those conferences took place, in July and October 1899, they broke up in disagreement and acrimony. The employers' position was that since lead poisoning statistics were falling there was no need for further interference in their trade. The *Staffordshire Sentinel* accused the Home Office of endangering the staple industry of the Potteries. In a leading article it maintained that notwithstanding 'comfortable theories from outsiders' and the views of London 'amateurs', leadless glazes remained at the experimental stage. [51]

Whitelegge and Home Office civil servants decided that the only way out of the *impasse* was to draw up a new set of rules that took no account of employer opinion. Whitelegge set about doing this and by 2 August 1900 he had produced a draft that offered the prospect of substantial relaxation of existing rules for any employer who used only leadless glazes. For all others the requirements would be for the regular medical examination of employees, including of adult males, and the suspension of those diagnosed as suffering from lead poisoning; use of only fritted lead after a period of six months and, after two years, the use only of fritted lead 'which yields to a dilute solution of hydrochloric acid [no] more than 2% of its dry weight of a soluble lead compound' (which became known as the 2% solubility standard). Initially the WTUL was sceptical of the Home Office's approach. It objected to the length of time that manufacturers were to be allowed to amend their working practices. It was also anxious about the risks of relaxing rules when, to its eyes, factory inspection was inadequate. However, its *Review* subsequently commented that the proposals were 'the best yet brought forward and the sooner they are formally promulgated the better'.[52] Predictably, the manufacturers disagreed. In their opinion, the 'quiet and patient' potters, who were 'as upright and as honest and as humane a body of manufacturers' as anywhere in the world, were being persecuted by the Home Office, the factory inspectorate and 'a very influential and busy-bodied lot unconnected with either the potting trade or any other trade except for their own advertisement'.[53] Even so, by the end of the year, following extensive negotiations, a fair measure of agreement had been reached on most points other than the solubility standard, on which manufacturers rejected anything below 5%. In these circumstances and much to the employers' chagrin, the Home Office decided to issue its original rules (regardless of subsequently agreed amendments), recognising that such a move would mean another arbitration. Troup explained that it was necessary to proceed in this way: 'otherwise the points already conceded by HO in hope of an agreement will merely be made the starting point for further weakening of the rules'.[54]

Arbitration

In January 1901 the Home Office issued the new 'draft amended special rules' to 604 pottery firms. By the end of March deadline, 329 companies had lodged objections. In addition one trade union, the United Society of Clay Potters, Printers and Ovenmen, had objected to the prospect of uncompensated suspensions for adult men found to be suffering from lead poisoning. It had proposed to employers the establishment of an insurance fund, financed by masters and men, to meet this difficulty and the Home Office agreed to support the proposal.

Arbitration on the special rules took place at Stoke-on-Trent in November 1901 before the lawyer, Lord James of Hereford, who was Chancellor of the Duchy of Lancaster in Lord Salisbury's government. On the fifth day of the hearing Lord James, having heard all the Home Office evidence, but none from employers or workers, halted proceedings to make a statement. He said that the state had assumed the duty of protecting operatives in dangerous trades, but 'the Home Office representing the State will recognise that such interference with the trade of this country must be regulated and controlled by considerations of a grave character'. Interference, he suggested, 'should not take place if it can be avoided'. While the interests of the employers might be 'personal, [and] the profit may be theirs', the well-being of their trade affected the whole country. As a result, interference should be avoided where possible. Lord James came to the conclusion that hasty decisions should be avoided and proposed a compromise whereby all rules other than those dealing with fritting, solubility and suspension of adult males would be settled along agreed lines. Discussion of the three outstanding rules would be postponed for eighteen months, that is, until May 1903, at which point further postponement would be possible. Lord James expressed the hope that in the meantime employers would improve conditions, that they would take on 'substantially the burden of the Compensation Act', that poisoning statistics would decline and that the Home Office would exempt from all other rules any producer who could meet the 2 per cent solubility standard.[55]

The Home Office was pilloried in parliament and the press for what many saw as its arbitration failure. The *Staffordshire Sentinel*, for example, stated that '[c]ommonsense has triumphed. The trade of the Potteries is not to be arbitrarily destroyed at the behest of the Home Office. The Home Office has sustained one of the most tremendous rebuffs that any public Department ever encountered'.[56] But while the department suffered an embarrassment, it did not lose a great deal by Lord James' decision. Three important rules were postponed but employers were on notice to produce safer glazes and to set up a compensation scheme. In the meantime the Home Office was free to encourage adoption of the 2 per cent standard by offering relaxation of the rules to those who achieved it. Any judgment of the department must take into account that it was not in a position to impose regulations. Given the diminishing scale of the poisoning problem (see Table 4.1), the determined resistance of the manufacturers, and the legal constraints under which it operated, the Home Office deserves less criticism than it received at the time. On the other hand, if the department had negotiated more effectively it could have avoided arbitration and secured an agreement for fritting and for a maximum level of solubility for glazes. That level would have been 150 per cent higher than it was seeking. However, this would have been preferable to the arbitration outcome of no maximum, particularly as Thorpe never justified his 2 per cent figure and indeed, on the eve of arbitration, produced a report suggesting that 2.9 per cent, a figure which represented a significant move towards the employers, was satisfactory.[57]

By February 1902 the Home Office had prepared its rules offering freedom from all other special rules for those who used only glazes conforming to the 2 per cent solubility standard. But at the beginning of 1903 only one manufacturer had taken advantage of this offer. Whitelegge wrote gloomily to Thorpe in January 1903 that 'there is reason to think that raw lead is used even more widely than in 1900'.[58] The compensation scheme also proved something of a damp squib. The Potters' Insurance Company was set up in mid-

1902 to provide non-contributory benefits to lead poisoning victims, their wives and children. In line with practice under the *Workmen's Compensation Act*, premiums were based on wages paid and were not risk-related. They were initially set at 1% of wages and compensation rates were broadly similar to those under the *Workmen's Compensation Act.* By November 1902 only 62 of 530 firms, employing 2325 of the 6372 persons in scheduled processes covered by the 1901 Rules, had joined the scheme. Troup found the number of participating firms 'rather disappointing' and 'not nearly so large as expected'. By February 1903, at which time there were still only 72 firms in the scheme, a mere four compensation claims had been considered.[59] The concern felt by directors of the Potters' Insurance Company about the poor take-up of insurance is indicated by their wish that factory inspectors should publicise the company. However, while Troup welcomed this suggestion, Whitelegge would not agree to act upon it. Thus, at the beginning of 1903, in which year the arbitration was due to be resumed, there had been little progress towards an industry-wide compensation scheme.

Lord James's final award (of December 1903) established a voluntary standard of 5 per cent solubility for lead glazes. But manufacturers remained free to use any type of glaze provided they gave due notice to the Home Office and accepted two conditions. These were that they would provide compensation for any worker who succumbed to lead poisoning and that the monthly medical examinations already established for women and young persons, should be extended to adult males employed in scheduled lead processes. Lord James wrote to Charles Dilke, 'I have done my best to protect the operatives without bringing the trade to a standstill'. His 'intention was that the rules should be very protective to the operatives – and I hope and think they are'.[60] For his part Dilke expressed relief that notwithstanding the pressure he was under from employers, Lord James had not been obliged to remove 'everything which would make it [his award] useful to humanity'.[61] Lord James told Dilke that the *Staffordshire Sentinel*, 'the employers [sic] organ is very jubilant and claims a great victory over the Home Office'. He could not understand this, however, for he regarded the award as a significant step forward. In particular, the '5 p-c of lead allowed is I believe quite innocuous'.[62] The *British Clayworker*'s comment on the award was that it 'would seem to be more satisfactory to the employer than to the worker, for the latter may still continue using poisonous material provided his employer is prepared to pay him a monetary compensation'.[63] Although the employers expressed dissatisfaction with the award, they grudgingly decided to accept it without further demur and the new rules came into operation in 1904. The establishment of the new code saw the end of the popular campaign against lead poisoning in potteries – although efforts by the Christian Social Union and the Women's Trade Union League to promote use of leadless ware continued unabated.[64] In practice most firms (377 of the 481 to which the rules applied) opted to keep using lead without restriction. Under the *Workmen's Compensation Act, 1906*, a measure which extended the 1897 'no-fault' arrangement to a small number of occupational diseases, victims of occupational lead poisoning had a claim for compensation against their employers provided they could demonstrate that their incapacity arose 'out of and in the course of employment'.

In 1908 a Departmental Committee of Inquiry (the Hatch Committee) was appointed to inquire into the continuing use of lead in pottery and earthenware manufacture. This appointment came about because the 1896-1902 drop in lead poisoning notifications had ceased thereafter (see Table 4.1). It enquired into the possibility of prohibiting the use of raw lead in glazes, but decided against such a step on the grounds 'that if the precautions which they had agreed to recommend in relation to lead processes are adopted [these were extensive but included provision of protective clothing, medical examinations, milk drinks, washing facilities, exhaust ventilation] and effectively carried out, they will, in conjunction with those now in force, reduce the risk to a level common to all industrial occupations'. The committee believed that observance of special rules had been 'far from satisfactory' and proposed a 'scheme of supervision by inspection of factories from within', i.e. self-regulation, as well as the adoption of various other specific measures. A number of these recommendations were incorporated in a new set of rules established in 1913.[65]

Conclusion

Comparison of the white lead and pottery trades indicates that while there were some common features in the regulatory processes they underwent, there were also a number of contrasts. These contrasts derived, in large part, from the differences between the two industries. White lead manufacturers did not have the economic power and cohesion that enabled their pottery and earthenware counterparts to combine so effectively against the Home Office. Whereas government bodies experienced little difficulty in imposing their views upon the white lead industry, the concerted opposition of

TABLE 4.1:
United Kingdom Industrial Lead Poisoning Statistics, 1896-1914

	Pottery & Earthenware		White Lead		Total (All industries)	
Year	Cases	Fatalities	Cases	Fatalities	Cases	Fatalities
1896	**432**	**n/a**	**239**	**n/a**	**1030**	**n/a**
1897	**446**	**n/a**	**370**	**n/a**	**1214**	**n/a**
1898	**457**	**n/a**	**332**	**n/a**	**1278**	**n/a**
1899	**249**	**16**	**399**	**n/a**	**1258**	**n/a**
1900	**200**	**8**	**358**	**6**	**1058**	**38**
1901	**106**	**5**	**189**	**7**	**863**	**34**
1902	**87**	**4**	**143**	**1**	**629**	**14**
1903	**97**	**3**	**109**	**3**	**614**	**19**
1904	**106**	**4**	**116**	**3**	**597**	**26**
1905	**84**	**3**	**90**	**2**	**592**	**23**
1906	**107**	**4**	**108**	**7**	**632**	**33**
1907	**103**	**9**	**71**	**0**	**646**	**26**
1908	**117**	**12**	**79**	**3**	**646**	**32**
1909	**58**	**5**	**32**	**2**	**553**	**32**
1910	**77**	**11**	**34**	**1**	**505**	**38**
1911	**92**	**6**	**41**	**2**	**669**	**37**
1912	**80**	**14**	**23**	**0**	**587**	**44**
1913	**62**	**11**	**29**	**2**	**535**	**21**
1914	**n/a**	**n/a**	**29**	**1**	**445**	**28**

Source: Annual Reports of HM Chief Inspector of Factories

Note that the figures refer to new cases reported in any given year. Consequently the cumulative number of cases would have been higher than indicated here. Where the interval between attacks suffered by one individual exceeded twelve months an individual might be included for more than one year. The figures include only those cases reported by medical practitioners under the terms of the *Factory and Workshop Act, 1895 (58 & 59 Vict. c.37)*. Although other cases sometimes came to the attention of factory inspectors, these were not tabulated.

the master potters ensured that they were able to resist many aspects of the proposed regulatory regime. The strength and effectiveness of their opposition suggest the need for scepticism in respect of the suggestion that late-Victorian and Edwardian factory regulation should be seen entirely in consensual terms.[66] There remained much scope for conflict.

The limited scope of the state to dictate to powerful industries is well illustrated in a letter that one of the leading pottery manufacturers, Bernard Moore, sent to the chief inspector of factories in 1901, that is, at the height of the lead controversy. Moore informed Whitelegge that he was inclined 'to let the Home Office bring in whatever rules they like. They could never be carried out and would either remain a dead letter or a great part of the potting industry would be driven to other countries'.[67] Moore's point was that the establishment of legal rules with enforcement machinery at prevailing levels was bound to fail without the co-operation of industry, while the introduction of tough rules strictly applied would have the effect of 'exporting' businesses and jobs. The factory inspectorate had recognised the truth of Moore's observation decades earlier and, accordingly, had developed its 'negotiated compliance' strategy of enforcement. The basis for dangerous trades regulation of the 1890s was the *Factory and Workshop Act, 1891*, a measure which, by conferring on manufacturers far-reaching powers of objection, recognised that regulation had to be by consent and that manufacturers should not be expected to go beyond the 'reasonably practicable'. Problems arose when some regulators tried to adopt a more confrontational approach, for this alienated many employers. The outcome was a reversion to a more consensual policy of regulating by means of discussion, bargaining and agreement. In 1910, the value of consensus regulation was endorsed by the Hatch Committee. The only dissenting voice on the Committee was that of Gertrude Tuckwell, president of the Women's Trade Union League (since 1905), who had campaigned for years for a total ban on the use of lead glazes. In a memorandum which followed the Committee's majority report she repeated her support for a ban on the use of lead. But, tellingly, she recognised that 'a very considerable increase in the staff of H.M. Inspectors' would be needed if a policy unacceptable to large numbers of producers were to be carried into effect.[68] Even so, the statistics of lead poisoning in potteries did decline from 1899, notwithstanding the continued growth of the industry in terms both of productive capacity and numbers employed

Before considering the impact of lead regulation, attention should be drawn to the input (or lack of it) of two groups: scientists and trade unions. As I have argued elsewhere, the extent of medical, scientific, or technical expertise within the factory inspectorate was extremely limited until the last years of the nineteenth century when a medically qualified chief inspector (1896), a medical inspector (1898), an inspector of dangerous trades (1899) and a few other specialist inspectors were appointed. Although independent scientists such as Thomas Oliver and the government chemist, Edward Thorpe, did contribute to the formulation of occupational health regulation in the 1890s it was only at a comparatively late stage that the expert came to play a decisive role. It seems likely that the absence of such expertise throughout the early years of the regulatory process contributed to the weakness and (on occasion) inappropriateness of the regulations introduced. In particular, the special rule debacle whereby different codes applied within the pottery and earthenware industry, was directly related to the fact that the manufacturers had a virtual monopoly of specialist knowledge. By way of contrast, government access to *bona fide* experts was extremely limited.[69] As for the trade unions, they have sometimes been accused of demonstrating little interest in occupational health and safety and even of conniving with employers to conceal employment risks.[70] This study provides little evidence to counter such a view. The Women's Trade Union League was active in the campaign against lead glazes in pottery manufacture, but this organisation was an 'umbrella' group rather than a trade union. It was run by middle and upper class women rather than by workers or those from a working-class background. It was, in addition, concerned about the notorious apathy of pottery workers towards unionisation.[71]

To turn to the question of impact. Assessing the impact of legal rules is a notoriously difficult undertaking, not least because of the shortcomings of the statistics on which any such assessment must be based. The chief inspector of factories acknowledged that the system for reporting cases of occupational disease was 'imperfect', that some medical practitioners were unaware of their legal obligations and that some cases never came to the attention of the factory inspectorate at all.[72] Although he did not mention the issue of definition, the absence of any criterion for defining lead poisoning must also have had a bearing upon the statistics. Whereas a factory accident was defined in relation to cause and effect in terms of the machinery or process which brought about the accident and the length of time off work to which it gave rise, diagnosis of lead poisoning was not only an intrinsically uncertain affair, it was one over which experts would inevitably differ. Nevertheless, these statistics were treated seriously by the factory inspectorate and Home Office, for whom they provided the basis for policy-making; they cannot therefore be overlooked by historians.

The assessment that follows is confined to the white lead trade since the homogeneity of that industry renders it more amenable to analysis. From what we know of the number of employers and premises it would appear that in the late-1890s by far the greatest incidence of lead poisoning was occurring in this industry. There were 399 white lead notifications in 1899 but thereafter the statistics declined dramatically with a pre-First World War low of 23 registered in 1912. How can such a drop be explained? There are up to four factors which, in isolation or combination, could account for this decline in poisoning notifications. It is likely, furthermore, that the same factors would also explain the decline in pottery and earthenware notifications. First, the statistics may be largely a product of changes in reporting requirements or behaviour. As such statistical fluctuations may have less to do with objective changes in the extent of illness and more with the process of collection. Second, technological change may have rendered the industry safer, thereby reducing the risks to which the workforce was exposed. Third, a poor state of trade with downward production and employment levels may have reduced the numbers at risk as well as the volume of toxic material to which workers were exposed. Fourth, the occupational health regulations introduced in the 1880s and 1890s, may have been effectual in rendering white lead works safer places. Let us, then, consider the significance of these four factors.

The only legislation affecting reporting was contained in section 73 of the *Factory and Workshop Act, 1901*. However, the 1901 act was mainly a consolidation of existing legislation; it effected no substantive change in reporting regulations. Hence, the statistics are strictly comparable from year to year. In other words, changed reporting regulations provide no explanation for the decline in lead poisoning statistics. This is not to say that reporting was always accurate, consistent and full. We know that medical practitioners did submit details of cases for which no returns were required under the terms of the legislation. It is also true that the symptoms of lead poisoning may be similar to those of other diseases or disorders including typhoid, intestinal obstruction and appendicitis. Year by year as many as 10 per cent of notifications were excluded from the official returns as subsequent inquiry revealed that for one reason or another they did not fall within statutory reporting requirements. In 1898 and 1900 the Home Office felt obliged to issue memoranda pointing out that:

> The opinion to be notified is not merely that the patient is suffering from lead poisoning, nor even that he is suffering from industrial lead poisoning, but that he is the subject of lead poisoning which the practitioner believes to have been contracted in a factory or workshop.[73]

If these memoranda had their desired effect, it is to be expected that subsequent returns of lead poisoning cases were compiled on a different basis from those of earlier years. Hence it cannot be assumed that annual notification showed a consistent degree of error. By the same token it is probable that the *Workmen's Compensation Act, 1906*, by giving the victims of certain occupational diseases a claim for compensation against their employers, led to the additional reporting of lead poisoning cases both by causing pre-existing cases to come to light and by encouraging the prompt replacement of suspected poisoning victims with new hands – amongst whom the incidence of disease tended to be high. Nevertheless, there is no reason to ascribe the long-term decline in lead poisoning statistics to changed reporting practices. Indeed, in the case of the *Workmen's Compensation Act*, this is more likely to have increased, rather than decreased, reporting levels.

A second explanation for falling statistics could be technological change. To some extent this factor is indistinguishable from the regulatory explanation for, as we have seen, the special rules which were applied to the white lead industry – especially those of 1899 – required structural alterations to premises in connection with the provision of ventilation.[74] Another quasi-technological change in white lead manufacture was the substitution of machinery for manual labour in some of the most dangerous processes, including packing, which probably had the effect of reducing exposure to lead dust. As far as manufacturing techniques were concerned, D.J. Rowe has noted that the lead industry as a whole 'did not experience dramatic change during the nineteenth century'. Although some white lead began to be produced by the chamber and precipitation processes – especially the former – Rowe observes that: 'In the late-nineteenth century all the objective accounts agree that in England there was no serious alternative to stack white lead'.[75] In 1914 the vast bulk of whitelead continued to be made by the traditional stack process. Some modifications in the setting of stacks were introduced, for example, by varying the amounts of tan used and introducing manure to encourage fermentation, but the essentials remained the same. Workers were most likely to suffer exposure to dust not during the corrosion process, but when stripping stacks and packing the finished product. While some progress towards mechanising these processes had been effected by 1914, they remained largely dependent upon manual labour. So, while there are some grounds for concluding that lead poisoning in white lead manufacture might

TABLE 4.2:
UK Imports of Pig and Sheet Lead (tons), 1896-1914

Year	Imports	Year	Imports
1896	**167,799**	**1906**	**208253**
1897	**167,441**	**1907**	**204,695**
1898	**194,479**	**1908**	**237,508**
1899	**198,377**	**1909**	**207,660**
1900	**195,380**	**1910**	**218,936**
1901	**218,060**	**1911**	**213,707**
1902	**231, 813**	**1912**	**205,375**
1903	**229,217**	**1913**	**204,136**
1904	**246,508**	**1914**	**224,916**
1905	**229,545**		

Source: Statistical Abstract for the UK

TABLE 4.3:
UK White Lead Exports and Imports, 1903-1913 (metric tons)

Year	Exports	Imports	Year	Exports	Imports
1903	**12,500**	**14,700**	**1909**	**15,400**	**12,900**
1904	**12,800**	**12,600**	**1910**	**16,400**	**11,700**
1905	**14,300**	**12,400**	**1911**	**16,300**	**13,600**
1906	**16,100**	**11,500**	**1912**	**18,700**	**14,200**
1907	**16,200**	**12,000**	**1913**	**14,968**	**13,059**
1908	**15,400**	**12,900**			

Source: D.J. Rowe, Lead Manufacturing in Great Britain (Beckenham: Croom Helm, 1983), 169

have fallen as a result of technological innovation, it is unlikely that technical change provides a complete explanation, particularly as such change cannot be divorced from the regulatory process that stimulated it.

The third reason for falling statistics might be that the white lead industry was contracting and therefore employing fewer workers. Assessment of the validity of this hypothesis is impeded by an absence of time series data for either employment or production. However, Table 4.2 presents figures for pig and sheet lead imports into the UK. Although these give no indication of the quantity of lead converted into carbonate, they do show that imports of the materials from which white lead was manufactured did not decline in line with poisoning statistics. Table 4.3 gives statistics for UK white lead imports and exports in the period 1903-13. While these show fluctuations consistent with the business cycle, they provide no indication of industrial decline of a degree that might explain the dramatic fall in poisoning notifications.

As for employment data, census figures for 1901 list 1,378 persons over the age of ten as being employed in lead manufacture in England and Wales.[76] The 1907 census of production for the UK showed that 1,472 persons were employed in white lead manufacture, at which point total white lead production was 42,700 tons pa. In addition 265 other persons engaged in white lead production worked for paint manufacturers. If their productivity equalled that of those included in other returns, it would seem that total white lead production in 1907 amounted to some 50,000 tons.[77] Unfortunately, in the absence of similar data for earlier or later periods, these figures provide no indication of the relative economic health of the white lead industry. The 1911 census figures do show a decline in the number of persons over the age of ten who were employed in lead manufacture (972 as against the 1,378 listed in 1901).[78] This might suggest that employment in the white lead industry was declining – though not in proportion to the decline in poisoning notifications. There is, however, reason to question whether all white lead workers were included in either the 1901 or the 1911 figures. Since white lead employment was often casual, with employees drifting in and out of the industry, there must always be doubt about the precise numbers employed in the trade. One thing is clear, however; notwithstanding the inadequacies of the statistics, there is no evidence of a collapse in employment or production sufficient to explain the fall in poisoning statistics revealed in Table 4.1.

We come now to the fourth factor potentially responsible for fewer poisoning notifications: regulatory intervention. We know that a considerable amount regulation was applied to the white lead trade in the 1880s and 1890s. This imposed stringent controls upon the industry in respect of production methods, persons eligible for employment, medical and inspectorial supervision and standards of hygiene. Both Thomas Oliver and the medical inspector of factories, Thomas Legge, believed that these regulations were responsible for the fall in lead poisoning notifications.[79] Of course, in the last analysis there is no final 'proof' that regulation was responsible for this change. It was, after all, the manufacturers and workers themselves, rather than factory inspectors or MPs, who exercised real control over the conditions in which white lead was produced. Furthermore, it is possible that the extent of ill-health would have declined anyway, perhaps in response to changing public attitudes towards public health which encouraged better standards of care on the part of employers and moderated the demands they made on their employees. Perhaps better standards of diet and general health made the workforce more resistant to poisoning.[80] Some anecdotal evidence suggests that the extent of poisoning was in decline before regulation was introduced. Nevertheless, it is barely conceivable that attitudes were not further influenced by the introduction of legal rules.

If regulation was significant in reducing levels of lead poisoning, it would suggest that by the 1890s it was soundly-based in terms of being acceptable to the industry and enforceable by the factory inspectorate. In the latter respect it may have been important that the industry was relatively small and highly concentrated, being located principally in East London and on Tyneside. This meant that it was possible for inspectors to monitor premises closely and regularly in order to establish close working relationships with occupiers and to ascertain that compliance with the law was occurring. The historical significance for legal compliance of long-term working relationships between inspectors and employers – as opposed to a more penal approach to enforcement – has been pointed out elsewhere.[81] Given the size of the inspectorate and the wide spread of some large industries in which some factories might be small and remotely-located, such relationships were not always developed. The white lead industry, however, appears to be one in which they were. Inspectors were expected to visit premises under special rules four times each year. In 1901, however, Cramp, superintending inspector of the southern division, reported that of

1,650 such works in his region, 1,595 were not inspected on four occasions. Included in the latter figure were such dangerous premises as potteries, paint and colour works. But all white and red lead factories were visited four times.[82] According to Inspector Jasper Redgrave, who was worried about over-visiting and over-inspection, one Midlands factory was visited twenty-four times in one year – largely in connection with accident and poisoning inquiries.[83]

That regulation succeeded by means of working relationships between regulators and regulatees and through recognition on the part of regulatees that regulation was appropriate and sensible, is indicated by the virtual absence of prosecutions for breach of white lead rules. Only in 1901 did the factory inspectorate bring such a prosecution. Yet prosecutions for breach of special rules and of occupational health regulations in general occurred regularly, if at a relatively low level. Thus, in the decade, 1899-1908, such prosecutions were brought at an annual frequency of about 48 cases (with a conviction rate of approximately 86 per cent). The fact that prosecution for breach of white lead rules almost literally never occurred does suggest general observance of the law. Hence, despite the absence of any conclusive proof, the balance of probability is that regulation did effect a marked improvement in occupational health in white lead factories. In her unpublished *Reminiscences* Gertrude Tuckwell, a long-time advocate of the prohibition of lead glazes, came to a similar conclusion in respect of lead poisoning in the pottery and earthenware industry. She noted that only fourteen cases of poisoning occurred in 1929 compared with the 'hundreds' of the 1890s. Her explanation for this decline ran as follows:

> ...the end of the dangerous trades... did not come by the abolition of all poisons as I had thought.... Good results were being obtained under the Home Office rules, increased inspection and the presence of a woman Inspector in the Potteries – that is to say by perfected administration and not by the abolition of the dangerous ingredient [i.e. lead] that we had asked for.[84]

Notes

1. Marguerite W. Dupree, *Family Structure in the Staffordshire Potteries* (Oxford: Clarendon Press, 1995), 217.
2. H.A. Mess, *Factory Legislation and its Administration, 1891–1924* (London: P.S. King, 1926), 51–2.
3. On Arlidge see Clare Holdsworth, 'Dr John Thomas Arlidge and

Victorian Occupational Medicine', *Medical History*, 42 (1998), 458–75.

4. More prevalent among men were: bronchitis, phthisis, rheumatic afflictions and stomach disorders. Among women stomach disorders, uterine maladies, phthisis, anaemia and bronchitis were more common.
5. J.T. Arlidge, *On the Diseases Prevalent Among Potters* (London: np, 1872), 3–4, 9.
6. J.T. Arlidge, 'Diseases Incident to the Manufacture of Pottery', *BMJ*, 26 Aug. 1876, 272.
7. *Minutes of Evidence taken before the Commissioners Appointed to Inquire into the Factory and Workshop Acts*, PP 1876 XXX, 553 and 586.
8. *Factory and Workshop Act, 1878, 41 Vict. c.16*, s. 38 and first schedule.
9. *Daily Chronicle*, 24 Nov. 1892. Only the Secretary of State's 1882 order prohibiting meal-taking in various workrooms afforded any legal protection against lead poisoning.
10. See Clare Holdsworth, 'Potters' Rot and Plumbism: Occupational Health in the North Staffordshire Pottery Industry', Liverpool University Ph.D. thesis (1995), chapter 6, where the establishment of special rules in pottery manufacture is assessed 'as a process of state formation', 182.
11. *Factory and Workshop Act, 1891* (*54 & 55 Vict. c.75, s.8*).
12. H.J. Tennant, 'Dangerous Trades. A Case for Legislation', *Fortnightly Review*, (Feb. 1899), 317; see *idem.*, 'Principles of Prospective Legislation for Dangerous Trades' in Thomas Oliver (ed), *Dangerous Trades. The Historical, Social and Legal Aspects of Industrial Occupations as Affecting Health, by a Number of Experts* (London: John Murray, 1902), 63–72. Until the passage of the *Factory and Workshop Act, 1895* workers had no right of representation at an arbitration. See Miss Gertrude Tuckwell, 'The More Obvious Defects in our Factory Code', in Mrs Sidney Webb (ed.), *The Case for the Factory Acts* (London: Grant Richards, 1901).
13. TUC Library Collections, University of North London. Women's Trade Union League. Minutes of Annual Meetings held at the Trades Union Congress, (Manchester, 25 Jan. 1899) and (Huddersfield, 3 Sept. 1900).
14. *Factory and Workshop Act, 1901* (*1 Edw. 7 c.22 ss.79–86*); Oliver, *op. cit.* (note 12), 4–5; 4 *Hansard*, 79 (2 March 1900), 1539–41.
15. See Mess, *op. cit.* (note 2) 52. Arlidge's book was based on the

author's 1891 Milroy Lectures given at the Royal College of Physicians in London.

16. *Royal Commission on Labour. The Employment of Women. Report of Clara Collet on the Staffordshire Potteries*, PP 1893–4 XXXVII, 609–11;
17. *Annual Report of HM Chief Inspector of Factories and Workshops*, (1891–2) PP 1893–4 XVII, 107–13. In his book Arlidge suggested that the rise of trade unionism obviated the need for protective legislation because workers could 'for the most part dictate to masters their own terms as to time and most of the circumstances of employment'. J.T. Arlidge, *Hygiene, Diseases and Mortality of Occupations* (London: Percival, 1892), 50. However, when he spoke to Cramp he credited the Factory Acts with improving potters' health and supported the extension of existing regulations to adult males.
18. *Daily Chronicle*, 24 Nov. 1892; 15, 21 Dec. 1892.
19. *Statutory Rules & Orders, 1892* (London: HMSO, 1892), 474.
20. Public Record Office (PRO) HO 45/9851/B12393E, Sprague Oram to Lushington, 24 Dec. 1892, 9 March 1893; A.P. Llewellyn (Secretary to North Staffordshire Chamber of Commerce) to Sprague Oram, 20 Jan. 1893; Lushington to Sprague Oram, 10 Feb. 1893; Cramp to Sprague Oram, 14 Feb. 1893; Draft invitations to serve on the Pottery Committee, dated April 1893; *Annual Report of HM Chief Inspector of Factories and Workshops*, (1891–2) PP 1893–4 XVII, 110–12; *Daily Chronicle*, 28 Dec. 1892; *The Potter*, Feb. 1893.
21. *Report on the Conditions of Labour in Potteries, the Injurious Effects upon the Health of the Workpeople and the Proposed Remedies*, PP 1893–4 XVII, 43–53. As Spanton makes clear in his autobiography, in which he gives a very brief account of the Committee's work, he and Arlidge were not entirely in sympathy with each other. W.D. Spanton (ed. E.E. Young), *The Story of My Life* (London: The Connoisseur, 1920), 38–9 and 93.
22. *Report on the Conditions of Labour in Potteries, the Injurious Effects upon the Health of the Workpeople and the Proposed Remedies*, PP 1893–4 XVII, 53.
23. *Civil Service Estimates*, PP 1892 LIII, 107; P.W.J. Bartrip and P.T. Fenn, 'The Measurement of Safety. Factory Accident Statistics in Victorian and Edwardian Britain', *Historical Research*, 63 (1990), 58–72.
24. Bodleian Library. Ms Asquith 71. Minute of 6 Dec. 1893; Earl of

Oxford and Asquith, *Fifty Years of Parliament* (London: Cassell, 1926), 213–14, 230–1.

25. Tuckwell, *op. cit.* (note 12), 126–7; see *Royal Commission on Labour*, PP 1893–4 XXIV, Evidence of William Owen of the Amalgamated Potters' Society, Burslem, 418.
26. PRO HO 45/9851/B12393E, A.P. Llewellyn to Asquith, 9 Jan. 1894; Resolution of Joint Committee and letter of 21 Feb.; *The Times*, 15 March 1894; *Staffordshire Sentinel* 15 March 1894; *Daily News*, 2 May 1894.
27. *Annual Report of HM Chief Inspector of Factories,* (1895) PP 1896 XIX, 159–60; *Women's Trade Union Review* (hereafter *WTUR*), 25 (April 1897), 3.
28. *Annual Report of HM Chief Inspector of Factories and Workshops,* (1898) PP 1900 XI, 119. Spanton, who had a good deal of sympathy for the manufacturers, later observed that if the special rules had been 'more warmly adopted' by them they might have avoided the 'far more stringent ones' subsequently enacted. *Op. cit.* (note 21), 93.
29. Mess, *op. cit.* (note 2), 52–3.
30. *Annual Report of HM Chief Inspector of Factories and Workshops,* (1895) PP 1896 XIX, 159–60.
31. *Daily Chronicle*, 22 Jan. 1898; 4 *Hansard*, 63 (29 July 1898), 475. See G. Tuckwell, 'Commercial Manslaughter', *Nineteenth Century*, 44 (1898), 257.
32. 4 *Hansard*, 54 (4 March 1898), 633; 63 (29 July 1898), 480; *Annual Report of HM Chief Inspector of Factories and Workshops,* (1896) PP 1897 XVII, 248; *Birmingham Post*, 2 June 1896.
33. *Annual Report of HM Chief Inspector of Factories and Workshops,* (1897) PP 1898 XIV, 57–63. The Paterson-Deane Report is discussed in Clare Holdsworth, 'Women's Work and Family Health: Evidence from the Staffordshire Potteries, 1890–1920', *Continuity and Change*, 12 (1997), 103–28.
34. *Historical Studies in Industrial Relations*, 2 (1996), 3–26.
35. Holdsworth, *op. cit.* (note 10), 158 and chapter 6; D. Stuart, *Millicent Duchess of Sutherland, 1867–1955* (London: Gollancz, 1982). In 1906 Shaw lectured at the Caxton Hall on the subject of 'Poisoning the Proletariat'. See *The Times*, 29 June 1906.
36. On Emma Paterson and the early history of the WPPL see K. Busbey, 'The Women's Trade Union Movement in Great Britain', *Bulletin of the Bureau of Labour*, 83 (1909); H. Goldman, *Emma Paterson* (London: Lawrence and Wishart, 1974); A. Godwin, 'Early

Years in the Trade Unions', in L. Middleton (ed), *Women in the Labour Movement: the British Experience* (Beckenham: Croom Helm, 1977), 94–112; S. Lewenhak, *Women and Trade Unions* (London: Benn, 1977), 67–82; S. Boston, *Women Workers and the Trade Union Movement* (London: Davis-Poynter, 1980), 30–60.

37. TUC Library Collections, University of North London. WTUL Ledger on Health and Work in the Potteries District. The *Workmen's Compensation Act, 1897 (60 & 61 Vict. c.37)* permitted some groups of injured workers to recover compensation from their employers for physical injuries arising 'out of and in the course of employment' without the need to prove negligence. But the act (until amended in 1906) did not cover victims of occupational disease.
38. PRO HO45/9852/B12393E, note of 7 May 1898; 4 *Hansard,* 54 (4 March 1898), 634, 642–3, 653–4, 660–1; 6; *WTUR*, 29 (April 1898), 12–14; *Statutory Rules and Orders 1898 no.349* (London: HMSO, 1898). In Dilke's later years he became a strong advocate of state intervention to mitigate working conditions. In this connection his most recent biographer detects the influence of his second wife, Emilia: 'it is difficult to believe that Dilke would have gone quite as far down the collectivist road had he not been married to a committed feminist and trade unionist'. See David Nicholls, *The Lost Prime Minister. A Life of Sir Charles Dilke* (London: Hambledon Press, 1995), 249.
39. *The Times*, 20, 24 May 1898; *Daily Chronicle*, 24 May 1898; 4 *Hansard*, 58 (23 May 1898), 339–40; 63 (29 July 1898), 480; PRO HO45 10117/B12393P, B.A. Whitelegge to Kenelm Digby, 28 March 1898; draft letter to Drs Oliver and Thorpe, sent 7 May 1898. Thomas Edward Thorpe (1845–1925) was the son of a Manchester cotton merchant. He studied chemistry at Owens College, Manchester and Heidelberg. He held chairs in chemistry in Glasgow, Leeds, and, for many years, the Royal College of Science. Between 1894 and 1909 he was the Government Chemist. As such, 'he conducted numerous investigations bearing on industrial and public welfare. Thomas Oliver (1853–1942) was born in Ayrshire. After studying medicine in Glasgow and Paris he became a physician in Newcastle upon Tyne. In 1880 he was appointed lecturer, later professor, in the city's medical school (then attached to Durham University). Repeated contact with cases of industrial disease stimulated an abiding interest in this field of medicine and as Goulstonian lecturer at the Royal College of Physicians, in 1891, Oliver's subject was lead poisoning. In 1893 he was a member of the

Departmental Committee on White Lead. This was the first of many official inquiries into industrial disease on which he served. Over the course of his career he published several important books on diseases of occupation. In the 1920s and 1930s Oliver was President of the Durham College of Medicine and Vice Chancellor of Durham University. See *Dictionary of National Biography, 1941–1950* (London: OUP, 1959), 640–1 and *New DNB* (Oxford: OUP, forthcoming).

40. *Staffordshire Sentinel*, 8, 15 June 1898; *Westminster Gazette*, 8 June 1898; *The Times*, 13, 18 June 1898; *Times and Echo* 11 June 1898; 4 *Hansard*, 59 (14 June 1898), 223; (17 June 1898), 584–5.
41. See PRO HO45/9853/B12393E for correspondence and other Home Office documentation relating to the arbitration. The *Women's Trade Union Review*, the organ of the Women's Trade Union League, argued that there had been significant weakening. *WTUR*, (Jan. 1899), 12–15.
42. *Annual Report of HM Chief Inspector of Factories and Workshops*, (1898) PP 1900 XI, 119–21; *WTUR*, (Jan. 1899), 11–15.
43. *Report on the Employment of Compounds of Lead in the Manufacture of Pottery*, PP 1899 XII, 281–91.
44. *Ibid.*, 282.
45. Colour and litho-dusters were involved in the decoration of ware. Oxford English Dictionary On-Line.
46. *Report on the Employment of Compounds of Lead in the Manufacture of Pottery*, PP 1899 XII, 285.
47. *Ibid.*, 281–91.
48. W. Dowling Prendergast, *The Potter and Lead Poisoning* (Stoke-on-Trent: n.p., 1898); W. Furnival, *Researches on Leadless Glazes* (Stone: W.J. Furnival, 1898). The idea of leadless glaze was hardly new, for Josiah Wedgwood had experimented with them (albeit unsuccessfully) in the late-eighteenth century. See Holdsworth, *op. cit.* (note 10), 12 and 192.
49. PRO HO 45/10117/B12393P, Home Office minutes on the Report of Drs Oliver and Thorpe.
50. PRO HO 45/10117/B12393P, Whitelegge's memorandum, 2 March 1899; *WTUR*, 34 (July 1899), 4.
51. HO45 10118/B12393P, Report of Conference between Home Office officials and deputation of pottery employers, 18 July 1899; *idem.*, Notes of Deputation from the Allied Manufacturers' (Pottery) Associations on the Proposed Special Rules, 31 Oct. 1899; *Staffordshire Sentinel*, 19 July 1899; *The Times*, 19 July 1899.

52. *WTUR*, 39 (Oct. 1900), 1.
53. *Staffordshire Sentinel*, 25 Aug. 1900; PRO HO45/10119/B12393P, Bernard Moore (china and porcelain manufacturer) to B.A. Whitelegge, 31 Jan. 1901.
54. PRO HO45/10019/B12393P, Troup's minute dated 24 Jan. 1901.
55. PRO HO 45/10120/B12393P, Minutes of Proceedings at an Arbitration under the Factory Act, 1891. Held before Lord James of Hereford (Umpire), Chester Jones, Esq. And A.P. Llewellyn, Esq., into the Special Rules Proposed by the Home Office for the Regulation of the Manufacture of Pottery 7–12 Nov. 1901. On Lord James and the arbitration see TUC Library Collections, University of North London. Gertrude Tuckwell Papers. Unpublished Reminiscences of Gertrude Tuckwell, 188–89.
56. *Staffordshire Sentinel*, 12 Nov. 1901. The WTUL regarded the arbitration outcome as a 'triumph'. See TUC Library Collections, University of North London. Gertrude Tuckwell Papers. Unpublished Reminiscences of Gertrude Tuckwell, 190.
57. PRO HO 45/10120/B12393P, Minutes of Proceedings at an Arbitration under the Factory Act, 1891. Held before Lord James of Hereford (Umpire) and Chester Jones, Esq., A.P. Llewellyn, Esq., into the Special Rules Proposed by the Home Office for the Regulation of the Manufacture of Pottery 7–12 Nov. 1901. Thorpe's evidence was more extensive than that of any other witness. See also, in the same file, Thorpe's 32 page submission: 'The Chemical Evidence in Support of Rules 1 and 2'.
58. PRO HO 45/10121/B12393P, draft letter, B.A. Whitelegge to Professor T.E. Thorpe, 22 Jan. 1903.
59. PRO HO 45/10121/B12393P, A.P. Llewellyn to Secretary of State, 10 July 1902.
60. British Library, Dilke Papers, Add. Mss.43892 ff.259, Lord James of Hereford to Charles Dilke, 10 Dec. 1903; 14 Dec. 1903.
61. *Ibid.*, copy of letter from Dilke to James, 2 Dec. 1903.
62. *Ibid.*, Lord James of Hereford to Charles Dilke, 14 Dec. 1903.
63. *British Clayworker*, Dec. 1903.
64. For newpaper cuttings on initiatives in this area, including exhibitions of ware and proselytising articles, see TUC Library Collections, University of North London. Gertrude Tuckwell Papers. Unpublished Reminiscences of Gertrude Tuckwell, reel 2 20f.
65. *Report of the Departmental Committee Appointed to inquire into the Dangers attendant on the Use of Lead and the Danger or Injury to Health arising from Dust and other Causes in the Manufacture of*

Earthenware and China and in the Processes incidental thereto including the Making of Lithographic Transfers, PP 1910 XXIX, 133.

66. Bernice Martin has argued that factory regulation was largely consensual by the late-Victorian period. See 'The Development of the Factory Office up to 1878: Administrative Evolution and the Establishment of a Regulatory Style in the Early Factory Inspectorate', unpublished and undated paper.
67. PRO HO 45/10119/B12393P, Bernard Moore to Whitelegge, 31 Jan. 1901. On Moore see Aileen Dawson, *Bernard Moore. Master Potter, 1850–1935* (Richard Dennis: London, 1982) esp. 98 where it is stated that Moore's 'contribution to the improvement of conditions in the pottery trade can be said to have been most important over a period of some thirty years'.
68. *Report of the Departmental Committee Appointed to inquire into the Dangers attendant on the Use of Lead and the Danger or Injury to Health arising from Dust and other Causes in the Manufacture of Earthenware and China and in the Processes incidental thereto including the Making of Lithographic Transfers*, PP 1910 XXIX, 223–24; also TUC Library Collections, University of North London. Gertrude Tuckwell Papers. Unpublished Reminiscences of Gertrude Tuckwell, 167–8, 190–1. Tuckwell was the WTUL's secretary from 1893–1905. From 1898 she was also secretary to the Christian Social Union.
69. Peter Bartrip, 'Expertise and the Dangerous Trades, 1875–1900' in Roy MacLeod (ed), *Government and Expertise. Specialists, Administrators and Professional, 1860–1919* (Cambridge: Cambridge University Press, 1988), 89–109. On Thorpe's work as government chemist see P.W. Hammond and H. Egan, *Weighed in the Balance. A History of the Laboratory of the Government Chemist* (London: HMSO, 1992).
70. BBC Television Documentary, 'Dust to Dust', 17 Aug. 1982; see Richard Schilling, *A Challenging Life. Sixty Years in Occupational Health* (London: Canning Press, 1998), 114–15. Examination of TUC Congress Annual Reports reveals the very limited amount of attention devoted to occupational health questions.
71. P.W.J. Bartrip, ' "Petticoat Pestering": the Women's Trade Union League and Lead Poisoning in the Staffordshire Potteries, 1890–1914', *Historical Studies in Industrial Relations*, 2 (1996), 8; R. Whipp, *Patterns of Labour. Work and Social Change in the Pottery Industry* (London: Routledge, 1990), 11, 15–24, 109–12. Although Whipp questions pottery workers' indifference towards unionisation,

he confirms that rates of trade union membership in the Potteries were consistently lower than those for the UK as a whole. See also Dupree, *op. cit.* (note 1), 300–03.

72. *Annual Report of HM Chief Inspector of Factories and Workshops,* (1896) PP 1897 XVII, 247; see also TUC Library Collections, University of North London. Gertrude Tuckwell Papers. Unpublished Reminiscences of Gertrude Tuckwell, 179–80.
73. *Annual Report of HM Chief Inspector of Factories,* (1900) PP 1901 X, 127.
74. *Annual Report of HM Chief Inspector of Factories,* (1898) PP 1900 XI, 259.
75. D.J. Rowe, *Lead Manufacturing in Great Britain* (Beckenham: Croom Helm, 1983), 192–3.
76. *Census of England and Wales. 1901. Summary Tables*, PP 1903 LXXXIV, Table 36: Occupations of Males and Females Aged 10 years and Upwards in England and Wales, 211.
77. *Final Report on the First Census of Production of the United Kingdom (1907)*, PP 1912–13 CIX, 252.
78. *Census of England and Wales. 1911. Occupations and Industries*, PP 1913 LXXVIII, Table 2: Occupations of Persons, Males and Females Aged 10 years and Upwards in England and Wales, 481.
79. Oliver, *op. cit.* (note 12), 33; Sir Thomas Legge, *Industrial Maladies* (London: OUP, 1934), chapter iv; Thomas M. Legge and Kenneth W. Goadby, *Lead Poisoning and Lead Absorption* (London: Edward Arnold, 1912), esp. chapters xii–xiv.
80. Such an explanation would be consistent with the 'McKeown thesis' which (in brief) argues that increased life expectancy in the late-eighteenth and nineteenth centuries had little or nothing to do with medical science or public health legislation, but everything to do with rising living standards in general and improvements in the working class diet in particular. While McKeown developed this argument in a number of books and articles, particular attention is drawn to Thomas McKeown, *The Modern Rise of Population* (London: Edward Arnold, 1976).
81. P.W.J. Bartrip and P.T. Fenn, 'The Evolution of Regulatory Style in the Nineteenth Century Factory Inspectorate' *Journal of Law and Society*, 10 (1983), 201–22.
82. *Annual Report of HM Chief Inspector of Factories,* (1900) PP 1901 X, 155.
83. *Ibid.*, 203.
84. TUC Library Collections, University of North London. Gertrude

Tuckwell Papers. Unpublished Reminiscences of Gertrude Tuckwell, 190–1.

5

A Kind of Dread: Arsenic and Occupational Health

Introduction

During the nineteenth century arsenic entered the public consciousness in a variety of ways. It was recognised as a criminal poison, a means of vermin control, a useful medicine, an important raw material in manufacturing industry and a source of domestic ill health resulting from its presence in the domestic environment. The *Arsenic Act, 1851* sought to control the retail trade in arsenic and thereby limit the availability of the poison to would-be murderers and suicides. Subsequently it was no longer legally permissible to purchase it in small quantities, with 'no questions asked', on the pretext of pest extermination. The act, for which the organised medical and pharmaceutical professions were chiefly responsible, imposed no restrictions on medicinal prescription of the poison. Before and after 1851 medical practitioners prescribed arsenic in the treatment of a number of diseases and ailments including migraine, syphilis, asthma, rheumatism, neuralgia, psoriasis, cholera and cancer.[1] Neither did the *Arsenic Act* limit agricultural or industrial usage of the poison. Widely employed in sheep dipping and for other farmyard purposes, arsenic remained an important weapon for the farmer in his war against rats, mice, wireworm, other 'vermin' and 'smut' (a fungal disease of cereals).

Industry also used arsenical compounds in many products, particularly as a dye and, to a lesser extent, as a preservative and insecticide. As a result, dozens, if not hundreds, of consumer goods in everyday use contained arsenic. These included clothes, soap, books, kitchen-ware, glassware, pottery and earthenware (glazes), paint and distemper, artificial and dried flowers, stuffed animals, playing cards, children's toys, paper and packaging, candles, handkerchiefs, fly-papers, lampshades, soft furnishings, artificial leaves and fruit, patent medicine and wallpaper. Periodically, between about 1857 and 1885, the threat to health posed by the poison in these products escaping into the domestic environment created public disquiet. As a result there were frequent demands for the introduction of controls upon the commercial use of arsenic. But these all came to nothing; farmers and manufacturers remained free to employ it as they wished while going about their legitimate business.[2]

Arsenic is an irritant mineral poison capable, even in minute quantities, of causing the death of humans who inhale or ingest it. The symptoms of chronic poisoning can include headache, dry throat, colic, loss of appetite, lassitude, hot and cold sweats, trembling, dimmed vision, shortness of breath, depression, uneven pulse, partial paralysis, cramps, vomiting and diarrhoea. External contact may lead to boils, skin blotches and burning sensations, especially around the nose and eyes. The widespread use made of arsenic in the nineteenth century meant that various occupational groups came into close contact with it. After all, self-evidently, workers were engaged in mining, processing and applying the arsenic that went into so many consumer goods. Accordingly miners, those involved in extracting the mineral from its ore, workers in manufacturing industry and those employed in the painting and decorating trades were among those exposed to a risk of poisoning. Although, in 1892, arsenic poisoning gained official recognition as an occupational disease, this accorded protection only to those workers in industries covered by the factory acts and, in the case of the arsenic extraction industry, the mines and quarries acts.[3] Others, including house painters and decorators remained unprotected. Before 1892 no one who worked with arsenic enjoyed any legal protection. It was a case of *caveat operarius* (let the worker beware).

Until the rash of political and legal activity on workmen's compensation and industrial disease in the late-Victorian and Edwardian periods, there was comparatively little medical, official, or popular interest in arsenic as an occupational health threat. Yet, in some quarters, the dangers of arsenic in the workplace had been recognised many years before. Thus, in the early-1830s Thackrah documented instances of arsenic poisoning among paper stainers and house painters.[4] In 1843 a meeting of the Medical Society of London discussed the case of a 'watch-dial enameller' who was poisoned by the arsenious acid vapour given off by the raw materials used in his enamelling work. Curiously, the same meeting heard that workers at a Swansea copper works, who experienced considerable exposure to arsenical fume, arsenic often being found in copper ore, rarely suffered ill effects or reduced lifespan. This, however, may have had something to do with the fact that anyone who showed symptoms of poisoning was sacked, leaving only the unsusceptible in employment. In 1845 an inquest jury brought in a verdict: 'That the deceased died from the mortal effects of his exposure to the poison of arsenic, while at work in a candle manufactory'. The candles in question, known as 'composites', were made from cocoa oil and stearin wax, the arsenic being added to give a waxier appearance.[5]

Occasional references to arsenic as an occupational disease may be found in the literature of the 1850s. In 1857 Alfred Swaine Taylor, the forensic scientist, told a select committee that arsenical wallpaper was 'very injurious' including to those involved in its production. Many decorators, he pointed out, refused to hang it. In response, Alfred Fletcher of the East London Colour, Chymical and Printing Ink Works, maintained that workmen in colour factories where arsenic was used, were 'in the regular enjoyment of perfect health'.[6] However, Taylor's point was endorsed by another forensic scientist and physician, William Augustus Guy. In his experience, paper stainers, that is, those who made wallpaper, book covers and the like, suffered greatly from their contact with arsenical compounds. Within a day of commencing employment a new worker would develop a painful rash which often spread over the whole body, turning into open sores. Guy had found that few were able to work with arsenical compounds for more than two or three days.[7] Until the 1860s, however, perhaps partly reflecting the low priority accorded to occupational health by the Victorian medical profession, arsenical poisoning in the workplace gained little attention either in the medical press or elsewhere.

By this time the dangers of arsenic poisoning resulting from its presence in consumer goods were already being vigorously debated in the press. Possibly it was the growing awareness of the dangers of arsenic in the home that awakened concern about the threat it posed in the workplace, but it is also likely that appreciation of occupational hazards increased as arsenical colours found new applications – especially in the clothing trades. For example, aniline (coal tar) dyes, many of which contained arsenic, were coming into vogue in the late-1850s. By the early-60s they had all but replaced vegetable dyes for clothes. Self-preservation may have inspired the middle-class campaign against domestic poisons but the Victorian moral conscience was important in converting this concern into a workplace question. Another factor, as we shall see, was feminism. Arsenically-coloured fashions were, primarily, made by women for women; they threatened the health of workers and wearers alike. Not surprisingly, therefore, the Ladies' Sanitary Association and Barbara Leigh Bodichon's *Englishwoman's Journal* both played parts in raising public and official consciousness about the perils of arsenic in the workplace. In the sixties women's political impotence meant that they could do little more than prompt men to act. But, handicapped though they were, they did this to considerable effect.[8]

Leaves and flowers

In 1860 Arthur Hill Hassall, who had spearheaded the *Lancet*'s campaign against the adulteration of food and drink in the fifties, wrote about occupational ill-health in artificial leaf and flower manufacture.[9] The use of artificial flowers and leaves as clothing accessories had become fashionable in the 1850s. To meet consumer demand hundreds of workshops quickly entered production. At this juncture such premises were not covered by the factory acts and were, therefore, not subject to inspection. They relied on arsenite of copper to produce the green hues and employed mainly girls and young women, the condition of whom was, according to Hassall, 'wretched in the extreme'.

Hassall was no sentimentalist. A year earlier he had defended the wallpaper industry against allegations that its products were responsible for illness among those whose homes contained arsenically-dyed papers. Since the arsenic in varnished papers could not be vaporised at room temperature and was unlikely to come off as dust, except in small quantities, there was, he argued, little need for concern. However, he took a very different view of the risks of the artificial flower and leaf trade. The workers in it, he observed,

> ...all labour and many in a severe form, under symptoms of arsenical poisoning. The poison is diffused throughout the atmosphere they breathe and is of course, inhaled; further, it acts as a local irritant and escharotic on the hands and other parts of the body to which it becomes mechanically applied.

He went on to relate two case histories and describe the symptoms of poisoning. These included 'general derangement of the health', debility, nervousness, headache, thirst, sickness, loss of appetite, diarrhoea, sore throat and gums, swollen, sore and watery eyes, sore and running nose and body ulcers. Yet, Hassall contended, all this suffering was unnecessary for even if suitable substitutes for arsenical dyes were not, as he suspected, available, 'simple and obvious precautions' to protect the workforce could easily be adopted.[10]

Many of Hassall's findings were soon to be confirmed in the *Englishwoman's Journal*'s popular account of arsenic poisoning among women and children in London's artificial flower industry.

The *Journal*'s article claimed that when manufacturers recruited workers they announced that they did not use emerald (i.e. arsenical) green. As a result, although workers were aware that their labour made them feel unwell, they did not realise that their health was being undermined by arsenic. But while the author of this piece, M.N(icholson), stated that the trade had claimed the lives of some workers, she differed from Hassall in calling not for legislative intervention, merely for women shoppers to eschew green wreaths and 'artifical flower devices', thereby ending consumer demand and closing the market.[11] Whatever the solution might be, the case for reform gained weight with the much-publicised death, following long illness, of a young London woman (aged 19) named Matilda Scheurer.

Scheurer had been employed in artificial leaf manufacture in which arsenite of copper (emerald green) was used to colour leaves and buds green.[12] Post-mortem examination showed her bodily tissues to be 'impregnated' with arsenic. Her employer, in whose service were 98 women, claimed that his employees had rejected his suggestion for the wearing of masks on the grounds of discomfort, but that they had worn muslin over their mouths. The *Lancet* regarded this precaution as 'most imperfect and inefficient'. The coroner's jury, which heard that Scheurer's sister had died in similar circumstances, returned a verdict of accidental poisoning by arsenite of copper used in employment. The *Lancet*, which maintained that arsenic had no place in industry, argued that its use should be 'rendered criminal', hinting that custodial sentences would be the appropriate punishment for employers who caused their workers to use it.[13]

Scheurer had been employed in a workshop off the Euston Road (Judd Street). Her death aroused the interest of Dr Hillier, the medical officer of health for St Pancras, who investigated. He uncovered a number of alarming facts, for example, that the factory was overcrowded and poorly ventilated and its workforce unaware that it was handling toxic materials. Moreover the employees were using methods of work that led not only to their inhalation of arsenical compounds, but to them becoming smothered with poisonous dust. It also appeared that Scheurer was not the first member of the workforce to have died from arsenic poisoning. When questioned, some workers testified to constant sickness, while a local surgeon stated that he 'repeatedly' saw patients from the factory who showed signs of chronic poisoning. Yet Hillier knew of no law that might be used to put an end to the conditions he had discovered.

Convinced that 'something ought to be done' he felt that the Home Office, as the department of state responsible for enforcing industrial safety legislation, should be notified. His report found its way to the Home Office and on Christmas Eve 1861 the home secretary, Sir George Grey, wrote to the clerk of the Privy Council enclosing an extract. This prompted the Council, in January 1862, to order William Guy (on whom see below, 144) to inquire into the 'alleged fatal cases of poisoning by emerald green; and the poisonous effects of that substance as used in the arts'.[14]

The timing of all this is somewhat curious, for in the early-1860s the domestic artificial flower industry was in deep recession following the removal, in 1860, of the protective duty on imports. Provided with the opportunity to purchase the superior products of France and Germany, consumers shunned the 'ugly monstrosities' devoid of skill and taste made by British firms. As a result, 'for a year or two the trade was so greatly depressed that many of those engaged in it never hoped to see a revival'. Subsequently, the domestic industry put its house in order and began to compete effectively against its continental rivals. As a result, by 1867 it had 'thoroughly revived and was being carried on in London on a larger scale than ever before experienced'. Ten years later it was reported as being bigger and more successful than ever before.[15] In other words, the likelihood is that the scale of the arsenic threat was far from being at its greatest when the government and others began to take an interest in it as a health hazard. This in turn suggests that this interest owed less to any objective criteria and more to a 'concatenation of circumstances' that briefly made arsenic poisoning in artificial flower manufacture a matter of notoriety.

The Scheurer case became something of a *cause celèbre* when it was 'picked up' by the Ladies' Sanitary Association (LSA). This association, one of many such bodies that existed in Victorian Britain, was founded in October 1857 with the object of diffusing sanitary information amongst 'the people', i.e. the working classes, by means of tracts and lectures. Originally linked with the *Englishwoman's Journal*, the LSA stressed a Christian rather than a feminist ethic. At its 1861 annual meeting it claimed to have a membership of 206 and to have distributed some 138,000 pamphlets on a variety of topics including the value of fresh air, good food, pure water, wholesome drink, warm clothing and 'the power of soap and water'. On this occasion the platform held several dignitaries amongst whom were Lord Shaftesbury, the Bishops of London and Oxford, the latter of whom served as chairman, and the author, Thomas Hughes. The Association's report was read by William Cowper MP (1811-1888), who was the grandson of a former prime minister (Lord Melbourne) and stepson of the incumbent (Lord Palmerston). As President of the Board of Health (1857-58) he had been a prime mover in the passage of the *Medical Act, 1858*. In 1861 he held the post of Commissioner of Works. Notwithstanding the LSA's name, not a single woman occupied a platform seat. It hardly needs to be said that their absence underlines the male domination of Victorian society.[16]

Although women were conspicuously absent from the seats of prominence at the LSA's 1861 meeting, the Association's joint secretaries were Georgina Cowper and Elizabeth Sutherland. Their tenure of these offices suggests that while men held the LSA's high profile positions, it was women who performed the real work. Georgina Cowper, the daughter of a vice-admiral, was the second wife of William Cowper, through whom she was connected to the highest levels of British society. Elizabeth Sutherland's social credentials were less exalted; she was married to John Sutherland, an important figure in Victorian 'sanitary science'. An inspector under the first Board of Health, he had been involved in the official inquiry into the hygiene of British troops in the Crimea. What all this indicates is that the Ladies' Sanitary Association was no obscure body, but one which, like the Women's Trade Union League of a later era (see Chapters 4 and 8), enjoyed the support of powerful and influential persons. Hence, when the LSA's secretaries wrote to *The Times* on the subject of occupational arsenic poisoning, following the Scheurer death, it was to be expected that their letter would attract much attention.

The letter, which was accompanied by a statement from a chemistry professor, A.W. Hofmann, on the prevalence and the perils of arsenic in consumer goods, bore the title, 'The Dance of Death'.[17] In it the LSA's secretaries drew attention to 'the melancholy fate of hundreds of young women and children, who, as artificial florists, are suffering in the most terrible manner from handling and inhaling the cruelly destructive poison with which they colour the brilliant green leaves now so much in fashion'. Prompted by *The Times*'s account of the Scheurer inquest, they, in the footsteps of Hillier, had investigated the green leaf trade. They found workshops in which women sat with towels wrapped around their faces in an effort to keep out the dust. Like Hillier, they too ascertained that Scheurer's death was no isolated occurrence. Finally, like Miss Nicholson, they called for people who wore clothing in which the colour was created by means of arsenical compounds to change their purchasing habits, if not out of regard for their own health, then out of concern for the sufferings of the workforce. This strategy of seeking to improve occupational health by means of changed consumer behaviour was, as we have seen, later to be employed by the Women's Trade Union League in its campaign against lead-glazed pottery. Cowper and Sutherland's letter, though brief, was influential.[18] When it appeared the Medical Officer of the Privy Council, John Simon, had already received instructions to investigate the facts of the Scheurer case and health aspects of arsenic use, but the LSA's allegations extended the scope of the inquiry and ensured that its findings would receive close scrutiny.

Simon's investigator, William Guy (1810-85) was Professor of Forensic Medicine at King's College, London and physician to King's College Hospital. In the early-1860s he was also medical superintendent of Millbank Prison. A pioneer statistician, Guy had a keen interest in sanitary reform and occupational health. Not only had he given evidence to a Royal Commission on pulmonary consumption among printers (to the Health of Towns Commission in 1844), he had published, in 1843-44, a lengthy, three-part paper on health and occupation. In addition he had recently written on arsenic poisoning among paper stainers (see above 139).[19]

In conducting his inquiry Guy studied documentary evidence such as Hillier's report, the letters of Cowper and Sutherland and Hofmann, plus newspaper and periodical articles and books, among which was Alfred Taylor's work *On Poisons*. He also visited premises in which emerald green was either made or used in the manufacture of goods and interviewed people (manufacturers, employees and medical practitioners) with personal experience of arsenical poisoning in general and the Scheurer case in particular. In order to evaluate the full extent of the arsenic threat he focused not only on the occupational context, but also reported cases of suicide by ingestion of the poison and alleged instances of accidental poisoning by exposure to manufactured goods and wrappings in which the poison was present. It is noteworthy, in view of the contemporary concern about accidental domestic poisoning and earlier anxieties about a supposed epidemic of secret poisoning, that Guy regarded these contexts as being of minor importance in comparison with occupational exposures.[20]

Guy found that those involved in making emerald green, a large part of which process was conducted in the open air, suffered only minor symptoms of ill health. On the other hand, 'the manufacturing occupations in which emerald green is used are many, the persons employed numerous and the effects produced often serious and sometimes fatal'.[21] Guy looked at four trades in which arsenical colours were employed: colour printing (chromo-lithography); ornamental paper production (for wrappings, labels and boxes); wallpaper manufacture; and artificial flower, leaf, fruit and seed making. Of these, he found that the first three gave rise to 'serious inconvenience and suffering...and occasionally of illnesses of some duration and severity' to employees. The dangers of the fourth, however, were of a different order.

According to the 1851 Census, artificial flower-making provided employment for 3510 individuals of whom nearly 3000 were women; almost half of the total female workforce was below the age of 20. A substantial part of the trade was located in London. Guy visited two metropolitan factories: Bergeron's, where Scheurer had been employed, which had recently re-located to large premises in Essex Street, Islington and that of Cliplow and Martin of Argyll Square. With a workforce of some 200 young women, the latter was around twice as large as Bergeron's. Guy spoke to about one-third of Bergeron's employees, including all those who had suffered severe symptoms of poisoning. One of his main objectives was to ascertain whether Matilda Scheurer and the other alleged victim of arsenic poisoning, Frances Rollo, had indeed died as a result of contact with emerald green. He concluded that there was 'no reasonable doubt' that Scheurer was such a victim. Although the Rollo case was less clear cut, Guy was satisfied that 'the symptoms of her last fatal illness, as far as they have been ascertained, are consistent with the supposition of arsenical poisoning'. More generally, he was convinced that the use of arsenic in manufacturing industry 'exposes a considerable number of men, women and children to serious suffering and even to some risk of life'.[22]

When he came to make suggestions for removing or reducing the dangers of poisoning Guy paid much attention to the means by which the health of the general public might be safeguarded, for example, by banning the sale of emerald green to toy makers and confectioners, or requiring clothes, papers and other goods containing arsenic to carry warning notices. As far as workers were concerned, Guy argued himself into a very muddled position. He did not feel that his discovery of only one death 'distinctly traceable to the use of emerald green as its sole cause' justified him in recommending a prohibition of those trades that made use of emerald green:

> no case can be made out to justify any special legislation of a highly restrictive character. The effects of emerald green, though disagreeable and even painful, soon subside and pass away without leaving any permanent disability or constitutional injury behind them. They show themselves, too, at an early period and in a form not to be mistaken; so that the men and women who work with the poison are able to abandon their employment, to suspend it for a time, or to substitute for it, as occasion may require, some other branch of their trade carried on under the same roof.[23]

Such an approach was, of course, consistent with the principles of *laissez-faire* whereby adult employees were perceived to be equal participants in the market place with their employers. If they preferred not to pursue a hazardous occupation they were free to shun it and take alternative employment. Consciously or unconsciously, Guy was also applying the legal concept of *volenti non fit injuria* – that in accepting employment the employee willingly accepted the risks that went with it – which contributed to the difficulties faced by those injured at work to recover damages from their employers. In so doing, he assumed, unrealistically, that workers were aware of the dangers to which they were exposed, capable of making the connexion between an illness and the employment which gave rise to it and able to obtain alternative employment, whenever the need arose, either in another department of their employer's business or elsewhere. Working with arsenic might be 'unhealthy and productive of very distressing consequences' but in Guy's view, age conferred on workers the ability 'to judge and to act for themselves'. Once over the age of 18 it was a case of 'let the worker beware'. Arguably, however, Guy was applying a double standard in his attitude towards public and occupational health, for while he was prepared to countenance protective measures for adult consumers (regardless of their theoretical ability to shun hazardous goods), adult workers were to be left to fend for themselves. Given that the higher purchasing power of the middle classes placed them at greater risk from dangerous consumer goods than the 'lower orders', whereas precisely the opposite applied in the context of occupational danger, it would seem that social class was as relevant a consideration as age in determining who should gain legal protection.

Although Guy expressed sympathy with the idea of introducing legal regulations that would require all industrial premises 'in which such operations are being carried on as seriously affect either the health of the community or the health of the persons employed' to meet certain standards in terms of space and cleanliness, he rejected it as impractical and undesirable. First, the small scale of the operations most in need of supervision would make enforcement (by means of registration and inspection) virtually impossible. Second, government intervention in 'the affairs of individuals' and 'the liberty of manufacture' was wrong in principle. Third, trade restrictions would allow foreign manufacturers to capture British markets. In consequence, Guy advocated reliance on 'enlightened public opinion' as the optimum way of improving occupational health. This would operate partly through consumer rejection of commodities containing poisons, partly through the mutual agreement of workers and masters that they had no wish to produce toxic goods but every desire to operate in safe conditions, and partly through the employer's 'dread of the public exposure and censure' if death could be traced to his neglect. Guy then listed the ways in which the dangers of emerald green could be voluntarily lowered or eliminated. These included stopping work at the first sign of symptoms, avoidance of overcrowding and observance of strict cleanliness. Only if voluntarism failed did Guy contemplate the introduction of 'legal interferences'.[24]

Supporters of *laissez-faire* principles usually recognised the need to make exceptions for minors; in this respect Guy was no exception, even though he acknowledged it rather grudgingly. 'The case of young children is somewhat different. They are more completely under the control of their parents on the one hand and their employers on the other; and they may be compelled to continue their occupation to the injury of their health and even to the risk of their lives'.[25] Accordingly, he felt it was 'not...unreasonable' to prohibit anyone below the age of 18 from working on processes which brought them into contact with emerald green. What Guy neglected to consider was how such a prohibition could be carried into effect except by means of the registration and inspection that he explicitly ruled out.

While Guy's report was largely endorsed by the Privy Council's medical officer, John Simon, the latter showed himself more willing to countenance the introduction of some legislative controls. In his fourth report (for 1861) he had recommended that all industrial premises that directly or indirectly endangered health ought to be regulated and inspected. Guy had considered this suggestion only to reject it.[26] The two men also differed in their appraisals of the need for arsenical dyes. Guy had accepted that emerald green possessed 'valuable and unique properties...inasmuch as it yields a colour which for brilliancy is not to be surpassed', Simon, on the other hand, termed it a 'not indispensable, branch of industry'. He favoured a ban on the employment of anyone showing signs of poisoning and a requirement for adequate ventilation and cleanliness. In both these areas Guy had preferred to see whether voluntary arrangements could bring about improvements without, or at least before, legal intervention.[27]

A few years later the question of arsenic in artificial flower making was raised by the Children's Employment Commission. One of the assistant commissioners, Henry Lord, who was a barrister and erstwhile fellow of Trinity College, Cambridge, investigated artificial flower and ostrich feather manufacture. In the course of his inquiry he took evidence from several London flower manufacturers including a Mr Lockyer of Messrs. Lockyer & Co., Shaftesbury Street, New North Road and a Mr Bannister of Messrs. Foster & Duncan of Wigmore Street. Lockyer stated that arsenical colours were 'very rarely used now', while Bannister claimed that emerald green 'had almost wholly ceased throughout the trade; Messrs. Foster never use it in their factory'.[28] Robert Taylor, a surgeon at the Central London Eye Hospital, was not so sure, although he agreed that arsenical colours were less used than was once the case and reported that it was some time since he had last seen a case of poisoning.[29] In his report Lord observed that arsenical green was 'very rarely used now'.[30] As for the Commissioners themselves, their report made no mention of arsenic poisoning in the artificial flower trade. Although it recommended that the trade should be brought within the factory acts, the *Factory Acts Extension Act, 1864* did not apply to it.

The paper trade

While Guy was conducting his inquiry another branch of industry in which arsenical compounds were used – paper staining – was being officially investigated by the Children's Employment Commission (CEC). Appointed, as we have seen (66–70), in February 1862, the Royal Commission on Children's Employment comprised three commissioners: H.S. Tremenheere, Richard Dugard Grainger and Edward Carleton Tufnell, plus, as assistant commissioners: Francis Davy Longe, John Edward White and Henry William Lord. They were directed to look at the employment of children and young persons not already regulated by law. This, of course, represented an enormous brief given that no manufacturing industry other than some branches of the textile trade were then under regulation.

Accordingly, it was decided to look first at those industries in which employers or workers had indicated a desire for legislation, plus those which had grown in importance since the inquiries of the previous CEC, 'some of which moreover, came within the category of "Noxious Trades" and were well known to cause serious injury to the health of the persons engaged in them'.[31] The commission selected paper staining as one of the trades in need of prompt investigation. Ostensibly, this was because 'many influential employers' in the trade had expressed a willingness to be placed under legislative restriction for the benefit of their workers. Probably a further factor was the growing public concern about the safety of arsenical wallpaper. The assistant commissioner charged with making the investigation was (again) Henry Lord.[32] He obtained details of 26 firms, 13 of which were in London, most of the others being in Lancashire, Yorkshire and Scotland. The total number of children and young persons employed in these premises was 1150, more than half of whom were under the age of 13; some of those employed being as young as 8. A large majority (954) of the children and young persons in the trade was male. Since Lord's remit was to investigate child labour he did not assemble full details of adult employment. He estimated, however, that some 700-800 adults worked in the 26 firms for which he obtained returns.[33]

Lord, who visited several paper staining factories, taking evidence from workers, proprietors and managers, reached mixed conclusions about the conditions of juvenile employment. Although he did not question 'the general testimony' that the trade was 'a healthy one', he did find the atmosphere of the factories to be 'hot and unwholesome'. Moreover, the work though not especially arduous, involved long hours (from 6.00 am to 10.00 pm or even later), as a result of which fatigue and ill health occurred.[34] The trade consisted of printing coloured patterns or designs on paper. This was done either by hand, using blocks, or mechanically, by means of steam-driven rollers. The colouring matter comprised emerald green 'in greater or less proportions'. Although Lord took a considerable amount of evidence on the hazards (or otherwise) of this material, his report virtually ignored the toxic aspects of paper staining.[35]

It was left to the commissioners themselves to review the evidence received in relation to arsenic poisoning. They believed that emerald green was dangerous only if it had been poorly manufactured and was, in consequence, powdery; if it had been imperfectly mixed with size (adhesive); if the workers were exposed to it for too long; or if cleanliness was not observed. Equally, they believed that the 'sources of danger, being well known in the trade, are watched and to a considerable extent, guarded against'. As a result serious cases of poisoning were rare while the one alleged fatality brought to Lord's attention, even if it was attributable to arsenic – and the commissioners were not convinced that it was – was 'exceptional'.[36]

Their review of the evidence satisfied the commissioners that there was 'no necessity for any special legislative regulations with a view to the protection of children and young persons from the effects of working with the emerald green'. Persuaded that the factory acts should be applied to paper staining, they anticipated that these would suffice to eliminate such dangers of poisoning as did exist. First, the half-time system, which provided for the education of factory children, would 'impose as a rule that which now exists as a very general precautionary practice; namely, an intermittent mode of employment whenever the work has anything to do with the emerald green'.[37] Second, inspection would ensure the observance of precautionary measures such as personal cleanliness, ventilation, use of respirators and proper mixing of good quality emerald green. This supposition, based on the assumption that factory inspection involved 'frequent' visits, shows the extent to which the commissioners were out of touch with social reality. The truth is that premises covered by the factory act might, literally, never see an inspector.[38]

The commission's report and the evidence on which it was based raise a number of questions, not the least of which is that the conclusions reached and recommendations made were grounded in a suspect methodology. The commissioners themselves had made no site visits but based their findings entirely on documentation supplied by their assistant commissioner. Since Lord's report paid virtually no attention to the emerald green question, they had to rely on the transcripts of the oral evidence he took. That they did so is apparent from the conflicting opinions of Lord and the commission on the subject of arsenical pigment. In his only reference to it Lord described it as being rarely used, but dangerous when it was employed. This was more or less the opposite of his superiors' conclusion that emerald green was regularly and safely used.[39] If we leave this conflict on one side, the question that remains is: how reliable was the evidence on which the commission based its report? This brings us to the issue of methodology.

When Lord visited a factory he interviewed workers, managers and proprietors. Even if his interviewees were seen separately it is unlikely that employees would have been critical of (or honest about) health standards knowing that their remarks could get back to their employers. In fact, interviewees were not even anonymous, for the CEC report identified all witnesses by name and place of occupation. Was it probable that the employees of John Godwin, at Godwin's Works, Chelsea would condemn emerald green when the proprietor said: 'This room of mine is papered with emerald green paper; look, I can rub it hard, I can lick it a dozen times with my tongue and nothing comes off'? This, it should be noted, was the same John Godwin who told Lord: 'I don't think the boys here work too much and they have time enough of an evening to get all the education they need'. Yet the hours of work in Godwin's factory were 7.00 am to 7.00 pm; some of his operatives were aged 10. Not surprisingly, the workers Lord interviewed all said how healthy they were. As was said of another branch of industry in which arsenical compounds were employed: 'The workers generally dread the occupation, but dread still more the alternative of being without work'.[40]

A further methodological shortcoming of the CEC investigation was its failure to take evidence from experts such as chemists, toxicologists and medical practitioners. Lord interviewed only one general practitioner (J.H. Wraith of Over Darwen) and, as we shall see, the commissioners ignored his unequivocal condemnation of emerald green.[41] Yet such evidence, coming from sources with no direct financial stake in the paper staining trade, might have been more objective than that taken from those who relied upon it for their living. Although paper staining raised obvious occupational health questions relating to the action of a mineral poison, the only expert to pronounce upon emerald green did so not in the course of the paper staining inquiry, but as part of his evidence on another industry (lucifer match manufacture) under the CEC's consideration (see Chapter 6). This was Dr Henry Letheby of the London Hospital who was a professor of chemistry and toxicology. Letheby, who has been described as an 'exceedingly accurate technological chemist', had frequently been consulted by medical practitioners in connection with cases of illness and death thought to be associated with exposure to arsenical goods, especially wallpaper. He considered Scheele's and Schweinfurth Green to be 'very dangerous pigments'.[42] In common with Simon, but unlike Guy, he regarded them as being commercially unnecessary. If they were used he thought the danger to workers might be reduced by the wearing of respirators but, in his opinion, 'the prime remedy is the total prohibition of the use of poisonous pigment'. In their report the commissioners alluded to the importance of Letheby's opinions but then proceeded to ignore them, preferring to highlight the views of the industrialists and workers engaged in the business of paper staining.[43]

Because the commission's methods of inquiry were seriously flawed, it is doubtful whether reliance should be placed on its findings. There is, however, another reason for viewing its report with scepticism, namely, the discordance between it and the evidence on which it was based. The report consisted of a précis of the evidence, liberally larded with quotations, leading to conclusions and recommendations that the evidence ostensibly supported. Yet comparison of the report with the full transcript of evidence suggests that, deliberately or fortuitously, the commissioners underplayed the arsenic problem, justifying this by means of selective quotation and omission. The point may be illustrated by reference to a few examples. First, the evidence of Edward Clarke, a block printer at a Whitechapel works. In order to demonstrate emerald green's minimal threat to the workforce, the commissioners quoted Clarke's comment that 'here we divide the labour; so if there is anything bad one is not so long over it'. Yet when this comment is read in context it is not even clear that it applied to emerald green. Furthermore, Clarke's opinion that emerald green was 'bad and no mistake' was excluded from the report altogether.[44] Second, while the report quoted the words of John Boden, a machine printer from Manchester: 'I have never known any permanent injury from working the emerald green', it excluded the remainder of his sentence: '...the irritations with some constitutions is so great that the whole skin peels off'.[45] As for the observation of an Over Darwen surgeon, J.H. Wraith, that working with emerald green was 'slow poison', the report overlooked this altogether.[46]

Limited intervention

The *Factory Acts Extension Act, 1864* was, as we have seen, the first outcome of the Children's Employment Commission.[47] It applied the terms of the existing factory acts to six further trades: earthenware, lucifer match, percussion cap and cartridge manufacture, plus paper staining and fustian cutting. All of these had been investigated by the CEC; all were 'selected because of the unhealthiness of the conditions under which they were then carried on'.[48] The bill, brought in by Lord Palmerston's Whig-Liberal Government in March 1864, encountered little opposition in its passage through parliament. Industrial arsenic poisoning was not debated. The act made occupational health a matter of legislative importance for the first time since the enforcement of the factory acts had become a practical possibility. As the factory inspector, Robert Baker, later said, '[t]he prevalence of dusts and gases generated during manufacture was first recognised in a legal sense by the Act of 1864'.[49]

But while it is clear that the 1864 act did turn inspectors' attention to questions of ill-health and ventilation, in the short term no part of that attention was focused on the question of arsenic poisoning, even though inspectors' reports did occasionally discuss conditions of work in paper staining. The few references there are to arsenic poisoning in the inspectors' reports of the 1860s and 1870s displayed complacency towards questions of risk and precaution. Thus, when Baker's sub-inspector George Blenkinsopp reported to his superior on female workers using lead and arsenic to colour paper, he revealed that he had found some people to be adversely affected by handling the poisons 'but, as far as I could ascertain, care is taken by the managers to remove any women or young persons who do not seem able to stand the work'. Similarly, another of Baker's sub-inspectors, W.H. Johnston, whose district covered south Birmingham, suggested that the only practical precaution against arsenical green was to rotate workers in order to minimise periods of exposure. That this was untrue even in the 1860s is demonstrated by reference to the report of the Children's Employment Commission where it was pointed out that observance of precautionary measures such as personal cleanliness, ventilation, use of respirators and proper mixing of good quality emerald green could reduce the risk of poisoning. To be sure, Johnston went on to argue that the use of arsenical compounds should be made illegal on the grounds of the health risks they posed to consumers and workers alike. But he demonstrated his ignorance of the question with his comment that scientists, if made aware of the problem, would find a solution. As we have seen, men of science, particularly those engaged in medical research and practice had been debating the issue without devising solutions for some years.[50]

Occupational health in factories and workshops received attention from the Royal Commission on Factories and Workshops which reported in 1876. Thomas Arlidge gave evidence to the commission on behalf of the Association of Certifying Surgeons, of which he was chairman.[51] He recommended that the responsibilities of these part-time officials, which then comprised accident investigation and the issue of age certificates, should be extended to cover issues of hygiene and sanitation. However, the commissioners rejected any idea of medical inspection. It would, they reported, 'be going beyond what Government can properly undertake, to carry on a continual medical inspection of all places of work. Such inspection might be with almost equal propriety extended to the homes of the poor'. The commissioners took some evidence concerning the problem of industrial arsenic (as well as lead and mercury poisoning). But their main recommendation for improving occupational health was for the cleanliness and ventilation clauses of the 1864 act to be extended to all places of work.[52]

Towards regulation

In 1878, when Robert Baker retired from the factory inspectorate, leaving Alexander Redgrave in sole command, occupational health remained more or less virgin soil as far as legal intervention in the running of businesses was concerned. Arsenic poisoning at work, after the brief flurry of attention in the 1860s, attracted little notice. But because of developments beyond the factory gate, it would appear that industrialists were forced to modify their production processes. These developments comprised the wave of adverse publicity about the dangers of arsenically-coloured consumer goods. Fearful of lost business and reduced profits as potential customers deserted them, manufacturers who had used arsenic began to abandon it in favour of safe, vegetable dyes. Hence, consumer demand, or the marketplace, appears to have played a part in achieving the healthier workplace that regulation had, hitherto, largely failed to produce.

Two witnesses made this point in their evidence to to the 1876 royal commission. Thus, William Clegg, of the paper stainers Carlisle and Clegg, while accepting that emerald green was dangerous, pointed out that there was a disappearing market for arsenical wallpaper: 'People will not have it so much. They very often compel us to use non arsenical green'. As a result, production was 'very materially diminishing'. William Hamilton, of Messrs Wylie and Lochhead, manufacturers of upholstery, furnishings and wallpaper, concurred. Green in wallpaper he told the commissioners, was 'used very sparingly now'. This chronology does not quite coincide with that of the domestic arsenic scare, the furore over which persisted into the 1880s. But this difference may be easily explained, for there would inevitably be a time lag between the phasing out of arsenical production and the replacement of arsenically-coloured products in people's homes. [53] Certainly, by the end of the 1870s Redgrave was persuaded that the British wallpaper industry had largely dispensed with arsenic. As a result, 'many colour makers' had ceased to manufacture arsenical green.[54]

It was not altogether clear, however, whether the same trend applied in other industries, for in the same report (1878-9) Redgrave wrote of a 'large and increasing demand... for illuminated almanacs and for every species of illuminated wrapper and box, whether paper or tin'. These, it appears, often contained arsenic. Though Redgrave's report also indicated continuing use of arsenic by artificial florists, one of his inspectors, Edward Gould was soon to report that 'artificial flower-making, in which poisonous ingredients used largely to enter, is now, probably owing to the introduction of new fashions requiring more sober tints, a comparatively harmless employment'.[55]

It is important to avoid reading too much into isolated observations in the chief factory inspector's reports. Occupational disease was not a high priority for the inspectorate until the 1890s. Neither, between Baker's retirement and the appointment of B.A. Whitelegge as the chief inspector of factories in 1896, did the inspectorate possess any medically-trained staff. Comments on arsenic and industrial arsenic poisoning were also irregular and inconsistent. On balance, the likelihood is that while industry's dependence on arsenical colours was diminishing, as many observers agreed, the decline was uneven both between industries and between manufacturers in the same industry.[56] Equally, it is apparent that demand for arsenically-coloured goods remained and that this demand was met by British producers as well as by imports.

In 1888, Inspector Charles Bowling, whose district covered East London and surrounding area, was still able to report on the 'evils arising from working among fine arsenical powder used largely in the production of emerald green and consequently in many colour and paper staining factories'. At a factory in Bromley in Kent (Hemingway's), he 'found a number of men employed in filling casks with this powder. The day being damp and heavy the air was filled with it. I could hardly breathe and for some hours after my visit suffered from soreness in the throat'. Change arsenical green for white lead and this is resonant of an incident described by Robert Tressell, in *The Ragged Trousered Philanthropists* (see above 81–2).[57] Bowling discussed the problem with Hemingway's manager who subsequently devised a means of loading casks without generating clouds of dust. Nevertheless, Bowling recommended to his chief, Redgrave, that health and hygiene rules already in force in whitelead works should be applied to premises in which arsenic was worked.[58] In May 1892, following the passage of the *Factory and Workshop Act, 1891*, which empowered the home secretary to certify particular trades 'dangerous or injurious to health' and then to make 'special rules' to render them safe (or safer), arsenic extraction (from ore) and the manufacture of paints and colours (along with white lead manufacture and the enamelling of iron plates) were certified as dangerous trades.[59] The resulting special rules for 'processes in the manufacture of paints, colours and in the extraction of arsenic' required the provision and use of washing facilities, protective clothing and respirators, a ban on smoking and the taking of meals in work rooms and the free supply to workers of 'sanitary' drinks and aperient medicines. The impact of these rules is hard to gauge. Certainly, Bowling was still coming across cases of arsenic poisoning in East End factories in the 1890s.[60] By the same token Arlidge reported in 1892 that while the use of arsenical colours in industry had 'greatly abated' since their dangers had been publicised, they were by no means, as newspaper reports of poisonings attested, 'wholly disused'.[61] However, in a period when the popular press acquired a taste for reporting the more lurid aspects of occupational disease, it is questionable whether newspaper articles provide an objective guide to health standards in British factories. In relation to arsenic the point is well illustrated by examining the case of the East End paint manufacturer, Berger.

In March 1893, fresh from its triumphant exposure of Bryant and May's cynical treatment of workers exposed to phosphorus (see below 196–207), the London evening newspaper, the *Star*, turned its attention to the plight of workers who made emerald green. Its account could scarcely have been more lurid:

> Purchasers of emerald green little know the terrible cost at which that composition is manufactured.... We read of men working in a cloud of fine green arsenic dust, which eats into everything it touches, penetrating even the walls of the factory and leaving patches of green outside. the results to the men are terrible – flesh burned to the bone, running sores provoked in the eyes, nose, ears and mouth, legs and arms rotting. Need we wonder that despairing workers should declare that they would have cut their throats sooner than embark on such a life if they had known what was in store for them? Human nature must be strangely changed if these ghastly particulars do not cause a thrill of horror and indignation to run through the land. Money is made out of the rotting of men's bodies at a pound a week. It is infamous.

And this litany of symptoms did not include the 'painful and long-sustained constipation and paralysis' that could also ensue. Indeed, so 'hideous' was the lot of the emerald green worker that even the sufferings of phosphorus-poisoned matchmakers paled into 'absolute insignificance'. Neither were employers doing anything to provide for employees who had fallen ill, the only recourse of the poisoned worker being the Poor Law. Yet employers in the industry were paying no more than £1 per sixty-hour week. The *Star*, stressing that there were numerous victims of 'emerald disease' in London's East End and no shortage of job applicants desperate for work regardless of the risks, called for Home Office action both to schedule paint mixing as a dangerous trade and to see that the sick were properly compensated. As it was, the newspaper alleged, the factory inspectorate was being duped, for although inspectors did sometimes visit these works, the dustiest processes were stopped while they were present.[62]

The *Star*, founded in 1888 with a cover price of just $^1/_2$ p, was an exemplar of what has been imprecisely called the 'new journalism'. It had achieved great success in its reporting of the Ripper murders in the year of its foundation and, by, 1892 was proclaiming itself the largest selling evening newspaper in the country.[63] Its reports on emerald green prompted James Hogan, the 'Anti-Parnellite, Home Rule' MP for Mid-Tipperary to table a parliamentary question for Asquith. They also prompted the attorney-general, Sir Charles Russell, MP for Hackney South, whose constituency included a number of paint and colour factories, to raise the matter personally with the home secretary. Hogan wished to know whether the recently-established special rules could be modified so as to render the trade safe or, alternatively, whether the manufacture of colours from poisons should be banned. Perhaps because the memory of the Bryant and May affair was so fresh, none of these politicians seems to have considered that the *Star*'s allegations might have been overstated or without foundation. When Asquith replied to Hogan, on 24 March 1893, he was able to state that two of the factory inspectors responsible for East London, Edward Gould and Henry Cameron, were well advanced upon an 'exhaustive inquiry' and that their report was expected within a week.[64]

In fact, the inspectorate had been monitoring health standards at Berger's Homerton plant since at least February. On 28 February, following 'certain allegations' particularly related to Lewis Berger, Cameron had carried out a surprise inspection of the firm. This had revealed allegations of unhealthy working conditions to be largely groundless. For example, in the packing room, in which emerald green was put in cans prior to its dispatch, Cameron found no evidence of dust or, indeed, any sign of a serious occupational hazard in the factory as a whole. Nevertheless, he recommended the installation of a Blackman fan. When he returned with Gould on 6 March, he found that a powerful fan had already been installed and that representatives of the engineering firm, Blackman Co., had visited Berger with a view to recommending a complete scheme of ventilation. On this occasion the two inspectors interviewed a Mr Ridler, the chief source of complaints about health standards at Berger, and Lewis Berger himself. They also toured the works and spoke to medical practitioners who, Ridler had alleged, had treated seriously ill emerald green workers. Yet in none of this did they turn up evidence of any serious health hazard posed by emerald green. Berger was found to be complying with the special rules, for example, in providing its workers with protective clothing and washing facilities. Although some workers were found to be suffering a degree of skin irritation as a result of external contact with arsenical dust, Cameron wrote that '...employment in emerald green though resulting commonly and indeed well nigh as an accompaniment, in serious discomfort and possibly, on occasions, in temporary illness...is never fatal in its results. The suffering is limited and of a passing character'. Since emerald green was being made in much smaller quantities than formerly – mainly as a pesticide for treating colorado beetle infestation – there seemed little reason to believe that workers' health would deteriorate.[65] These findings were confirmed when Cameron and Gould returned to Homerton later in the month. Visits to local hospitals and to the homes of alleged victims revealed either that the alleged sufferers did not exist or that they had been diagnosed as suffering with non-occupational maladies such as laryngitis or enteritis. Of the six local medical practitioners consulted, not one had encountered a serious case of poisoning from emerald green.[66]

Although the two inspectors considered that the 1892 special rules would remove such health hazards as were experienced in emerald green manufacture, they (somewhat illogically) recommended an extension of the rules to the effect that workers should be provided with weekly warm baths and that the use of respirators and protective overalls should be mandatory. When Herbert Gladstone read the reports of Cameron and Gould, which he termed 'very satisfactory', he noted that the dangers of emerald green had been 'much exaggerated'. The Home Office turned down

Sprague Oram's suggestion that the emerald green issue should be investigated by the Chemical Works Committee, but endorsed the compilation of additional special rules. For his part Asquith suggested that emerald green manufacture should be kept 'under close and constant supervision' with 'special reports made from time to time as to the working of the rules'.[67]

In 1895, on the recommendation of the Association of Factory Surgeons Asquith introduced a bill, one section of which required the reporting of all cases of four specific diseases, including arsenic poisoning. This clause, virtually ignored in the parliamentary debates, promised the identification of those premises, hitherto located only on an *ad hoc* basis, in which serious occupational illness occurred, thereby enabling the extent of a health hazard to be gauged before the introduction of regulations. Asquith's original intention was more restrictive. He had proposed to ban the use of arsenic (and lead) in the tinning or enamelling of metal holloware cooking utensils (saucepans). This plan was criticised in the bill's second reading debate, one MP maintaining that the time was approaching when 'the Government would have seriously to face the question of whether they were to allow the markets of this country to be flooded with articles of foreign manufacture, made under conditions prohibited in respect of British goods'. The clause was weeded out by the standing committee on trade.[68]

With the passage of the 1895 act, the first phase of the regulatory process was over. Ironically, by this time, the worst was probably past in respect of arsenic poisoning (and the other three occupational diseases – lead and phosphorus poisoning and anthrax – made notifiable). Certainly, the literary evidence suggests as much. For example, the Dangerous Trades Committee, the interim report of which appeared in 1896, the year in which the 1895 act was implemented, maintained that as a result of changes in the nature of the manufacturing process, arsenical poisoning in the wallpaper industry had become 'of rare occurrence'.[69] The implementation of the 1895 act and the consequent generation of poisoning statistics (under the terms of section 29), provided an opportunity to test such observations, including against hard data.

From 1896-1914

The *Factory and Workshop Act, 1895* came into operation on 1 Jan 1896. The inspectorate soon began to receive information about the four reportable industrial diseases (five from 1899 when mercury poisoning became notifiable). Fifty-one years after the beginning of factory accident notification, the data that began to flow in (trickled might be a better word for some disease categories) provided the basis for the first quantitative picture of occupational disease in Britain. Table 5.1 indicates the number of cases of industrial arsenic poisoning of which the factory inspectorate was given notice in the period 1896-1914. These figures, which apply only to those occupations covered by the factory acts, would certainly differ from the hypothetical but unobtainable data of arsenical poisoning among all British workers (including agricultural labourers). While the 1896-1914 statistics could and did, include arsenical poisonings among those employed in manufacturing sheep dip, they excluded those that arose in the course of its application.

TABLE 5.1:
Occupational Arsenic Poisoning. Cases Reported to Factory Inspectorate, 1896-1914 (fatalities in parenthesis)

Year	Paints, Colour and Extraction	Other	Industries Total
1896	**1**	**0**	**1**
1897	**0**	**0**	**0**
1898	**0**	**0**	**0**
1899	**0**	**0**	**0**
1900	**7**	**15 (3)**	**22 (3)**
1901	**3**	**9 (1)**	**12 (1)**
1902	**5**	**0**	**5**
1903	**3**	**2**	**5**
1904	**3**	**2**	**5**
1905	**0**	**1**	**1**
1906	**2**	**3**	**5**
1907	**4**	**5 (2)**	**9 (2)**
1908	**16 (1)**	**7**	**23 (1)**
1909	**4**	**0**	**4**
1910	**5**	**2**	**7**
1911	**7**	**3 (1)**	**10 (1)**
1912	**0**	**5**	**5**
1913	**1**	**5**	**6**
1914	**0**	**2 (1)**	**2 (1)**
Total	**61 (1)**	**61 (8)**	**122 (9)**

Source: *Reports of the Chief Inspector of Factories and Workshops*

The official statistics show that between 1896 and 1914 (inclusive), industrial arsenic poisonings occurred at an average rate of only 6.4 per year. The average incidence of fatal poisonings was below 0.5 cases per year. Although not included in the table, the official statistics were sub-divided by age (ie whether the victim was an adult or a 'young person') and gender. Over 85 per cent of those reported as suffering from arsenic poisoning contracted at work were adult men; adult women constituted the next highest category (about 11 per cent). Whether this age/gender breakdown merely reflected the demographic profile of the workforce is unclear for there are no employment statistics for those trades in which arsenic figured. As a result, there are no means of establishing 'attack rates', that is, the proportion of arsenical workers who were poisoned. The statistics are and were, therefore, of very limited value. Indeed, the medical inspector of factories, who was chiefly responsible for analysing the data and investigating cases, seems to have been at a loss what to make of them. Usually his annual report included a perfunctory reference to individual cases with no attempt to consider trends or reflect upon the value of the data.

Even so, such statistical evidence as we have suggests that industrial arsenic poisoning had become a minor problem in the late-Victorian and Edwardian period. On four occasions only did the annual number of reported cases even reach double figures; on three occasions there were no reported cases at all. Less than 0.8 per cent of all reported industrial poisonings were arsenic cases. Of course, it is possible that the reported statistics failed to reflect objective reality. Perhaps as a result of ignorance, deliberate concealment, or misdiagnosis, the reported statistics may provide a less than complete record of reportable cases. There is some evidence in inspectors' reports to indicate that this was the case, not only for arsenic, but for all the notifiable diseases. Hence, in 1897 the chief inspector of factories admitted that '...the whole system [of reporting] is still imperfect and beyond doubt many cases are never reported to the Factory Department at all'.[70] At first there was doubt as to whether all reported diseases should be recorded or only those that came via the certifying surgeons. The 1896 tables were based exclusively on the surgeons' reports, but from 1897 all reported cases were included in the tables. As far as arsenic poisoning is concerned it is probably fair to say that this adjustment made no difference for only one case was reported in the period 1896-9 (inclusive) and this for 1896.

Subsequently, the inspectorate paid little attention to the possibility of under-reporting. Usually, it appears, it was content to regard the statistical information received as indicative of objective reality. This suggests either that inspectors were extraordinarily naive in their approach to this sort of data, or that the low incidence of poisoning notified confirmed the evidence of their own inspections that the health of operatives in factories in which arsenic was employed was generally satisfactory. An isolated hint of under-reporting is to be found in the chief lady inspector's report for 1907. On this occasion Rose Squire reported on the ill health of women workers employed as packers of toxic material destined for export as pesticide. What she saw as arsenic poisoning, the Poor Law medical officer and certifying surgeon diagnosed as 'general debility resulting from poor living'. There is, of course, no means of determining which of these views was the more accurate.[71]

While the inspectorate clearly regarded the number of arsenic cases as low, it generally attributed this not to under-reporting but to a declining use of arsenic and the introduction of safer working conditions in those industries in which it continued to be employed. As we have seen, a consumer-led reduction in the use of arsenical had begun as early as the 1880s, or even the late-1870s.[72] In 1896 the Dangerous Trades Committee noted that the wallpaper industry had 'undergone very considerable change in the last 25 years', notably in its rejection of arsenical colours. Although this chronology may have been slightly inaccurate, the observation was generally valid:

> ...the march of science and the increased interest in the public health have introduced many effective reforms in this trade, the most noticeable being the almost universal substitution of vegetable for mineral colouring materials. This was proved to the satisfaction of the Committee by the official analyses of diverse colouring materials taken away by them at the time of their visits.[73]

This verdict received endorsement in 1900 when the factory inspector, Commander H.P. Smith, who had served on the Dangerous Trades Committee, examined the wallpaper industry. He found that the Wallpaper Manufacturers Ltd., a combine dating from 1899 which rapidly acquired the lion's share of the British wallpaper market, had instructed all its branches 'to avoid the use of arsenical colours and materials of all kinds and we believe in all cases the manufacturers of colours used in the manufacture of paper-hangings undertake that such colours and materials shall be arsenic free'. Smith's view was that 'now arsenical colours appear to be used by very few firms and by those few they are used at rare intervals, the persons applying them never being continuously engaged at this work'. In conclusion, he judged that paper colouring 'can hardly properly be described as a "dangerous" industry'.[74] The medical inspector of factories concurred, adding that arsenical colours had been rejected not only in the wallpaper trade, but in artificial flower manufacture too. Indeed, Scheele's Green, once so common throughout British industry, was, by the beginning of the twentieth century, mainly used to control Colorado beetle and fruit tree pests.[75]

Even so, the Home Office pressed ahead in the establishment of a system of voluntary self-regulation. This system had its origins in the third interim report of the Dangerous Trades Committee. In this document, published in 1899, the committee had made certain recommendations for improving safety standards in the use of Bessemer converters in steel works. When White Ridley, at the Home Office, received the report he sent it to the manufacturers asking them how they intended to respond. The result was that the manufacturers adopted the recommendations voluntarily. This outcome was so satisfactory that the Home Office followed the practice in respect of several other dangerous trades, including wallpaper. The department's scope for doing this was significantly increased by the terms of the *Factory and Workshop Act, 1901*. Hitherto, manufacturers had effectively been able to negotiate the rules under which they were required to operate. The 1901 act ended their right to force arbitration; they could still object to Home Office proposals, suggest modifications to them and and even insist upon a public inquiry but, unlike in the past, the power to modify health requirements rested entirely with the secretary of state. This important difference allowed the home secretary, in effect, to say to manufacturers: if you do not act as I suggest you will have to act as I demand. In September 1901 voluntary regulations came into operations with the agreement of the occupiers of all wallpaper factories. These gave effect to the recommendations of the Departmental Committee on Dangerous Trades, as amended by further inquiry and consultation with the industry. [76]

Two main conclusions may be drawn from the above account. First, it appears likely that the introduction of reporting regulations in respect of occupational arsenic poisoning came when the full extent of the problem was on the wane. Certainly, the industry itself seems to have been in decline. Thus, when the *Star* published its revelations about the occupational health hazards of emerald green, in Spring 1893, a defender of the industry suggested that 'the quantity of emerald green made now is not one-third what it was 12 years ago'.[77] However, this point about a diminishing health hazard should not be pressed too far for we have no means of accurately gauging the full extent of the Victorian arsenic problem either in occupational or public health. Nevertheless, the qualitative evidence appears to indicate that this was the case. Second, the problem was 'solved', or at least, greatly mitigated, less by parliamentary inquiry, legislation and a system of inspection – which was so often the pattern of Victorian social regulation – more through the operation of the market place. Consumer demand for safer goods led to changed methods of production with, almost incidentally, benefits for workforces.

Notes

1. See John S. Haller Jnr., 'Therapeutic Mule: the Use of Arsenic in Nineteenth Century *Materia Medica*', *Pharmacy in History*, 17 (1975), 87–100; Peter Bartrip, 'A "Pennurth of Arsenic for Rat Poison": the Arsenic Act, 1851 and the Prevention of Secret Poisoning' *Medical History*, 36 (1992), 53-69; Judith Knelman, 'The Amendment of the Sale of Arsenic Bill', *Victorian Review*, xvii (1991), 1–10.
2. See P.W.J. Bartrip, 'How Green was My Valance: Environmental Arsenic Poisoning and the Myth of Victorian Domesticity', *English Historical Review*, cix (1994), 891–913.
3. On arsenic poisoning at a processing plant see Public Record Office (PRO) LAB 14/41. Arsenical Poisoning. Prevalence at Arsenic Works, Calstock, Cornwall, 1899 and PRO LAB 14/42. Arsenical Poisoning. Arsenic Works, Calstock, Cornwall: Local Government Board Report on Persons Disabled while at Works, 1899.
4. C.T. Thackrah, *The Effect of Arts, Trades and Professions and of Civic States and Habits of Living, on Health and Longevity: with Suggestions for the Removal of Many of the Agents which Produce Disease and Shorten the Duration of Life* (London: Longman, Rees, Orme, Brown, Green and Longman, 2nd edn, 1832), 106–8.
5. *Lancet*, 2 Oct. 1843, 98–101; *Dorset County Chronicle and Somerset Gazette*, 16 Jan. 1845. I am grateful to Judith Knelman for drawing my attention to the candle factory case. See *Lancet*, 4 Nov. 1837, 211–12; 11 Nov. 1837, 242–4; 18 Nov. 1837, 267; 16 Dec. 1837, 424–28.
6. *Select Committee of the House of Lords on the Sale of Poisons etc. Bill (H.L.)*, PP 1857(2) XII, Minutes of Evidence, 658; *Medical Times and Gazette*, 14 Feb. 1857, 177; *Journal of the Society of Arts* V (23 Oct. 1857), 652–53; (6 Nov. 1857), 678; *The Times*, 9 Jan. 1858.

7. W.A. Guy, 'Effects of Arsenite of Copper on Paper Stainers' *Archives of Medicine*, I (1857), 86–8.
8. C. Willett Cunnington, *English Women's Clothing in the Nineteenth Century* (London: Faber & Faber, 1937), 19, 34; Anne Buck, *Victorian Costume and Costume Accessories* (Carlton, Bedford: Ruth Bean 1984 edn), 37; Penelope, Byrde, *Nineteenth Century Fashion* (London: Batsford, 1992), 62; Asa Briggs, *Victorian Things* (London: Batsford, 1988); Henry Carr, *Our Domestic Poisons; or, the Poisonous Effects of Certain Dyes and Colours Used in Domestic Fabrics* (London: William Clowes, 1879); Edward Hyam (trans), *Taine's Notes on England* (London: Thames and Hudson, 1957 edn); Simon Garfield, *Mauve. How one Man Invented a Colour that Changed the World* (London: Faber and Faber, 2000), 77–8. Barbara Leigh Bodichon (née Smith) (1827-91) is perhaps best known for her association with Girton College, of which she was a generous benefactor).
9. On Hassall and food adulteration see John Burnett, *Plenty and Want. A Social History of Diet in England from 1815 to the Present Day* (London: Scolar Press, 1979 edn), chapter 10; Ingeborg Paulus, *The Search for Pure Food: a Sociology of Legislation in Great Britain* (London: Martin Robertson, 1974), 16, 22–3; E.G. Clayton, *A Memoir of the late Dr. A.H. Hassall* (London: n.p.,1908).
10. *Lancet*, 15 Jan. 1859, 70; 23 July 1859, 951 Dec. 1860, 535.
11. *Englishwoman's Journal*, VII (July 1861), 308–14; see *ibid.*, letter from S.E.M. (Aug. 1861), 428.
12. Emerald green, which was also known by a variety of other names (see note 42 below), was made by combining arsenious acid (white arsenic), soda, sulphate of copper, acetic acid and, water. The process is described in detail in PRO HO 45/9849/B12393B. Memorandum on the manufacture of emerald green.
13. *The Times*, 26 Nov. 1861; *Lancet*, 30 Nov. 1861, 530;
14. *Fifth Report of the Medical Officer of the Privy Council, Appendix III*, PP 1863 XXV, 126–7.
15. *Reports of the Factory Inspectors, Half Yearly Report of Alexander Redgrave*, PP 1877 XXIII, 206.
16. *Englishwoman's Journal*, III (April 1859), 73–85; (Aug. 1859), 380–87; VI (Dec. 1860), 236–41; VII (May 1861), 191–97; *Lancet*, 4 May 1861, 450; Mary Anne Baines, 'The Ladies' National Association for the Diffusion of Sanitary Knowledge', in G.W. Hastings (ed), *Transactions of the National Association for the Promotion of Social Science* (London: John Parker, 1859), 531–2. On Cowper see *Dictionary of National Biography. Supplement* (London:

Smith, Elder, 1909), XXII, 499–500. Ladies' charities and the men associated with them were satirised by Wilkie Collins in *The Moonstone* (1868) where reference is made to the imaginary 'Mothers' Small-Clothes-Conversion Society' and the 'British Ladies'-Servants'-Sunday-Sweetheart-Supervision Society'. On women and philanthropy see F.K. Prochaska, *Women and Philanthropy in Nineteenth Century England* (Oxford: Clarendon Press, 1980).

17. On Hofmann see Anthony S. Travis, 'Science's Powerful Companion: A.W. Hofmann's Investigation of Aniline Red and its Derivatives', *British Journal of the History of Science*, xxv (1992), 27–44. See also Garfield, *op. cit.* (note 8).
18. *The Times*, 1 Feb. 1862.
19. W.A. Guy, 'Contributions to a Knowledge of the Influence of Employments upon Health' *Journal of the Royal Statistical Society*, (1843), 197–211 and 283–301, (1844), 232–43; *Royal Commission on the State of Large Towns and Populous Districts*, PP 1844 XVII, Evidence of W.A. Guy, 365–71. On Guy see *Lancet*, 19 Sept. 1885, 554; *BMJ*, 19 Sept. 1885, 573; *Dictionary of National Biography* (London: Smith, Elder, 1908), VIII, 835–6; G.H. Brown (comp.), *Munk's Roll. Lives of Fellows of the Royal College of Physicians of London* (London: RCP, 1955), IV, 36; C. Fraser Brockington, *Public Health in the Nineteenth Century* (Edinburgh and London: E. & S. Livingstone, 1965), 238–40 Sir John Simon paid a generous tribute to Guy in his *English Sanitary Institutions* (London: John Murray, 1897), 139.
20. *Fifth Report of the Medical Officer of the Privy Council, Appendix III*, PP 1863 XXV, 126–38.
21. *Ibid.*, 138.
22. *Ibid.*, 153, 158.
23. *Ibid.*, 159.
24. *Ibid.*, 159–62.
25. *Ibid.*, 159.
26. *Ibid.*, Report, 10–13; *Fourth Report of the Medical Officer of Health of the Privy Council*, PP 1862 XXVII, 494–5. See R. J. Lambert, *Sir John Simon and English Social Administration* (London: MacGibbon & Key, 1963), 334.
27. *Fifth Report of the Medical Officer of Health of the Privy Council*, PP 1863 XXV, Report, 13; Appendix, 156.
28. *Fourth Report of the Children's Employment Commission. Appendix, Reports and Evidence of the Assistant Commissioners*. PP 1865 XX, 262–68.

29. *Ibid.*, 269.
30. *Ibid.*, 261.
31. *First Report of the Children's Employment Commission*, PP 1863 XVIII, 7.
32. *Ibid.*
33. *Ibid.*, 58–9.
34. *Ibid.*, 59–60, 72.
35. *Ibid.*, 215–39.
36. *Ibid.*, 72–4.
37. The half-time system provided for the education of factory children during their normal hours of work by a person provided and paid for by the employer. It dated from the Health and Morals of Apprentices Act, 1802 and was re-enacted in the subsequent legislation. Ostensibly it took children out of the workplace and into the classroom for part of the working day. The original clauses were described by a mid-century inspector (Robert Baker) as 'a total failure'. He also argued that the half-time provisions of the *Factory Act, 1833* were 'faulty in detail'. In 1866, however, he estimated that more than 70 000 children were being educated in 'first-class schools' under the factory acts. *Reports of Factory Inspectors, Half-Year Ending 31 Oct. 1866*, PP 1867 XVI, 413–50.
38. *First Report of the Children's Employment Commission*, PP 1863 XVIII, 74. On factory inspectors' enforcement problems including their numerical limitations in relation to the number of premises under inspection see P.W.J. Bartrip, 'British Government Inspection, 1832-1875: some Observations' *Historical Journal*, 25 (1982), 605–26 and P.W.J.Bartrip, 'State Intervention in Mid-Nineteenth Century Britain: Fact or Fiction' *Journal of British Studies*, xxiii (1983), 63–83.
39. *First Report of the Children's Employment Commission*, PP 1863 XVIII, 72–4, 215.
40. *Ibid.*, 238; *The Times*, 1 Feb. 1862.
41. *First Report of the Children's Employment Commission*, PP 1863 XVIII, 221.
42. Scheele's Green (which was the same as arsenite of copper or emerald green) was named after the Swedish chemist, Karl Scheele, who invented it in 1775. Schweinfurth Green, named after the Bavarian town in which it was produced in large quantities, was another arsenical compound. In fact, there were a number of different names for the same arsenical pigment (eg Paris green, French green, emerald green etc). As Hunter points out, manufacturers kept coming up with new and attractive names in order to suggest that

they had a new, innocous dye rather than the same old poisonous one. Donald Hunter, *The Diseases of Occupations* (London: English Universities Press, 1955), 292.

43. *First Report of the Children's Employment Commission*, PP 1863 XVIII, 72, 141–3. On Letheby see *Dictionary of National Biography* (London: Smith, Elder, 1908), XI, 1010; *Practitioner*, 208 (1972), 401 05.
44. *First Report of the Children's Employment Commission*, PP 1863 XVIII, 73, 230.
45. *Ibid.*, 73, 222.
46. *Ibid.*, 221.
47. 27 & 28 Vict. c.48. For the act's occupational health and hygiene provisions see above 70–1.
48. *Report of the Commissioners Appointed to Inquire into the Working of the Factory and Workshops Acts with a View to their Consolidation and Amendment*, PP 1876 XXIX, lxxiii.
49. *Reports of the Factory Inspectors, Half-Year Ending 31 Oct. 1871*, PP 1872 XVI, 130; see *Report of the Commissioners Appointed to Inquire into the Working of the Factory and Workshops Acts with a View to their Consolidation and Amendment*, PP 1876 XXIX, lxxiii.
50. *Reports of the Factory Inspectors, Half-Year Ending 31 Oct. 1869*, PP 1870 XV, 288, 295; *Half-Year Ending 30 April 1877*, PP 1877 XXIII, 209–10; *First Report of the Children's Employment Commission*, PP 1863 XVIII, 74.
51. On the ACS see Stephen Huzzard, 'The Role of the Certifying Surgeon in the State Regulation of Child Labour and Industrial Health, 1833-1973', University of Manchester, MA thesis, (1976).
52. *Report of the Commissioners Appointed to Inquire into the Working of the Factory and Workshops Acts with a View to their Consolidation and Amendment*, PP 1876 XXIX, lxxi–iii.
53. *Minutes of Evidence taken before the Commissioners Appointed to Inquire into the Factory and Workshop Acts*, PP 1876 XXX, 171–3, 705.
54. *Report of the Chief Factory Inspector, PP 1880 XIV*, 139.
55. *Ibid.*, 139–49; *Report of Chief Factory Inspector*, PP 1881 XXIII, 121.
56. See Bartrip, *op. cit.* (note 2) 891–913.
57. Robert Tressell, *The Ragged Trousered Philanthropists* (London: Lawrence & Wishart, 1955 edn), 453; Peter Bartrip, 'Expertise and the Dangerous Trades, 1875-1900' in Roy MacLeod (ed), *Government and Expertise. Specialists, Administrators and Professionals, 1860-1919* (Cambridge: Cambridge University Press, 1988), 89–109.

58. *Annual Report of HM Chief Inspector of Factories, (1888)* PP 1889 XVIII, 465. On whitelead see P.W.J. Bartrip, *op. cit.* (note 57) ; Barbara Harrison, '"Some of them Gets Lead Poisoned": Occupational Lead Exposure in Women, 1880-1914', *Social History of Medicine*, 2 (1989), 171–95; D.J. Rowe, *Lead Manufacturing in Great Britain. A History* (Beckenham: Croom Helm, 1983).
59. *Statutory Rules & Orders, 1892* (London: HMSO, 1892), 472–73.
60. *Annual Report of HM Chief Inspector of Factories and Workshops (1891-2)*, PP 1893-4 XVII, 87–90.
61. J.T. Arlidge, *The Hygiene, Diseases and Mortality of Occupations* (London: Percival, 1892), 434–5.
62. *Star*, 13, 14, 15, 16, 20 March, 3 June 1893.
63. Alan J. Lee, *The Origins of the Popular Press in England, 1855-1914* (London: Croom Helm, 1976), 128. The characteristics of new journalism included sensationalism, cross-class appeal, coverage of all aspects of life, focus on 'human interest' stories, use of interview and presentational devices ranging from typographical inventiveness to the innovative use of headlines and sub-heads with a view to promoting what we would now call 'reader friendliness'. See Lucy Brown, *Victorian News and Newspapers* (New York, OUP, 1985); Joel H. Weiner (ed), *Papers for the Millions, the New Journalism in Britain, 1850s to 1914* (London and New York: London, 1988); Carolyn Malone, 'Sensational Stories, Endangered Bodies: Women's Work and the New Journalism in England in the 1890s', *Albion*, 31 (1999), 49–71.
64. 4 *Hansard*, 10 (24 March 1893), 1034; *The Times*, 25 March 1893; *Star*, 25 March 1893.
65. PRO HO 45/9849/B12393B. Report of Henry Cameron, 6 March 1893. See J.F. McDiarmid Clark, 'Eleanor Ormerod (1828-1901) as an Economic Entomologist: "Pioneer of Purity even more than of Paris Green"', *British Journal for the History of Science*, xxv (1992), 431-52; John F. Clark, 'Beetle Mania: the Colorado Beetle Scare of 1877', *History Today*, xii (1992), 5–7.
66. PRO HO 45/9849/B12393B. Report of Henry Cameron and Edward Gould, 5 April 1893.
67. PRO HO 45/9849/B12393B. Notes of 8 and 16 April 1893.
68. 4 *Hansard*, 31 (1 March 1895) 178, 180; 32 (22 April 1895) 1461; *58 & 59 Vict. c.37*; *Factory & Workshops Bill, PP 1895 III*, 109–62, esp.122, 150.
69. *Departmental Committee Appointed to Inquire into and Report upon Certain Miscellaneous Dangerous Trades, Interim Report*, PP 1896 XXXIII, 9.

70. *Annual Report of HM Chief Inspector of Factories and Workshops (1896)*, PP 1897 XVII, 247.
71. *Annual Report of HM Chief Inspector of Factories and Workshops (1907)*, PP 1908 XII, 590.
72. Hyam, *op. cit.* (note 8), 19–20, 46, 263–4; John Gloag, *Victorian Comfort. A Social History of Design from 1830 to 1900* (Newton Abbot: David & Charles, 1973 edn), 48 and 122–23; Doreen Yarwood, *The English Home* (London: Batsford, 1979), 40 and 206; Briggs, *op. cit.* (note 8), 22–3; Byrde, *op. cit.* (note 8); Bartrip, *op. cit.* (note 2), 898.
73. *Interim Report of the Departmental Committee Appointed to Inquire into and Report upon Certain Miscellaneous Dangerous Trades*, PP 1896 XXXIII, 9; see also, appendix III, 31.
74. *Annual Report of HM Chief Inspector of Factories and Workshops (1900)*, PP 1901 X, 89–91, 101.
75. *Ibid.*, 469; *Annual Report of HM Chief Inspector of Factories and Workshops (1902)*, PP 1903 XII, 304; Clark, *op. cit.* (note 65), 431–52; *idem.*, *op. cit.* (note 65), 5–7.
76. *Third Interim Report of the Departmental Committee on Dangerous Trades*, PP 1899 XII, 161–4; *1 Edw. 7 c.21* ss.79–86; *Annual Report of HM Chief Inspector of Factories and Workshops (1900)*, PP 1901 X, 11, 89–102; *Annual Report of HM Chief Inspector of Factories and Workshops (1901)*, PP 1902 XII, 53.
77. *Star*, 16 March 1893.

6

'The Poorest of the Poor and the Lowest of the Low': Lucifer Matches and 'Phossy Jaw'

> Girls born and bred in the slums of our large cities, reared upon improper and insufficient food, anaemic, undergrown and ill-clad, do not form a desirable class from which workers for such a dangerous industry should be drawn and yet, unfortunately, it is too often such that one sees in large numbers in the boxing and other departments of match factories.[1]

Chemistry, Congreves and Commissions

Phosphorus is a non-metallic element (chemical symbol P, atomic number 15), which, though highly combustible and toxic, is nevertheless essential for plant and animal growth. It was discovered, in 1669, by a German alchemist experimenting with urine, in which it is present in minute quantities. A century later it was found to be an important ingredient of bones. Karl Scheele, the Swedish chemist and inventor of the green arsenical pigment that bore his name, found a way of manufacturing it in large quantities by using bone ash and nitric acid. In a later, simpler, process, sulphuric acid was substituted for nitric. Phosphorus is now obtained from phosphate rock. In the nineteenth century its western European manufacture was concentrated in two factories: Messrs Albright and Wilson Ltd., at Oldbury, near Birmingham, in the English Midlands and Messieurs Coignet *et fils* of Lyons, France. The only other British producer was Eden Jones & Co. (later Proctor), of Bristol, though this firm seems to have ceased production during the second half of the century. Hence, by the 1890s, Albright and Wilson had a virtual monopoly of the British market.[2] Phosphorus manufacture seems to have posed few health hazards to workers. In the 1860s the larger of the two British phosphorus manufacturers employed only 60-70 people, few of whom appear to have been exposed to danger. An 1880 report from the factory inspectorate referred to 7 poisoning cases in 29 years at Albright and Wilson, which then employed some 260 men. Five of these cases had occurred in a single year (1871).

Phosphorus was of considerable importance in Victorian chemistry laboratories, especially in the production of organic compounds. But it had fewer commercial applications than arsenic and lead. Like arsenic it was employed, in the form of phosphor-bronze, as a rat poison. It had medicinal applications, especially in the treatment of nervous disease, in which it was valued for its restorative and stimulant powers, and fever. It was also an ingredient of saccharin, distress flares, luminous goods (because of its phosphorescence) and, of greatest relevance to this chapter, matches.[3] In most of the trades and occupations in which phosphorus was used: pharmacy, science, medicine and pest control, poisoning was unusual either on account of the small numbers employed, the modest quantities of phosphorus used, or the precautions that were adopted.[4]

Robert Christison's *Treatise on Poisons* accorded the material little attention, presumably because poisoning from it was seldom encountered in medical practice in the 1820s. So while he found that minute quantities could destroy human life, he observed that '[i]ts effects on man have not often been witnessed'. Nevertheless, Christison was able to describe a case in which 'a stout young man', who took a grain and a half, died twelve days later following stomach and bowel pains, incessant diarrhoea and vomiting. He also noted that while it had been the custom to prescribe small doses of phosphorus in medical practice, that 'the uncertainty and occasional severity of its operation have very properly expelled it from modern pharmacopoeias'. Finally, Christison recorded phosphorus's reputation as a 'powerful aphrodisiac', pointing out, in a rare shaft of humour, that '[n]o such symptom was remarked in the fatal case just related', that is, of the 'stout young man'.[5] Two decades later Alfred Swaine Taylor confirmed most of Christison's observations: 'It is not often that we hear of cases of poisoning by phosphorus or its compounds.... So few cases of poisoning by phosphorus have occurred, that we are scarcely in a position to generalise upon its effects'. Because phosphorus was readily detectable by smell and taste, it was seldom employed for criminal purposes, other than suicide attempts. The one significant difference between the Christison and Taylor accounts is the latter's reference to recent suggestions of a link between chronic phosphorus poisoning and the manufacture of phosphorus matches.[6]

Without doubt phosphorus poisoning was most prevalent in 'lucifer' matchmaking, a trade that consumed almost all the phosphorus produced in Britain – about 60 tons p.a. in the 1890s. In the early-1860s match production, exclusive of those who worked in their own homes, provided employment for some 2500-2650 people in around 57 factories. Subsequent 'rationalisation', which

TABLE 6.1:
Location of and Employment in Lucifer Match Making in 1896

Regional Location	Number Employed
England & Wales	**3813**
Scotland	**261**
Ireland	**237**
Total	**4311**

Category of Employee	Number Employed
Women	**2283**
Men	**617**
Young Persons (Female)	**1015**
Young persons (Male)	**390**
Half Timers (Female)	**0**
Half Timers (Male)	**6**
Total	**4311**

Source: *Report to the Secretary of State for the Home Department on the Use of Phosphorus in the Manufacture of Lucifer Matches*, by Professor T.E. Thorpe, PP 1899 XII, 459

T.H.S. Escott attributed to factory legislation, meant fewer but bigger factories and a highly competitive industry, the greater part of which was London-based.[7] By the mid-1890s 25 match factories employed around 4300 people, about three-quarters of whom were women (see Tables 6.1 and 6.2).[8] Nearly 70 per cent of this workforce was employed by three firms: Bell and Bryant and May, both of London, and the Diamond Match Corporation in Liverpool. Of these three companies Bell was the oldest, the first match factory anywhere in the world having been established by Richard Bell & Co. in Wandsworth, London in 1832. The Diamond Match Company was an American firm which set up in Britain only in 1895; it amalgamated with Bryant and May in 1901. From 1884, when it became a public company, Bryant and May embarked on two decades of rapid expansion which made it the dominant force in the British match industry.[9]

Although matches were not a nineteenth century invention – they are known to have existed in the sixteenth – it has been claimed that the 'first really practical friction matches' were produced at Stockton-on-Tees by an apothecary, John Walker, in 1827. The

TABLE 6.2:
Regional Concentration of the Match Industry in 1896

Location	Number of Factories
London	**8**
Belfast	**3**
Leeds	**2**
Manchester	**2**
Aberdeen	**1**
Bristol	**1**
Cork	**1**
Dublin	**1**
Glasgow	**1**
Gloucester	**1**
Hull	**1**
Liverpool	**1**
Llandaff	**1**
Swansea	**1**
Total	**25**

Source: *Report to the Secretary of State for the Home Department on the Use of Phosphorus in the Manufacture of Lucifer Matches,* by Professor T.E. Thorpe, PP 1899 XII, 459–60

practicality of Walker's matches, which were supposedly invented by pure serendipity, has been disputed. According to William Hepworth Dixon, their ignition required considerable pressure with the result that their heads tended to fall off. He contends that 'the first completely successful friction match' was made in France, of phosphorus, in 1831. However, the validity of this contention is also disputed. What is clear is that Walker's matchheads were made not from white (sometimes known as yellow or ordinary) phosphorus, but from chlorate of potash, sulphide of antimony and, to provide adhesion to the splint, gum arabic. As such, they posed no health risk to those who made them.[10] Also beyond dispute is the fact that the market for friction matches 'took off' during the 1830s.[11]

The phosphorus match, whether it was a 'Congreve', 'wax-vesta', 'vesuvian', or 'fusee', rapidly superseded its potash-antimony counterpart, becoming 'a necessity for all classes'. Safety matches, which could be ignited only on a box coated with a strip of non-toxic red or amorphous phosphorus – patented by Albright and Wilson in

1851 – were available from 1855, if not earlier. While these offered an alternative means of ignition, which was harmless to workers, they failed to oust the strike-anywhere, white phosphorus match. Their limited popularity appears to have been due to their slightly higher cost, public preference for the convenience of the strike-anywhere article and certain practical shortcomings (i.e. ignition strips that absorbed moisture, thereby losing their power to ignite, or wore out while matches remained in the box). In other words, at least until a comparatively 'late' stage neither the market nor the consumer came to the rescue of the beleaguered worker threatened with occupational ill health. Consequently, it fell to the state to intervene.

One aspect of the early history of matches that merits attention is the crime and protest dimension. The 1830s and 1840s saw an upsurge of rural incendiarism or arson, especially in East Anglia. Although this phenomenon has been linked with economic deprivation, social alienation, resentment over the New Poor Law and political impotence, it has seldom been placed within its technological or commercial context. Yet it is surely not fanciful to associate this spate of arson attacks with the recent availability of an instantaneous, cheap, easily-portable and readily-concealable means of producing fire. As John Archer has pointed out, the advent of the match was

> an absolute boon to would-be incendiaries... The essence of a successful incendiary was his speed and stealth and the 'Lucifer' match with its effective ignition allowed him to strike the match and then escape across the fields. The 'Lucifer' or strike-anywhere match thus opened up a whole new vista for the angry labourer.[12]

While the match did not provoke arson attacks or establish arson as a form of social protest, it certainly facilitated incendiarism. As *Punch* said, when commenting on a sentence of transportation imposed upon a 10 year old boy for firing a stack of straw in Huntingdonshire: 'We are shocked at the powers of mischief which the lucifer match places in the hands of the reckless and malignant'.[13] No longer was it necessary, as in an 1802 case of incendiarism described by E.P. Thompson, for the arsonist to take 'a hod of coals from her fire to the [hay] stack' and to return with bellows when the rick failed to ignite.[14]

Phosphorus matches were dangerous because of their unpredictable ignition. They sometimes produced showers of sparks when struck, or burst into flame unexpectedly, for example, when dropped or left in heat. As a result, smokers who carried them loose in their pockets could receive a nasty shock. Francis Kilvert recorded an example of this in his diary entry for 5 July 1874:

> During afternoon service Frederick Vincent rushed out of Church in a flame of smoke leaving the congregation half smothered in a dense smoke. When he came back I went to him to know what had happened. He said he had sat upon a fusee which had exploded in his pocket and burnt him.[15]

Because they could ignite 'by rubbing or almost touching anything a little rough', 'A Chymyst' informed *The Times* in 1842, phosphorus matches were 'much too dangerous for general use'. It is clear that many domestic, agricultural and factory fires were started by their accidental combustion. One report suggested that in the ten years, 1833-42, 63 lucifer match factories caught fire in London alone. Indeed, 'A Chymyst' expressed surprise 'that half London has not burnt down' as a result of fires started by matches. Not for nothing were phosphorus matches known as Congreves, after the rocket pioneer, Sir William Congreve. There were suggestions that they should be banned or, by the imposition of a government stamp, sold only at a price which placed them beyond the means of the young and feckless. Although these ideas came to nothing, legislation enacted in 1844 provided, in the interests of fire prevention, that after a period of 20 years it would be unlawful for any lucifer match factory, new or existing, to be sited within 50 feet of another building or 40 feet of a public thoroughfare.[16]

Fire was not the only danger posed by phosphorus matches, for at least one early manufacturer warned users against inhaling their noxious smoke. A greater risk, perhaps, was the ingestion, deliberate or accidental, of match heads. As early as 1842 the *Provincial Medical Journal* reported the death of a child, aged six months, as a result of sucking the tips of lucifer matches. A year later the *Lancet* reported a similar case.[17] Tragic though such deaths obviously were, it is unlikely that it was the purchasers of lucifer matches (or their families) who suffered most from phosphorus poisoning. Indeed, it has been noted that phosphorus matches, provided 'very great satisfaction to the consumer' for some seventy years. Far greater risk was faced by matchworkers whose constant contact with poisonous vapours exposed them to the possibility of contracting one of the ghastliest of all occupational diseases. This was phosphorus necrosis, or, as it was commonly known, 'phossy jaw'.[18]

Caused by exposure to oxidising phosphorus, necrosis affected the jaw bones of workers in the match industry, particularly those affected by dental caries or gum disease. The living bone literally rotted *in situ*, causing terrible pain, potentially horrible disfigurement and, if untreated, death. Only surgical excision of the affected parts, an operation with terrible implications for the sufferer, and removal from exposure, could save the lives of those who were severely afflicted. But, as John Brown pondered in relation to a factory accident victim pulled alive but dreadfully maimed from machinery, 'saved to what end'? In extreme cases it might be to face a precarious future with little or no jaw bone and the mere ruin of a face with 'bare bone grinning out, a living death's-head', as an official investigator of the 1860s described one victim. Not without reason did Hunter cite phosphorus matchmaking as 'the greatest tragedy in the whole story of occupational disease'.[19]

At least until the 1860s, when Bryant and May became manufacturers – they had previously been importers of Swedish matches – the British match industry was of comparatively modest dimensions. It was labour intensive and under-capitalised; often the small-scale match entrepreneur was a former 'dipper' (see note 32) whose workforce might chiefly comprise members of his own family. As an observer of the 1860s noted, matchmaking was open to anyone, no matter how slender their means, character, or intelligence. Such businesses tended to have only a transient existence. When the industry was investigated in the early-1840s, by the Children's Employment Commission (CEC), the sub-commissioner, R.D. Grainger, encountered an unmechanised trade carried on in appalling conditions, often by under-nourished, ill-clad and illiterate children aged as young as seven or eight. Although Grainger's brief report and synopsis of evidence contained few references to phosphorus and none to necrosis of the jaw, which was first described only in 1845 (1846 in the UK), it did carry frequent references to 'disagreeable', 'oppressive' and 'noxious' fumes and to the generally unhealthy and unpleasant conditions of work in a business which, like the cottage industry of matchbox making and the street trade of selling lucifers, attracted only those who were truly desperate for work. As William Sutton, an overseer in a Lambeth factory, pointed out: 'There is always a very unpleasant and unwholesome smell in the shop, which is injurious to the lungs. The boys when they first come cannot stand it and "are often afterwards ill with a sick headache"'.[20]

Of course, the CEC, as its name indicates, was concerned only with the problem of juvenile labour. While children in the match factories did come into contact with phosphorus and could hardly avoid its fume and dust if employed in the vicinity of its use, the task of dipping match splints in the phosphorus 'composition' usually fell to adult males. In line with the *laissez-faire* conventions of the day, the state treated them as free agents in the employment market who had no need of statutory protection. As such they were perceived to be at liberty to bargain with employers on a basis of full equality, to assess the health and safety hazards of the workplace and accept or reject work as they saw fit. It was these 'free agents' who came into most regular contact with phosphorus. As Sutton pointed out, '[t]he boys who are employed about the matches when first dipped in the brimstone do not suffer so much as the men who are employed in dipping them in the composition of phosphorus'.[21]

A growing awareness

The CEC's report led to no statutory intervention in the lucifer match industry. Not only did hygiene and sanitation remain matters of discretion for individual masters, but also an employer's liberty to hire whomsoever he desired, regardless of age or any other consideration, remained unimpeded. The imposition of legal restrictions on the industry, as in the case of paper staining and pottery, dated from 1864 (the *Factory Acts Extension Act*) and followed two further official inquiries into the trade, one by the Medical Office of the Privy Council, the other by another CEC. By this time the link between phosphorus necrosis and lucifer match manufacture had been amply demonstrated in several epidemiological studies. The pioneer work in this area was undertaken on the continent, particularly in those areas where match manufacture was carried out on a large scale. Britain, with its modestly-sized match industry contributed little.

From 1845 German and Austrian, followed by French, investigators began to establish a causal connection between phosphorus match manufacture and necrosis of the jaw. As a result, as early as October 1846, the Imperial Provincial Government of Lower Austria, having previously appointed a commission of inquiry, issued a civil ordinance to combat phosphorus necrosis. These continental developments did not go unnoticed in Great Britain. Thus, the British physician, G.W. Balfour, who visited Vienna in 1846, reported in the *Northern Journal of Medicine* that the 'attention of surgeons in Germany has, not long since been drawn to a peculiar form of necrosis of the jaw-bones – produced by long continued exposure to the action of the fumes of phosphorus'. Meanwhile, in July 1846 J.F. Heyfelder's paper, 'Necrosis of the Maxillary Bones produced by the Vapours of Phosphorus', which had appeared in the October 1845 issue of *Archives Generales de Medicine*, was briefly summarised in the *Edinburgh Medical and Surgical Journal*. Generally, however, the scientific papers emanating from Vienna, Nuremburg, Strasbourg, Berlin, Paris and Lyons attracted little immediate attention in Great Britain. This began to change after Ernst von Bibra and Lorenz Geist, the first a chemist, the second a physician, published *Die Krankheiten der Arbeiter in den Phosphorzundholzfabriken, ins besondere das Leiden der Kieferknochen durch Phosphordampfe. Vom Chemischphysiologischen, Medicischchirurgischen und Medicinisch-Polizeilichen Standpunkte* (The Diseases of Workers in Phosphorus Match Factories...) (Erlangen, 1847).[22]

This substantial volume which ran to almost 350 pages, not only summarised all previous work in the field but constituted, as the *British and Foreign Medico-Chirurgical Review* put it, 'an original and satisfactory investigation...worthy in every way of the present state of natural and strictly medical science'. Based partly on a painstaking study of sixty-eight cases, the monograph was, for many years, the definitive work on phosphorus necrosis, containing 'full and detailed accounts of the disease, its origin, its symptoms and its effects, with profitable suggestions for its prevention.' Even so, it would probably have attracted little attention in Britain had it not been 'picked up', summarised in English and praised by the British medical press, notably the *British and Foreign Medico-Chirurgical Review*, though also, later and more briefly, in the *Dublin Quarterly Journal of Medical Science* and the distinguished *Edinburgh Medical and Surgical Journal*.[23]

As it was, von Bibra and Geist alerted the British medical profession to the existence of phosphorus necrosis as an occupational disease of matchmakers. In so doing they encouraged British practitioners and researchers to investigate and report upon conditions in the UK industry. Hitherto, notwithstanding one surgeon's observation that the disease 'had previously been noticed not to be uncommon in those working in phosphorus', British medical men had written virtually nothing about phosphorus as an occupational disease. Subsequently a regular flow of articles began to appear in the UK medical press, though still in nothing like the volume of continental periodicals. At the same time monographs also began to tackle the question. All of this work acknowledged the debt to German investigators.[24]

First, Alfred Swaine Taylor, doyen of forensic scientists, noted in his book, *On Poisons*, that continental research had linked chronic poisoning among matchworkers with inhalation of phosphorus vapour. He went on to suggest, however, that the subject 'still demands inquiry'. A year later, in 1849, Edward Stanley, President of the Royal College of Surgeons, referred, in his path-breaking book on bone disease, not only to German work but to cases that had been treated at the London and St Bartholomew's Hospitals. In this, the first work on bone disease by a British surgeon, Stanley expressed himself ready to accept that the phosphorus used in lucifer match manufacture was responsible for necrosis of the jaw. 'It seems well ascertained', he wrote, 'that the disease is the result of long exposure to the fumes of phosphorus acid, giving rise to inflammation of the periosteum of the jaw, in conjunction with extreme depravation of the general health'. Later in the same year a Nottingham surgeon, Henry Taylor, reported two cases of necrosis in the city's matchworks to the *Lancet*.[25]

By 1850 John Simon was lecturing to medical students at St. Thomas's Hospital on 'Disease of the Lower Jaw produced by Phosphorus Fumes'. While noting that the subject of his lecture had 'not yet passed into the text-books of surgery' he was in no doubt that

> [d]uring the last five years, several successive papers by various German and French surgeons have concurred to establish the fact, that persons exposed to the vapours of phosphorus – as, for instance, in the manufacture of lucifer-matches, are liable to contract a disease under which more or less of their jaws becomes necrosed and exfoliates [comes away].[26]

Clearly, therefore, by 1850, a causal connection between lucifer matchmaking and phosphorus necrosis had been scientifically established; it had also been recognised in Great Britain. In the next few years James Bower Harrison reported on cases of phosphorus necrosis among Manchester matchworkers. To this account the editor of the *Dublin Quarterly Journal of Medical Science*, in which it was published, added a postscript on the position in the Irish capital. A popular account of the hazards of match making (based on Harrison's article) appeared in Charles Dickens's *Household Words* in 1852.[27] However, even by the end of the fifties, most accounts of match manufacture and phosphorus necrosis had been published in specialist journals and monographs. The subject had yet, as Thomas Wakley, the editor of the *Lancet*, observed in 1857, to make much of an impression in surgical textbooks.[28] Neither was there much idea about the dimensions of the problem. Wakley, for example, referred only to 'occasional' cases of necrosis being treated by hospitals. James Harrison, Henry Taylor and others had proposed precautionary measures for the protection of workers, but, as Harrison observed, such measures 'require not merely being known, but being enforced'. This implied a need for regulation and inspection or, at least, for an official inquiry. Clearly, the time had come for the question to be investigated and put before parliament.

Bristowe and White

Although an official report by Waller Lewis in the 1850s on the Regulation of Noxious Trades and Occupations in France had included material on occupational health in the French match trade, it was Dr John Bristowe's 1862 report on the phosphorus industries, published, like William Guy's on arsenic, in John Simon's Fifth Report (as Medical Officer of the Privy Council), that first brought the existence of 'phossy jaw' to the attention of parliament.[29] Thirty years after it appeared Thomas Arlidge considered that Bristowe's account remained the best appraisal of occupational health in the phosphorus industries. Indeed, even in the 1960s Bristowe's account of the aetiology of phosphorus necrosis was said to represent 'exactly the state of present-day knowledge'.[30] It therefore merits detailed consideration here, as does the lengthy report of John White, published a year later, for the CEC.

John Syer Bristowe (1827-95) was born in Camberwell into a well-established medical family. In his youth he was an accomplished boxer with literary and artistic ambitions. He received his medical education at St Thomas's Hospital in London and went on to become a general physician, with a particular interest in neurology, at the same hospital. It was probably at St Thomas's that he made the acquaintance of John Simon and acquired an interest in public health. In any event Bristowe spent many years as a metropolitan medical officer of health. Aside from his report on phosphorus he undertook several other official inquiries on public health questions. These included a second investigation, in 1865, for the Medical Office of the Privy Council, this time on rag-borne infection amongst paper makers and collaborations on cattle plague and sanitary conditions in English hospitals. Towards the end of his life he served on the Royal Commission on Vaccination. He also published important books on general medicine and the nervous system.[31]

In the course of his inquiry into phosphorus match making Bristowe visited most British match factories ranging from 'shoe-string' operations, using a mere 3lbs (1.36 kg) of phosphorus to produce as few as 70 gross (10,080) of boxes per week, to the largest manufacturer, employing a workforce of nearly 500 people and consuming some 160lbs (72.58 kg) of phosphorus per week. While he found that in size, layout and standards of ventilation, workshops varied considerably, he also ascertained that in all factories most work processes exposed operatives, in some degree, to phosphorus fumes. These processes included mixing the phosphorus composition, as well as dipping, drying, cutting, sorting and boxing the matches. Those most at risk were the mixers, dippers and driers producing blue-tipped matches, in unmechanised, single-room premises.[32] In addition to his inspections of premises, Bristowe interviewed proprietors and workers, studied the medical literature and held discussions with members of the medical profession.[33]

What did these inquiries reveal about the hazards of the match trade and matchworkers' general state of health in the early-1860s? First, Bristowe confirmed the general opinion that phosphorus alone was responsible for necrosis, and also that the greater the exposure, the greater was the risk. The degree of risk depended not only on the nature of a worker's tasks but the standards of hygiene and care observed. Second, Bristowe questioned whether, as the received wisdom insisted, decayed teeth were a precondition of necrosis. Although dental caries was all but universal among the working classes, his observations persuaded him that gum sores alone could account for the onset of the disease. Third, he found that with the exception of one disease, phosphorus necrosis, matchworkers' general state of health was 'quite average'. Fourth, he concluded that while there was 'ample proof of the occurrence of necrosis of the jaw' it was 'far less' prevalent 'than most persons would have supposed'. In fact, Bristowe obtained 'authentic' information of only 59 cases, 24 of which had originated in one large Manchester factory (of Dixon, Son and Evans). This total was, he considered, probably with justification, low in relation to the numbers employed in matchmaking during the period of the industry's existence. Although he accepted that he had not identified every case, he doubted whether the true extent of the disease's incidence 'exceeds very materially the number which I have recorded'.[34]

Although there are no extant data that allow Bristowe's assessment of incidence to be challenged, a statistical point raised many years later by that pioneer of occupational health, Ludwig

Teleky, does call it into question. Teleky doubted the accuracy of early-twentieth century official statistics on phosphorus poisoning because they showed a fatality rate which was far higher than would be expected. Whereas the usual rate in necrosis cases was between 15 and 20 per cent, figures published by the factory inspectorate indicated a mortality rate of around 36 per cent. Since the reporting of fatalities was likely to be more accurate than for non-fatal cases, the probability is that phosphorus cases were more frequent than the post-1896 records suggest. It should be remembered, however, that the small number of reported cases does compromise the validity of statistical relationships such as this. Bristowe's statistics indicated a mortality rate of over 37 per cent. If Teleky's estimate of 15-20 per cent was valid and Bristowe's 21 deaths accurate, the number of cases in Bristowe's survey may well have been between 105 and 139.[35]

Bristowe tried to obtain as much information as possible about the 59 ascertained necrosis victims, including gender, age when symptoms were first observed, duration of employment before attack, occupation within the factory and the disease's progress or victim's fate. However, either because factories had closed or changed hands, because his questions were answered evasively, or because the information provided was unverifiable, he amassed few firm details. It appeared that in some cases sufferers had worked in matchmaking for years before succumbing to necrosis, while in others they had fallen ill within months of entering the industry. As for the age of victims when first attacked, Bristowe ascertained only that most were between the ages of 18 and 30, that four were over the age of 40 and that 'several' were between the ages of 12 and 16. All of this was so imprecise and incomplete as to be of very little use in determining such matters as risk and susceptibility. Only in respect of victims' gender, type of work, seat of disease and outcome did Bristowe secure anything like full information. This is presented here in tabular form (Table 6.3, overleaf).[36]

Useful as these data are, for example, in suggesting the apparently low incidence of phossy jaw, identifying the disproportion between male and female sufferers (a reflection, Bristowe believed, of the composition of the workforce), the high rate of fatality and the riskiest occupations, it leaves many questions unanswered. This was because Bristowe provided, presumably because he did not possess them, few statistics of employment and industrial output. Although he estimated 2500 persons employed in match production, this does not help determine the incidence of necrosis. Not only had Bristowe's 59 cases occurred over an unspecified period, perhaps as long as 30

TABLE 6.3:
Fifty-Nine Necrosis Victims Identified by Bristowe

Category	Sub-Category	Sub-Total	Total
Gender	Male	44	
	Female	15	**59**
	Dipper/Mixer/ Grinder	36	
	Boxer/Picker/Cross-cutter	20	
	Unknown	3	**59**
Affected part	Lower Jaw	39	
	Upper Jaw	12	
	Both Jaws	5	
	Unknown	3	**59**
Outcome	Deceased	21	
	Recovered	25	
	Still Affected	12	
	Unknown	1	**59**

Source: *Fifth Report of the Medical Officer of the Privy Council*, PP 1863 XXV, 162–205

years, but we have no way of knowing what proportion of matchmakers was exposed to phosphorus.[37]

In the absence of crucial data and with no explicit proposals for the establishment of legally-binding precautions, Bristowe's account is open to interpretation as an exoneration of the match industry and a justification for the continued application of a *laissez-faire* policy. As its author pointed out, not only was the number of phosphorus poisonings very low, but also the firm where almost half of them had occurred, appeared to have put its house in order. Hence, in the five years preceding his inquiry no further cases had arisen among its workforce. In addition, the health of match workers free from necrosis was by no means sub-standard, that is, compared with their peers in other occupations. Bristowe favoured the introduction or extension of 'precautions, of the simplest and most obvious description', outlining what he felt to be needful (ventilation and modifications in factory layout in order to minimise the number of 'at-risk' workers). Such steps, he anticipated, could 'render the occurrence of jaw disease...a rare and quite exceptional occurrence'. As a result, there appeared to be no urgent necessity for legal regulation of working conditions or for a ban on the use of phosphorus.[38] Bristowe did hint that he favoured legislation compelling manufacturers to use only non-toxic, 'amorphous' phosphorus, but with no evidence adduced to demonstrate the extent of necrosis, it is hard to avoid the conclusion that Bristowe's preference for legal compulsion was based less on objective analysis of risk, more on the emotional case made by a few disfigured survivors of an obviously awful, but perhaps rare, disease. For his part Simon felt that since the application of 'reasonable precautions' could render lucifer matchmaking a not 'unwholesome occupation', use of amorphous phosphorus, while desirable, need not be made compulsory.[39]

Bristowe's inquiry into the phosphorus industries, which, of course, concentrated on match manufacture, coincided with the CEC's investigation of lucifer match production. As we have seen, this Commission, appointed on Lord Shaftesbury's motion, also investigated *inter alia* the pottery and paper staining industries. The lucifer match inquiry was carried out by John White, a barrister and fellow of New College, Oxford. Probably because he was a lawyer, rather than a medical practitioner, White concentrated less than Bristowe on phosphorus poisoning. In any case, his brief was to assess the case for the imposition of restrictions on the employment of minors. As such he was as much interested in the children's general welfare and educational attainments as in their state of health. Like Bristowe, White visited every match factory in the United Kingdom. Like his predecessor, Grainger, twenty years before, he encountered a trade carried on in the poorest and most populous areas of towns and cities, notably the East End of London, chiefly by uneducated and near destitute children, juveniles and women. Though his findings confirmed most of Bristowe's account, there were some differences, for example, in their assessments of the general state of matchworkers' health. White characterised this as poor, Bristowe as good. As for the extent of phossy jaw, White had no more to offer than Bristowe:

> The disease is found less in this country than abroad, where it has been so serious as to draw to itself the attention not only of the medical profession and other bodies, but of Governments. The cases also seem to have been less frequent the last few years than formerly and are often said to have occurred only amongst the few persons who prepare the phosphorus composition and put it onto the matches, who are chiefly, though not entirely, adults. But some cases

in England and very many abroad, as reported in several medical works, show that the evil spreads far beyond these.[40]

White's report was descriptive rather than prescriptive. He (briefly) outlined the history, location and nature of the match industry along with its effects upon the well being of the workforce. Beyond this he summarised and contextualised his witnesses' evidence, often allowing them to speak for themselves. Some of these witnesses, who included medical men, businessmen, workers, necrosis victims and scientists, held views on the prevention of poisoning. Foremost among them was Professor Henry Letheby, who was medical officer of health for the City of London as well as Professor of Chemistry and Toxicology at the London Hospital's school of medicine. Letheby, who had pioneered the study of phosphorus poisoning in Britain and possessed some 20 years experience of health conditions in the match industry, had several suggestions for reducing risk. These included the isolation of dangerous processes – as it was, these were often carried on alongside relatively safe tasks – proper ventilation, worker cleanliness, exclusion from work of persons with carious teeth and the use of prophylactics such as alkaline drinks and mouth washes. Bizarrely, he also suggested that workers on dangerous processes should have an open tin of turpentine suspended from their necks as they worked, thereby enabling them to inhale an atmosphere which, Letheby believed, 'will entirely check the evolution of phosphoric fumes'.[41]

Some of White's other witnesses made suggestions similar to Letheby's, emphasising in addition the potential benefits to workers' health of good diet, compulsory changes of clothing, a ban on the taking of meals in workshops, use of respirators and restrictions on the length of time spent on dangerous processes. Most important, however, were suggestions that the substitution of amorphous for white phosphorus provided the best opportunity for solving the problem. Letheby recognised that safety matches would be slightly dearer than the existing variety and that they were somewhat less serviceable than their lucifer counterparts. But these shortcomings, he maintained, were insignificant in relation to their advantages in terms of health and safety; not only were they non-toxic, but they were less inclined to ignite as the result of inadvertent friction or a rise in temperature. Letheby argued that a government ban on white phosphorus, by preventing a manufacturer from undercutting a rival who had voluntarily switched to using amorphous phosphorus and side-stepping the problem of consumer resistance to safety matches, would rapidly win public acceptance.[42] When this solution, which Bristowe had also proposed, was adopted phosphorus poisoning in the match trade rapidly became a thing of the past. However, it took over forty-five years, in the course of which there was much needless suffering and death, before this came about. Although Francis May, of Bryant and May, who were patentees of a safety match, told White that he favoured the use of amorphous phosphorus, other producers were unenthusiastic. For example, Samuel Bell of Bell and Black, Bow Bridge, Stratford found amorphous phosphorus difficult to ignite and doubted whether it would ever be a practicable alternative to the white variety.[43]

The CEC reported that 'this terrible infliction [necrosis] is, to a very great extent, if not entirely, within the reach of measures of prevention'. The commissioners recommended the introduction of most of the sanitary precautions suggested by various witnesses. In addition they proposed, as they already had in connection with pottery manufacture, that a medical inspector be appointed with responsibility to draw up special rules for health and safety tailored to the requirements of each factory. The one thing they did not propose was a ban on white phosphorus and compulsory use of the amorphous variety. In so doing, they overlooked the most vital aspect of Letheby's evidence and backed a strategy of containment rather than proscription. This set the tone for tackling the problem of phosphorus poisoning in matchmaking for the remainder of the century.[44]

Legislation and inspection, 1864-1891

Most of the recommendations of the Children's Employment Commission in respect of lucifer match making were embodied in the *Factory Acts Extension Bill, 1864*.[45] As we have seen, the main aims of this measure were to extend the terms of the existing factory acts, which applied restrictions on the employment of child labour, to several non-textile industries and to emphasise the importance of industrial health and hygiene. This emphasis was not entirely innovatory. The obligation to ventilate factories and maintain a state of cleanliness (for the control of disease) dated from the *Health and Morals of Apprentices Act, 1802*. However, over the years the factory inspectorate had come largely to overlook the health provisions of the factory acts. As Alexander Redgrave wrote in 1864, 'although the enactments of 1802 would be valid now in cotton and woollen factories the inspectors have no special directions to enforce them and they have been treated as obsolete'.[46] Effectively, therefore, the

1864 bill marked a fresh departure. The bill envisaged minimum standards of ventilation and cleanliness. It also proposed a ban on children, young persons and women taking meals in any part of a match factory.

As was the case with the other trades included in the bill, manufacturers, rather than the medical inspector proposed by the commissioners, were to compile 'special rules' to achieve the desired hygiene and sanitation goals. This raised the prospect of a strictly limited measure of protection. Not only was containment rather than the proscription of dangerous materials to be the watchword, the containment measures were to be compiled by the regulatees themselves rather than by independent arbiters. Furthermore, since a large part of the match industry was still conducted on domestic premises, which lay beyond the jurisdiction of the factory acts, a significant portion of the trade would remain beyond the reach of the legislators.[47]

As noted elsewhere, the *Factory Acts Extension Bill* gave rise to little contention in its passage through parliament. Beyond the observations that match manufacture gave employment to 'the poorest of the poor and the lowest of the low' and that such employment was 'exceedingly prejudicial to health and induced a most distressing and painful disease of the jaw', the debates included few references the match industry.[48] In the Lords the Earl of Harrowby, for motives that were not specified, suggested that matchmaking should be excluded from the bill's terms. However, this suggestion, which was firmly opposed by Lord Shaftesbury, came to nothing. The *Factory Acts Extension Act*, with lucifer matchmaking included in its list of newly-regulated industries, received the Royal Assent on 25 July 1864. It was then for the factory inspectorate, undermanned and under-resourced as it was, to decide on how to proceed. In the event, for more than a quarter of a century inspectors paid little attention to health problems in the match trade. When they did report about them it was generally in uncritical vein. In view of the events of the 1890s and 1900s, when it emerged that some manufacturers were systematically concealing poisoning cases, it would appear either that earlier inspections had been inadequate or that standards of health within the industry declined in the last years of the century. On balance, the former appears to be the likelier explanation.[49]

Redgrave's first report on the trade, produced in 1865, gave the large match factories in his district a 'clean bill of health'. Their 'principals', he noted in a phrase intended to convey their unimpeachable integrity and flawless respectability, were 'men of capital'. In this connection it is instructive to note that in 1844 Engels had used the words 'capital', 'capitalist' and 'capitalism' as pejoratives, arguing, for example, that 'capital...is the weapon with which...social warfare is carried on'. The victims of this war were the poor. Redgrave's interpretation of these terms was, obviously, more or less the complete inverse of Engels; he viewed capitalism as an instrument of social *welfare*.[50] If the word 'capital' loomed large in Redgrave's lexicon of inspection, so too did the notion of respectability. With other inspectors Redgrave tended to assume that a respectable or successful manufacturer was bound to be a responsible one. Considerations of 'respectability' loom large in the history of occupational health regulation, as they do in the history of nineteenth and twentieth century social policy as a whole. Not only could respectable firms expect a degree of immunity from the full rigour of the law, but also 'undeserving' employees were likely to receive a diminished measure of legal protection. Yet that most 'respectable' of firms, Bryant and May, run by Quakers in modern, spacious and purpose-built premises, was shown in the 1890s to have a disgraceful record in occupational health.[51]

At any event, in 1865 Redgrave reported that the rooms in which manufacturers of capital and respectability produced their matches were 'generally roomy and fairly ventilated and [that] various contrivances [were] erected in all for reducing the evils attached to the use of phosphorus'. He particularly congratulated Bell and Black of Bow Bridge for the excellence of their dipping arrangements, expressing confidence that in the future, there and elsewhere, even more attention would be paid to workers' health. He was less complimentary about the smaller match factories that he had inspected. He had found these to be damp, dark, dirty, dangerous and unhealthy. They were beyond redemption; he could only recommend their closure under the recently-implemented clause of the *Metropolitan Buildings Act, 1844*. Passed, as we have seen, in an attempt to control the fire and explosion hazards posed by lucifer factories, Redgrave anticipated that the act could improve occupational health. Used as he suggested, it is clear that it would also have benefited the larger manufacturers by terminating the businesses of their smaller competitors. Whether, in the light of later events, which indicated that 'show factories' could actually be unhealthy factories, this would also have been to the worker's advantage is debatable.[52] Nevertheless, Redgrave continued throughout the remainder of his inspecting career, a period of some twenty-six years, to praise new premises and to assume that 'lofty and airy' rooms were synonymous with and high standards of health.[53]

In Redgrave's inspection district match factories were to be found in Aberdeen, Glasgow, Leeds, Liverpool, Newcastle, Norwich and, particularly, in London. His long-time colleague (adversary might be a better word given the terms of their relationship), Robert Baker, was responsible for a district that included match factories in Birmingham, Bristol, Leicester, Manchester, Belfast and Dublin. Although Baker and Redgrave agreed on little (in fact they despised each other and seldom conferred), Baker and his sub-inspectors, shared Redgrave's opinion that phosphorus poisoning, insofar as it was a problem, was confined to the small, 'back-street' factories.[54] Generally, however, notwithstanding his medical background, Baker was more concerned with factory workers' morals than their health. He particularly deplored women's industrial employment, even deprecating the inhalation of phosphorus, a process which, it might be thought, was 'morally neutral' (at least as far as the inhalers were concerned), on the grounds that it tended 'to destroy the delicacy of the female character'.[55]

The Royal Commission on Factories and Workshops, which sat in the mid-1870s, provided an opportunity for monitoring a decade's progress in mitigating the dangers of lucifer match manufacture. The commissioners took evidence on matchmaking from only two sources, match manufacturers and factory inspectors; no workers were examined. The two producers questioned were John Jex Long, who had been in business in Glasgow since 1852 and Wilberforce Bryant, of the east London firm of Bryant and May. Perhaps unsurprisingly, both witnesses described an industry free from health problems. Thus, Long who provided his employees with a medical attendant, had never encountered a case of jaw disease. His workers, though poor, were healthy; ventilation and other technological innovations had rendered match factories safe:

> I do not think there are any ingredients used now that are at all unhealthy. In the beginning of the trade, when it was in its infancy, the principal part of the substance used was phosphorus. There is a very small portion, comparatively speaking, of phosphorus used now; the largest portion is chlorate of potash, which is comparatively innocuous.[56]

It was almost superfluous for Bryant to make the same points, for the commission's chairman, Sir James Fergusson, in a remarkable abandonment of objectivity, welcomed the witness by pointing out Bryant and May's excellent health and safety record. Bryant had only to agree and elaborate. This he did by extolling the virtues of his company's new premises and stating that in his firm too phosphorus had ceased to be much used. Only when asked whether he had ever had a case of jaw disease in a child worker did Bryant become less than convincing: 'We had one case, I think, of a child and I think there was one of a young woman, although I forget whether we had two; but they had worked in small places before they came to us; the disease was not contracted in our factories at all'.[57]

As for the views of the inspectorate, Alexander Redgrave's evidence, provided as part of his overall assessment of the impact of factory legislation, was startlingly complacent:

> Take, for instance, the children employed in lucifer-match making, which is a very unhealthy trade; the children employed in that trade now work under altogether different conditions. You never hear now of any case of that dreadful disease which used to be so fatal amongst them, the eating away of the jaw from the constant manipulation of phosphorus, that has entirely ceased.[58]

While the (erroneous) claim that phosphorus poisoning had 'entirely ceased' is the most striking aspect of this testimony, hardly less noteworthy is Redgrave's choice of the phrase: '[y]ou never hear now' of phosphorus poisoning. Unless this was merely an ill-considered response to an unexpected question posed in the course of oral examination, the implication is that the inspector's role was passive, that it was limited to the receipt of information, rather than encompassing an active process of discovery. If so, it does much to explain both the shortfall in inspectors' knowledge of events on the shop floor and also the ease with which manufacturers were able to circumvent occupational health regulations. This is not necessarily to say, of course, that individual inspectors were negligent or inefficient. Rather, their professional approach may have been governed by the resources at their disposal; these may have been insufficient for a more proactive approach to inspection.[59]

Although Baker was more or less silent on the question of lucifer matchmaking, several other inspectors broadly supported the Redgrave line. Robert Coles, an assistant inspector whose district covered most of Lancashire and Cumberland and contained three large match factories, claimed that health standards in the industry had improved since 1864. He did concede, however, that the trade was 'still prejudicial to health'. Rickards, a sub-inspector (the rank beneath assistant) whose district stretched from Hull in Yorkshire to Colne in Lancashire, had few match factories in his region, but those which were present were, he observed, 'not...badly conducted...they belong to very respectable firms'. He thought they made 'fair provision' for ventilation, noting that, 'I have never seen any disease from phosphorus in any lucifer match establishment that I have been in'.[60]

However, Rickard's point reveals more about inspectorial naiveté and the shortcomings of the inspection process than the objective state of health of British match workers. It was followed by the following exchange:

> Question: That [the absence of personal encounters with phossy jaw victims] would be a strong proof that they [match factories] were well conducted...
> Answer: Yes, I think so and I have never seen a recent case in any of my inspections.[61]

In all probability the 'invisibility' of 'phossy jaw' victims is accounted for by employers' refusal to keep them in work.[62] This, at any rate, was shown to be the case in the 1890s when affected workers tried to conceal their symptoms knowing that they would otherwise face dismissal; there is no reason to suppose that the position in the 1870s was any different.

Certainly, it is well documented that in the seventies and other decades a factory inspector's presence in a town, news of which quickly spread, or approach to a factory, precipitated a mass exodus of ineligible workers through a works' back door:

> A sub-inspector, paying his necessarily infrequent visits to a quarter where small brickfields are numerous, may see children being actually huddled off in various directions, like small fish out of a broken net. In a nail and chain, or a straw plait village, his approach is telegraphed and provided for and he may hear that overwork and unlawful employment is going on in a quarter where on his own visits he has seen nothing wrong.[63]

It is unlikely, given the appearance of 'phossy jaw' victims, at least those who had been severely affected, that, even if they returned to work having recovered from their disease, they would have been at their duties when the inspector called. Hence, the assumption that an absence of phosphorus victims in a factory meant an absence of poisoning cases has to be viewed with scepticism. The superintending inspector (a senior official), Robert Cullen was surely nearer to the truth when he gave the Factory and Workshops Commission his views on why phossy jaw sufferers were so rarely encountered. When he delivered his evidence Cullen's official base was Huddersfield, but he had only recently moved south from north-east Scotland where, in Aberdeen, there was a match factory.

Cullen had noticed, in the course of inspecting the Aberdeen premises, that children assisted with the dangerous dipping process. Yet while he formed the impression that the factory was unhealthy, he never encountered a case of jaw disease. Unlike his fellow inspectors, who tended simply to infer, whatever the indications to the contrary, that such a state of affairs proved satisfactory standards of health and hygiene, Cullen was unconvinced: 'I did not understand that [paradox] for some time, but I found out that the people there changed their employment so very often that they were not long enough in this factory to contract the jaw disease; that was the only explanation that I could find of it.'[64] In this instance the absence of 'phossy jaw' provided no indication of successful prophylaxis, but merely a guide to employment practices.

What did the commissioners make of all this? The brief answer is: very little. They virtually ignored the question of occupational health, concentrating instead on hours of work and education along with the need to consolidate the factory acts and improve their administration. The only recommendation aimed at advancing health standards in match factories was for a ban on meal taking (except in wood cutting rooms). As we have seen Thomas Arlidge's suggestion for the appointment of medical inspectors was summarily rejected as being an unwarranted extension of state intervention in the workplace.[65] With such official attitudes to the fore, including within the factory inspectorate, it is hardly surprising that the phosphorus question progressed so slowly. Only after Redgrave's retirement in 1891, following thirteen years as Chief Inspector of Factories, did phosphorus poisoning (and other occupational diseases) begin to be recognised for the perils they were.

Although Redgrave was not blind to the problem of occupational ill health – as we have seen he actually did much to stimulate public and official recognition of the perils of the white lead trade – it was his successor, R.E. Sprague Oram, who first included a section on 'Dangerous and Unhealthy Processes' in the chief inspector of factories' annual report. In the short term the main outcome of the Royal Commission Appointed to Inquire into the Working of the

Factory and Workshops Acts, so far as it affected occupational health in the match trade, were the two clauses in the *Factory and Workshop Act, 1878* which banned children (ie. those aged under 14) from dipping matches and prohibited women, children and young persons (aged 14-18) from their taking meals on factory premises other than wood-cutting rooms.[66]

Thomas Arlidge and the international dimension

Arlidge's *The Hygiene and Diseases of Occupation* (1892) included a section on phosphorus poisoning. Because the book was not an in-depth treatment of any particular disease but a survey of a wide field, Arlidge's discussion of the subject was brief, covering fewer than five pages. It also contained little that was not already well known, for it was based largely on Bristowe's 1863 account. It is unlikely that Arlidge, a lone investigator, had visited any match or phosphorus factories for he stated that: ' Having no better authority, we shall chiefly rely upon this [Fifth Report of the Medical Officer of the Privy Council] very satisfactory official document'.[67] It was mainly when assessing prevailing levels of risk, that is, some thirty years after the publication of Bristowe's report, that Arlidge offered opinions and observations of his own. These were reassuring. He believed that improvements in factory construction and the introduction of amorphous phosphorus had rendered match manufacture comparatively safe. Provided workers were fit and well when they entered the occupation, that they observed high standards of cleanliness and worked in well-ventilated rooms, 'even match-making is not incompatible with a good share of health and with life of average duration'. If all this ran contrary to continental experience, it confirmed much of what Redgrave had asserted some fifteen years earlier.[68]

Arlidge's section on phosphorus was far from the most impressive portion of his book. Taken on its own it would have done little to stimulate public interest in occupational health. *The Hygiene and Diseases of Occupation*, on the other hand did raise awareness about health in the workplace and one consequence of this was a focus of attention on matchmaking and 'phossy jaw'. Once necrosis was on the national agenda the international dimension soon began to loom large for, in an alleged era of 'splendid isolation', the British government and its officials showed much interest in how other nations were tackling the hazards of phosphorus necrosis. Indeed, it is clear that foreign experience and considerations of international trade had a significant impact upon British policy and practice. This was partly because the British appreciated that they might be able to learn something from others. Perhaps more important, however, was the realisation that in an era of overseas challenge to Britain's domination of global commerce, the regulation of the British industry might damage international competitiveness. Since it was international co-operation that ultimately led to a ban on the use of white phosphorus in match making, it is inadequate to view British developments in isolation.

British government interest in European developments began as early as the 1850s when Lord Palmerston, during his comparatively brief tenure of the Home Office (1852-5) instructed Waller Lewis, medical officer to the General Post Office, to compile a concise digest of French law and practice relating to the regulation of 'noxious trades and occupations'. Palmerston's reputation as a statesman rests largely upon his achievements in foreign affairs, but his initiative on occupational health provides further evidence of his stature as a home secretary. Not only did he identify an almost completely neglected area of social policy, but he took the unusual step of ordering an appraisal of overseas practice. Lewis was an unashamed admirer of France's regulatory régime which, he believed, protected workers without imposing onerous burdens upon employers. He judged French standards of occupational health to be considerably higher than Britain's. As part of his inquiry Lewis visited a number of match factories, reporting on the hygiene standards he observed in them. His report might have initiated British moves to tackle some of the 'old, objectionable and unhealthy [manufacturing] methods still all but universally employed in this country'. But when it appeared, in July 1855, Palmerston had already quit the Home Office for 10 Downing Street where his immediate priority was to bring the Crimean War to a successful conclusion. Under Palmerston's successor, Sir George Grey, Lewis's report came to nothing.[69]

In 1874 the prospects for non-toxic matches received a boost when Denmark banned the use of white phosphorus in match manufacture. But the Danish match industry was tiny compared with that of some of its European neighbours. The only one of those neighbours to emulate the ban, Switzerland in 1879, maintained it only until 1881.[70] In 1893 the Foreign Office requested HM Embassy in Berlin to report on the law affecting German match manufacture. Prussian regulations dated from the 1850s, long before intervention in the British industry was being seriously considered. In 1879 the Reichstag had petitioned the chancellor, Bismarck, to prohibit the use of white phosphorus in match manufacture and to increase the duty on imported matches. A commission of inquiry considered such extreme steps would jeopardise German exports and threaten the industry's viability. It therefore recommended the introduction of various health and safety measures for the protection of workers and the public. Regulations of 1884-5 and 1893 introduced a range of safety provisions aimed at facilitating safe production.

In 1895, a year in which representatives of the factory inspectorate visited the Amsterdam Museum for the Prevention of Accidents and Disease in Factories and Workshops, the chief lady inspector of factories, Adelaide Anderson, visited Germany and Austria reporting, *inter alia*, on rules of production and conditions in lucifer match manufacture. Three years later the Newcastle physician, Thomas Oliver, visited French match factories at Aubervilliers, Pantin and Marseilles. He discovered that, at least as far as the official figures were concerned, France's record on phosphorus poisoning was far worse than Britain's running, in 1896, to several hundred cases. However, he also found that there had been a recent decline in the incidence of illness owing to changes in the selection of workers, an increase in the minimum age of employment, the introduction of medical and dental supervision, suspension of workers suffering ill health, and improved methods of manufacture. In fact, Oliver concluded that the French government had 'left no stone unturned to introduce new methods of manufacture and to replace white phosphorus by harmless substances'. Not only had it primed this process with public money, it was employing chemists and inventors who were 'constantly making experiments'. As a result, the government 'has to some extent already succeeded in manufacturing a "strike anywhere" match free from white phosphorus'. It hardly needs to be said that Whitehall eschewed such interventionist policies. Indeed, when self-proclaimed inventors of yellow phosphorus-free matches wrote to the Home Office with offers to divulge their 'secrets' (for a fee), as several did in 1898, all received similar responses – that such matters were of no interest to the British government.[71] Notwithstanding this 'blinkered' attitude, by the end of the century, partly as a consequence of the 1898–9 Home Office inquiry into the 'Use of Phosphorus in the Manufacture of Lucifer Matches' British officials had personally visited or otherwise acquired information on match factories and match-making regulations throughout the greater part of the continent of Europe.[72]

The Star, Bryant and May and special rules

In his annual report for 1891-2 the newly-appointed chief inspector of factories, R.E. Sprague Oram, looked at a number of dangerous and unhealthy processes carried out in British factories and workshops. These included quarrying, iron-paint enamelling and the manufacture of white lead, paints and colours, di-nitro benzole, china and earthenware, chemicals and lucifer matches. He quoted from the evidence that Redgrave and Rickards had given to the Factory and Workshop Commission in the 1870s to support the view that necrosis of the jaw had hitherto 'been considered almost a thing of the past'. But while Sprague Oram agreed that 'the disease is fortunately not widespread', he rejected the basis – personal encounters with victims in the course of inspections – by which his predecessors had reached their conclusions. He realised that the consequences of phosphorus necrosis were

> ...so fearful that the victims are not to be found in any hospital, but are immediately removed from work and attended by the firm's medical advisers and supported at the expense of the firms. Hence, in an ordinary inspection of these works, H.M. Inspectors or others would not come across any cases of apparent suffering from this manufacture.[73]

It followed that means other than regular factory inspection were needed if the true extent of phosphorus necrosis were to be established.

Sprague Oram's comments on what became of necrosis sufferers who came to a firm's attention were so explicit that they suggest he had a particular event or events in mind, even though his report identified no individuals or companies. This was indeed the case; Sprague Oram's observations were the product not of armchair theorising but of information received, largely via the pages of the crusading *Star* newspaper, much of which was subsequently corroborated by a member of the chief inspector's staff and by Clara Collet, one of the lady assistant commissioners serving on the Labour Commission. In January 1892 the *Star* gave details of a necrosis sufferer, a Mrs Fleet, who had worked at Bryant and May for a period of five years. Initially sent home with a toothache she ended up by having four teeth and part of her jaw removed. Fleet's pain and suffering had been intense, though her employers had at least supplied the services of the company doctor and a payment of £1 per week for the 31 weeks of her incapacity. However, these payments ceased with her return to health, even though neither Bryant and May nor any other match manufacturer would hire her on account of her facial disfigurement. Mrs Fleet provided information about other Bryant and May workers who had suffered phosphorus necrosis. The *Star*'s reporter identified some of these but was unable to obtain interviews with any of those still in receipt of payments, the implication being that there was a risk of benefits being withdrawn if recipients spoke to a journalist.[74]

As the *Star*'s story developed in the course of the month other revelations were made. First, it appeared, that of all the matchworkers in the East End only Bryant and May's were succumbing to necrosis. This was said to be a consequence of the layout of the Bryant and May factory, in which the dipping room was sited below other departments with the result that phosphorus fume percolated throughout the premises. The practice of boxing damp and therefore fume-emitting, matches may also have been a factor. Second, it emerged that Bryant and May failed to provide their workers with soap and towels. Third, medical opinion obtained by the *Star* suggested that necrosis victims were in need of hospitalisation rather than treatment in their own homes. Fourth and perhaps most important, when the newspaper published an incomplete list of Bryant and May shareholders (with details of their holdings), it became known that MPs, numerous clerics, a senior Home Office official (Godfrey Lushington) and even the Prime Minister (Lord Salisbury) owned shares in the firm. One of the implications was that the government and its civil servants had a vested interest in minimising the burden of regulations imposed on a firm in which they had investments.[75]

The *BMJ* was shocked, not least because the revelations concerned 'the well-known firm of Bryant and May' whose factory, thirty years earlier, had been praised by Bristowe and Simon as a model of its kind. Phosphorus necrosis, an editorial pointed out, had been recognised for some fifty years. By the same token, the means of prevention (ventilation, cleanliness, substitution of white phosphorus for the amorphous variety) had also been long known. The editorial's restrained conclusion was that if there was any basis to the *Star*'s allegations 'it implies that the firm [Bryant and May] has lagged behind in the march of improvement'.[76] In these circumstances Sprague Oram instructed three factory inspectors, Henry Cameron, J.B. Lakeman and Jasper Redgrave (son of Alexander) to investigate more fully. When Redgrave discovered the existence of some necrosis cases his chief requested him to follow up by obtaining victims' names and addresses and visit them in their homes. Redgrave reported that '[i]t has been with some difficulty that the persons actually under treatment and in receipt of their wages have been approached and they are not at all ready to give information, either from loyalty to their employers, or from fear as to the probable loss of their allowances'. Thus, one woman, who first denied her identity, bolted when the inspector expressed scepticism. Despite such difficulties Redgrave acquired information about eleven possible cases, seven of which he investigated and verified himself. All the victims had worked for Bryant and May; all had received free medical treatment and money in lieu of wages; not one had been hospitalised. Redgrave termed one of those he visited 'a sad spectacle'; another he described as presenting 'a pitiable appearance'. On the basis of Redgrave's report Sprague Oram concluded that the evidence obtained 'is such as proves the necessity for adopting every reasonable means for getting entirely rid of so fearful a malady'.[77]

Meanwhile Clara Collet, one of the Labour Commission's 'lady assistant commissioners', as part of her investigation of metropolitan working conditions, was also investigating the extent of necrosis among East End matchworkers. During May 1892, accompanied by the trade unionist, Tom Mann, she made a number of unannounced visits to the premises of Bryant and May, Bell and other factories. In addition, she visited the London Hospital and the homes of some of the people known to have suffered from necrosis. Collet and Mann, a letter from whom was published with Collet's report, modified some of the *Star*'s allegations and disproved others but, by and large, they substantiated and amplified the newspaper's reports. For example, Collet obtained details of a considerable number of necrosis cases, including at least 33 women who had been employed at Bryant and May since 1880. She also hinted at the existence of a 'dark figure' of unknown dimensions. While she concluded that workers' carelessness, along with their poor state of general and dental health, were contributory factors in the occurrence of necrosis she also, with Mann, criticised the preventive measures taken by employers.[78]

Events then moved rapidly – so rapidly that Sprague Oram's contention that necrosis was uncommon begins to look more like an exercise in understatement than an objective judgment. On 2 June 1892 the home secretary, Henry Matthews, acting on Sprague Oram's recommendation, used the powers conferred upon him by the *Factory and Workshop Act, 1891* to certify lucifer match manufacture as being dangerous to the health of workers.[79] What this meant was that the home secretary, or chief inspector of factories acting as his proxy, acquired the power to propose such special rules or require the adoption of such special measures for the industry as appeared to be appropriate from a health and safety viewpoint and 'reasonably practicable'. As has been noted above, the 1891 act limited executive powers of dictation by giving employers a right of objection to any rules proposed. Since objections could be and sometimes were, pushed as far as a formal arbitration, the special rule procedure tended to develop either into a negotiating process in which employers (though not employees or their representatives) participated as equal partners and/or the promulgation of weak rules which employers, as least, the more successful among them, would have little difficulty in accepting. In either case the benefit to the endangered worker was likely to be limited.[80]

Special rules for lucifer match making were agreed, without recourse to arbitration, in August 1892. They applied to all premises other than those in which amorphous phosphorus alone was used. They required the processes of mixing, dipping and drying to be carried out in (a) separate part(s) of the factory. Employers were required to ventilate mixing, dipping and drying operations so as to prevent phosphorus fumes from penetrating other parts of the factory. They were also obliged to provide workers with washing facilities and to take steps to see that they were used. All cases of toothache or jaw swelling were to be medically examined, at the employer's expense. If symptoms of necrosis were discovered, the factory inspectorate was to be notified. No person who had had a tooth extracted was to work on mixing, dipping, or drying unless in possession of a medical certificate stating that the jaw had healed. No person who had suffered from phosphorus necrosis was to be employed in a match factory unless certified as fit by a qualified medical practitioner.[81]

Clearly some of these rules could involve employers in considerable expense but, by threatening to throw the sick out of work they were likely to penalise employees as much as employers. It was also questionable whether the rules would effectively protect workers' health. They included, for example, no requirement to ventilate mixing, dipping and drying rooms in such a way as to safeguard those who worked in them. Yet mixers, dippers and driers were the most vulnerable members of the workforce. Provision of washing facilities was of little relevance for the prevention of necrosis since inhaled fume was the main causal factor. Furthermore, notwithstanding the availability of a safe alternative, there was to be no restriction on the use of white phosphorus, the source of all the trouble. The emphasis was to be solely upon mitigating, though with little promise of success, the effects of a hazardous and unnecessary raw material. The *Star* dismissed them as 'absurdly slight and scrappy'.[82]

Lowell Satre observes, not without reason, that '[o]n the whole rather little came from this [the *Star*'s] exposé'.[83] In the short term this may have been true, for the 1892 rules were inadequate and, to some extent, inequitable. Attested cases of necrosis (two between August 1892 and October 1893) and many more that were concealed (see next section), continued to occur on Bryant and May's premises. On the other hand, these rules, which owed much to the *Star*'s investigations, did set the regulatory train in motion. Slightly tougher special rules were established in 1894, following the investigations of the Chemical Works Committee. In 1895, phosphorus necrosis became one of the first four notifiable occupational diseases. In 1908, following the Berne Convention of 1906, the UK imposed a total ban on the use of white phosphorus in match manufacture.

Cover up and exposure

Sprague Oram probably hoped that the establishment of special rules would resolve a question that had reflected little credit on the factory department. Consistently minimising the scale of the problem, the inspectorate had performed poorly in rooting out abuses at Bryant and May. Indeed, there were grounds for supposing that the press was more familiar with industrial conditions than HM inspectors of factories. Faced with such a situation the chief inspector might have attempted to boost public confidence in his office by adopting an aggressively pro-active line in his subsequent dealings with the matchmakers, especially Bryant and May. Alternatively, he could have endeavoured to minimise the problem by treating it as a 'storm in a teacup' whipped up by sensationalist journalism. He opted for the latter when, in early 1893, the Skeeles case came to light.

During 1892 Alice Skeeles, then aged 19, was employed in Bryant and May's boxing department. At some time toward the end of the year – she said it was in August or September, though Bryant and May claimed it was not until December – she began to complain of toothache. When Cornelius Garman, one of the company's doctors, examined her he failed to diagnose phosphorus poisoning. Even so the company told her to stay away from work and on 6 December began paying her, as was their practice in necrosis cases, a weekly allowance. The initial payment of 8/6 (42.5p) per week was increased to 15s (75p) when, three weeks later, Garman ordered her 'to keep to her bed'. Payments were discontinued in early February when Skeeles declined to remain under the care of Bryant and May's physician. On the grounds that necrosis had not been definitively diagnosed, the company made no report of the case to the inspectorate. But when Skeeles became a patient in St Bartholomew's Hospital necrosis was promptly diagnosed. The press was alerted and soon some familiar questions were being asked, not only about the conduct of Bryant and May, but also about the utility of the special rules and the justification for the continued use of such a hazardous material as white phosphorus.[84]

Notwithstanding the involvement of bodies such as the Bow and Bromley Women's Liberal Association (a Liberal Government was, of course, in power), Sprague Oram dismissed all this as 'agitation...fostered' by the Salvation Army which itself had match-making interests – it operated a safety-match factory in the East End – and was, therefore a competitor of Bryant and May. Yet it was clear to all with eyes to see that Bryant and May's record was at best suspect, including with regard to the reporting of 'phossy jaw'. Indeed, this was recognised to be the case by the inspector, James Henderson, who, on a visit to the factory told the managing director that the company's reason for not reporting the Skeeles case was unacceptable. The chief inspector, however, was not unduly perturbed. Though he was well aware of previous 'cover-ups' and under-reporting Sprague Oram placed reliance on the first annual statistical returns (under the terms of the *Factory and Workshop Act, 1895*), which, he concluded, showed necrosis cases to be 'so extremely rare as to render the prohibition of the manufacture of [white phosphorus] Lucifer Matches' unnecessary. He held to the view that 'the evils stated to exist in the trade generally have been much exaggerated'. A 'special inspection' of Bryant and May appeared reassuring. The three inspectors who carried it out, in April 1893, reported that 'as long as gelatinous phosphorous is allowed to be used this factory is conducted on such hygienic principles as should ensure fair conformity with the said special rules now adopted'. Later events rendered this verdict particularly ironic. In the meantime the inspectors recommended that the special rules should receive a longer trial before modifications were considered.[85]

An opportunity for further consideration came later in 1893. Twelve months after the introduction of the special rules, Asquith requested the Chemical Works Committee to extend its investigations to cover lucifer match production. On Sprague Oram's recommendation the task was largely entrusted to the two newly-appointed lady factory inspectors, May Abraham and Mary Paterson.[86] Abraham, who occupied a seat on the committee undertook the greater part of the inquiry. She visited all the UK's match factories bar one in Scotland which was examined by her colleague. The other committee members took a back seat, though they did visit some London factories. The results of these investigations were reassuring. Apart from the Skeeles case and one involving a woman named Winter – who was also a Bryant and May worker – no new poisonings were brought to light. Probably this was because the method of inspection employed by the Committee was limited to factory visits, the value of which even Sprague Oram had questioned, and did not utilise the more probing techniques employed by the *Star*. Nevertheless the Committee concluded that 'danger from that disease [necrosis] exists to all workers where white or yellow phosphorus is used'. As a result it recommended alterations and additions, especially in terms of better ventilation and periodic medical examination.[87]

New special rules were compiled. These required all match producers who used white phosphorus to be in possession of documentation from the factory inspectorate certifying that their works were being conducted in accordance with the rules. While this would ensure that all premises had to be inspected once, there was no provision for follow-up visits. The significance of this change was, therefore, limited, especially as, in practice, the factory inspectorate more or less ignored its requirements.[88] Potentially more important in terms of a move towards regular monitoring was the requirement (in Rule 6) for a monthly inspection of workers to be carried out by a certifying surgeon empowered to suspend, or insist on the transfer to 'safe' work, of any employee 'showing symptoms of incipient necrosis'. The possibility of follow-up studies into the health of former employees was provided for in the requirement that a register of 'at risk' employees, recording names and addresses along with dates of appointment to and departure from their jobs.

Owing to employers' objections that the rule was unnecessary, since necrosis had virtually disappeared, that employees would be alarmed, suffer mental anguish and physical injury, and be unwilling to work in match factories, this rule was suspended. The decision, it should be pointed out, was supported by Herbert Burrows, the treasurer of the Matchmakers' Union (and a member of both the Social Democratic Federation and Women's Trade Union League). He believed that implementation of the rule would lead to job losses and accepted that '[i]n the present state of society advantages [better health protection] have to be balanced against disadvantages [higher unemployment]'. To be sure, when a few years later, a dentist engaged on an official inquiry advised Bryant and May to cease employing, on health grounds, a girl with decayed teeth, 'the poor thing cried and begged not to be discharged'. Burrows was, therefore, surely right to suggest that workers preferred to face the possibility of occupational disease rather than the probability of unemployment.[89]

At any event, in the short term, the most important requirement of the 1894 rules was for the ventilation of mixing, dipping, drying and boxing rooms which, somewhat curiously, had been omitted from the earlier rules. Otherwise, the new rules were little different from those they replaced. A few years later an assistant under-secretary at the Home Office drew some significant conclusions about the suspension of rule 6, linking it directly with the scandals of 1898 involving Moreland and, particularly, Bryant and May. It

> only produced the result, that in order to prevent the imposition of the rule, several firms, viz, Bryant and May in London and messrs Moreland of Gloucester, appear to have adopted a systematic method of concealing necrosis cases, by having them treated by their own doctor, omitting to report them and giving the workpeople pensions contingent upon their keeping their illness secret.[90]

In other words, the scandals of 1898 were a direct consequence of the special rule process, for the Home Office, having announced its intentions, showed exactly how they could be side-stepped. This was an open invitation for the unscrupulous to flout the law.

The impact of the 1894 regulations is hard to gauge owing to the impossibility of ascertaining the real incidence of necrosis. In the first year of their operation only two cases of necrosis came to light and one of these was the notification of an earlier case. The new case occurred in a Liverpool factory. As Satre points out 'Bryant and May's public image shone very brightly' until tarnished by further newspaper revelations in 1898.[91] As far as the factory inspectorate was concerned, there was still ambivalence about the hazards of match manufacture. In 1894 May Abraham, H.S. Richmond (Liverpool District) and W.A. Beaumont (Bradford District) all gave the industry a 'clean bill of health', reporting no cases of necrosis and full compliance with special rules. But, as we have seen, such observations might reveal more about the inspectorate's methods of investigation than about the true extent of occupational ill health in the match (or any other) industry. In any case the position was rather less satisfactory in 1895 when Richmond reported the Liverpool case (in which a girl employed in boxing matches had had a large portion of her jaw removed at Stanley Hospital). It is instructive to note that when Richmond visited this girl she revealed that she had concealed her first symptom, toothache, for fear that she would lose her job. Although this was the only instance of necrosis reported by the inspectorate, Adelaide Anderson, one of the second *tranche* of lady inspectors, appointed in 1894, revealed that the ventilation and washing facilities of some factories could be unsatisfactory. Furthermore, her colleague, Lucy Deane, reported on the problems of adapting old premises to bring them into compliance with the requirements of the special rules.[92]

From 1896 it was obligatory for necrosis cases to be reported to the factory inspectorate (see Table 6.4). Two cases were reported in 1896 and again in 1897. While such numbers were not calculated to ring alarm bells at the Home Office, in 1898 the press, especially the two radical newspapers, the *Star* and the *Daily Chronicle*, began to

TABLE 6.4:
Cases of Phosphorus Poisoning Reported to the Factory Inspectorate, 1896-1914

Year	Number	Year	Number
1896	2	1906	0
1897	2	1907	1 (1)
1898	21	1908	1
1899	8 (1)	1909	3
1900	3	1910	0
1901	4	1911	0
1902	1 (2)	1912	0
1903	0	1913	0
1904	1 (1)	1914	0
1905	3 (1)		

Source: *Reports of HM Chief Inspector of Factories*

Notes: Figures in brackets represent fatalities. The 1898 figure includes 10 cases from earlier years which had been excluded from the 1896 and 1897 statistics. The 1902 figure for fatalities clearly incorporates at least one case which had been first reported in an earlier year. The manufacture and import of matches containing white phosphorus was prohibited from 1 January 1910

publish revelations of further of dark deeds at Bryant and May. It emerged that the company had 'hushed up' a case of necrosis involving one of its employees, using the threat of withdrawn sick pay as a means of silencing the victim's relations and dissuading them from seeking independent medical treatment. When the worker in question, Cornelius Lean, died Bryant and May's in-house physicians recorded acute cellulitis as the cause of death. But the bereaved family was no longer obliged to remain mute. As a result of, initially inadvertent, 'whistle-blowing' to public officials and the press, a post-mortem examination and coroner's inquest were convened. When examination of the deceased's lower jaw showed evidence of extensive necrosis, the inquest verdict was inevitable: 'death from phosphorus necrosis caused through working in a lucifer match factory'. Even Bryant and May's medical officers had to agree.[93]

Naturally, all this was 'grist to the mill' for the popular press. But was the Lean case an isolated one, as Sir Matthew White Ridley, the home secretary told parliament on 3 May, or was it, as the *Star* suggested, merely the 'tip of the iceberg'? Within days of Ridley's Commons statement the press was providing details of other victims. Under pressure from MPs, particularly Charles Dilke, the Home Office was forced to discard its mask of complacency and institute investigations of its own. Initially Bryant and May insisted that, the Lean case apart, they had had no case of necrosis for five years. But a few days later, after their surgeon had acknowledged 47 cases (9 fatal) over a 20-year period (4 more were subsequently uncovered), their managing director had no option but to admit that he had lied. It was a case said the chief inspector of factories (by this time this was B.A. Whitelegge), of 'wholesale and deliberate concealment' over a period of years. He recommended prosecution in order that an example could be made of the firm.[94] Although he feared that some of the informations might fail for technical reasons, the principal clerk at the Home Office, C.E. Troup, who had been appointed head of the Department's new parliamentary and industrial department in 1896, agreed that Bryant and May should be prosecuted.[95] He felt that even if they escaped conviction on some charges they would at least incur adverse publicity. On the other hand, he could not recommend proceeding against Garman. Not only did it appear that Garman might have notified the company of the necrosis cases, but his evidence would be needed by the prosecution if Bryant and May were to be convicted.[96]

On 1 June 1898 the case against Bryant and May came to court. The firm was prosecuted for breach of the special rules covering phosphorus poisoning, for not reporting a case of necrosis to the factory inspectorate and for failing to report the case to the certifying surgeon. Following a guilty plea the magistrates fined the firm a total of £20, which was the maximum possible, plus costs of £5 9s (£5.45). The *Daily Telegraph* opined that

> maximum punishments prescribed by the law of the land do not necessarily satisfy the conscience of the community. This one assuredly does not. It would be difficult to conceive a grosser instance of the deliberate and systematic defiance of an enactment passed in the interests of humanity and for the protection of a class who are virtually helpless to protect themselves than that of which the defendant company were convicted.... To a large and wealthy body of traders it cannot be a matter of great moment whether they are fined £20 or £100 and the heavier punishment would not fit the offence any better than the lighter. It is not really a case for a fine at all. Public policy demands that such outrageous violations of a humane and salutary law should entail consequences of a really deterrent nature and this they will never do until those who are guilty of them are made answerable, not in purse, but in person. They should be punished by a sharp term of imprisonment without the option of a fine; and the offenders who now escape so easily would think twice before committing the same offence again.

When it reviewed the outcome of the case the *Westminster Gazette* used the opportunity to direct some barbed comments at the paraphernalia of factory regulation and inspection. For five years 'the whole machinery of detection and prevention', the *Gazette* maintained, had been 'completely baffled'. There had been 'a complete break-down of departmental machinery, which may well make us anxious about the entire administration of the Factory Acts'. It called for more London-based inspectors and also, 'a much larger proportion of women'. Other newspapers echoed such thoughts.[97]

Another blue book

The immediate question that faced the Home Office after the court case was what to do next. To do nothing was out of the question, for a firm the factory inspectorate had previously attested to be of good standing, had been shown to have systematically lied and cheated while some of its employees had died or suffered appalling ill health. Questions in parliament, articles in the press and the agitations of interest groups imposed fierce pressure upon the home secretary to act promptly and decisively. Troup weighed up the options. One possibility was to obtain parliamentary sanction to make special rules that conceded employers no right of arbitration. Another was to appoint a committee to consider the prohibition of white phosphorus in match making. The verdict was for an official investigation by a small group of experts. In June 1898, less than a month after Bryant and May's conviction, Professor T.E. Thorpe, principal chemist in the Government Laboratory and Dr Thomas Oliver, physician to the Royal Infirmary, Newcastle-upon-Tyne – who were later joined by George Cunningham, senior dental surgeon to the London Hospital – were appointed to do for the match industry what they had recently been appointed to do in respect of lead glazes in pottery.[98]

With news of another necrosis case in which the special rules had been ignored, this time involving the Gloucester firm of S.J. Moreland (makers of 'England's Glory' matches), it was a timely decision. Indeed, the failure of the court to impose an adequate penalty on Moreland – the fine was a mere 10s (50p) plus costs of £2 6s 6d (£2 32 $^{1}/_{2}$p) – notwithstanding what Whitelegge termed a 'serious case of poisoning' necessitating the surgical removal of a part of the victim's jaw bone, underlined the limitations of existing law in protecting the vulnerable.[99] Reports from the lady inspectors, whom Whitelegge had instructed to undertake a systematic inquiry into British matchworks, confirmed and amplified these limitations. Widespread ill health among workers, evasion of special rules by employers, ignorance of reporting obligations on the part of medical practitioners; these were merely some of the shortcomings noted by Adelaide Anderson and her staff.[100]

Although an influential deputation, which met the home secretary on 21 July, called for a total ban on the use of white phosphorus in matchmaking, the minister was not lacking for contrary advice. For example, a *Times* leader urged the government to retain a sense of proportion, resist calls for a ban on white phosphorus, desist from 'hasty and sweeping legislation' and avoid 'the expense of increasing the already vast army of Government inspectors'. White phosphorus, it maintained, was 'not necessarily dangerous to health'; personal cleanliness and the observance of a few simple rules could render it virtually safe. At the same time the feminist, Millicent Garrett Fawcett (1847-1929), who was a Bryant and May shareholder, leapt to that firm's defence. After making a tour of its works she described it as a good employer that had simply made the mistake of breaching the factory acts, a fault for which it had been punished by the courts.[101]

Dogged at all turns by Treasury niggardliness, Thorpe, Oliver and Cunningham embarked upon a comprehensive investigation which took them to many parts of Europe, including Holland, Belgium, Norway, Sweden, France, Germany and Austria. Their terms of reference were to determine the nature and extent of the dangers of using white phosphorus, possible ways of reducing those dangers and the practicalities of banning its use. The three men did not conduct a joint inquiry or issue a joint report. Instead, each went his own way and compiled his own report. Thorpe concentrated on scientific aspects of the question, Oliver on the medical, and Cunningham on the dental. Whatever the theoretical attractions of this approach, the practical outcome was a very long, repetitive and indigestible set of documents. It fell to the chief inspector of factories to draft an introduction drawing the different strands of the reports together.

Although Whitelegge, without identifying specific companies, referred to the concealment of 'certain cases of phosphorus necrosis among workpeople', his introduction placed little emphasis upon the connection between Bryant and May's misdeeds and the decision to appoint expert investigators. Somewhat disingenuously, he laid more stress upon the 'generally...unsatisfactory' conditions of British match factories and on continental developments relating to the banning or substitution of white phosphorus. Whitelegge's reluctance to vilify an individual company followed the practice which he had adopted in his 1898 annual report, for at no point in this had either he or the recently appointed medical inspector of factories drawn attention to Bryant and May's culpability. The inspectorate's reticence in this respect suggests that it had no policy of using adverse publicity as a means of encouraging compliance with the law (though a few months earlier, see above 206, Troup had extolled the value of bad publicity in changing manufacturers' behaviour). It may also indicate Whitelegge's satisfaction with the company's concerted efforts to improve things in the aftermath of the court case. To be sure, his inspectors' frequent visits ascertained that Bryant and May had moved quickly to establish a free dental surgery, to provide overalls and clogs for 'at-risk' workers, to improve ventilation, and to provide better washing facilities.[102]

The main question at issue in the Home Office inquiry was whether the use of white phosphorus in match manufacture should be banned, as it had been in Denmark since 1874, or its continued usage made subject to much tougher restrictions. Although Whitelegge accepted that, at least for the domestic market, satisfactory safety matches, produced without risk to workers, were available, he opposed prohibition. This opposition was based chiefly on the fear that a ban might damage Britain's export markets. Although he accepted that their loss might be justified if 'grave injury' to workers' health were inevitable, Whitelegge explained that the findings of the Home Office's independent experts did not point to this conclusion. Rather, those findings indicated how occupational health in the match trade could be maintained without resort to a ban.[103]

Whitelegge's summary accurately represented the opinions of the Home Office's expert investigators. Although Thorpe doubted consumers' need for white phosphorus matches, he felt that prohibition would be impossible without international co-operation. Otherwise, since there was a domestic market for strike-anywhere matches, a simple ban on British production would merely deliver that market to foreign manufacturers. Cunningham endorsed much of this, adding that the loss of employment to 'large numbers of an industrial and deserving class', which would be the consequence of prohibition, meant that every possible precaution ought to be explored before such a decision was taken. Oliver concurred observing that a British ban would export a health problem to the workforce of those countries that stepped in to meet demand. All three experts favoured the establishment of additional special rules. However, while Thorpe was confident that regular dental and medical inspection combined with efficient ventilation and improved washing facilities could solve the necrosis problem, Oliver was less certain. 'There is', he stated, 'no doubt that so long as ordinary white phosphorus is used in matchworks, even with all known precautions, absolute freedom from risk cannot be guaranteed to the workers. Total prohibition of the use of white phosphorus is therefore the simplest and readiest way to obviate danger'. Hence while both he and Cunningham, opposed prohibition as an immediate and unilateral measure, neither dismissed it out of hand.[104]

From Bow to Berne

The outcome of the Thorpe-Oliver-Cunningham inquiry was that in November 1899 the factory department issued new special rules to replace those established in 1894. Arbitration became necessary when the Home Office refused to modify them to meet all the criticisms of firms that objected to their terms. This took place during March 1900 in London with the barrister, Chester Jones, presiding. Although the arbitrator accepted some dilution of the proposed code, Whitelegge believed the revised rules to be 'still far in advance of those previously in force'. Dilke and others, on the other hand, criticised them on the grounds that initially weak proposals had been further weakened by the arbitrator. Their originality lay mainly in the requirement for periodic dental inspection. This development was not always to the liking of workers who, in some cases were ordered to have as many as fifteen teeth extracted. It even prompted some Glasgow employees to take strike action. Bryant and May found a large number of their women workers absenting themselves from work and ongoing problems in securing sufficient women to maintain production at a level sufficient to satisfy orders.[105]

Soon after the establishment of the new rules factory inspectors began to note a steady drift of firms away from white phosphorus match production. By 1907 only eight factories continued to manufacture matches with white phosphorus.[106] At first sight this drift seems to have been brought about by a combination of three factors; first, the cost of complying with special rules, second, the influence of public opinion and third, acceptance that safety matches constituted a viable alternative to those made with white phosphorus. However, closer examination suggests that the third of these factors was more a consequence than a cause of this process. In other words, a hostile public and an increasingly oppressive regulatory regime led matchmakers finally to realise that the use of a safe alternative was preferable to the continued employment of white phosphorus. Meanwhile critics such as Dilke stressed the continuing need for the phosphorus match trade to be banned by international agreement.[107]

The possibility of an international ban was first mooted by the Derby MP, Geoffrey Drage and others, in 1898. In 1900 the home secretary, Matthew White Ridley, expressed doubts about the chances of such an agreement being reached: 'for those acquainted with the trade knew that they had everything to lose and nothing to gain by such an international arrangement'. It was, the minister continued, 'no use trying to find a solution of the difficulty in that direction'.[108] Yet within a few years the question was on the agenda at the International Labour Conferences held in Berne in 1905 and 1906. The practice of holding international conferences on the regulation of labour was initiated at Berlin in 1890. Thereafter, regular gatherings, usually focusing upon some specific aspects of industrial policy, were held in a number of European cities. For example, in 1891 an International Congress on Accidents to Workmen took place in Berne. The British, though involved from the start, tended to be no more than lukewarm about these meetings, as they often were about initiatives for international collaboration in other areas of social and scientific endeavour. Thus, the Home Office viewed the application of a factory inspector for financial help to attend the Berne Congress of 1891, at which he had been invited to deliver a paper, with extreme frostiness.[109]

In December 1904 the Swiss government issued invitations to the fifteen nations of western and central Europe to send representatives to an International Conference on Labour Regulation to be held at Berne in May 1905. Every invitee accepted though the British government, unlike some others, sent only civil servants, rather than ministers, as its representatives. These representatives, Henry Cunynghame (1848-1935), who was an assistant under-secretary in the Home Office and Malcolm Delevingne (1868-1950), who was a principal clerk in the same department, were barred from entering into any binding agreements. The purpose of the conference, which was held in May 1905, was to give preliminary consideration to two proposals for harmonising two areas of international industrial practice. One was for limiting the hours of women nightworkers; the other was for a ban on the use of white phosphorus in the manufacture of matches. This was to be effective from 1 January 1911, but only if it were accepted by all fifteen countries attending the conference, plus Japan. In the event three, Britain, Norway and Sweden, withheld acceptance.[110]

Of course, Britain's representatives were not authorised to sign any agreement, no matter what its terms, but the general position of the British government was that no ban on white phosphorus would be acceptable unless it was supported by proper means of enforcement, was signed by all producer countries and dealt with the question of imports. There were also doubts about the necessity for a manufacturing ban in the UK where, it was thought, the necrosis problem had been more or less solved by means of regulation. Since the Swiss proposals not only overlooked the enforcement and import questions, but omitted all mention of one major producer, the United States, they were doomed to failure.

By coincidence, the end of the Berne Conference coincided with the confirmation of several new necrosis cases at Moreland's Gloucester factory, thereby raising questions about the success of Britain's regulation. This prompted Dilke to criticise the government for its refusal to co-operate with other nations in a ban on white phosphorus. Mere controls, he argued, would never elicit total compliance: 'take the case of a poor woman, who had a decayed tooth extracted and concealed the fact in order not to be put off her miserable work. Such cases would always happen'. He urged the Home Office to reconsider its position. But Akers-Douglas, who had been home secretary since August 1902, declined. To have signed the convention, he maintained, would have been to destroy a part of British industry and to hand a competitive edge to other countries at a time when the special rules for match manufacture were working well.[111]

Meanwhile the Swiss were organising a second conference on the same subjects for September 1906. Britain's representatives were Herbert Samuel, under-secretary of state at the Home Office and, again, Delevingne. While British government misgivings remained, Samuel and Delevingne were authorised to enter into an agreement for a ban on the use of white phosphorus in match production provided all the other states present at the 1905 conference, plus Japan, agreed to do likewise. This did not happen. Not only did Norway decline to send any representatives, but the governments of Sweden, Spain, Portugal and Japan refused to contemplate prohibition. As for Austria, Hungary and Belgium, they adopted the same position as Britain. The remaining seven powers – Denmark, France, Germany, Holland, Italy, Luxembourg and Switzerland – decided that they would sign a convention. However, since Luxembourg had no match industry and all the other signatories apart from Italy had already introduced unilateral bans on manufacture and import, the initial significance of this decision was minimal. For its part, the British government decided to consider the revision of its special rules.[112]

While Britain was not alone in sabotaging the possibility of a more general international ban, the government's attitude provoked criticism in parliament. Hence, the Earl of Lytton suggested that '[i]f this country is to take part in these Conferences at all it would surely be better for the Government to send its representatives to them in rather a different spirit from that which has animated them in the past'. Instead of being a 'reluctant imitator' or 'tardy follower' of continental governments, it should be a 'willing initiator'.[113]

In 1907 the death from necrosis of a Moreland matchworker prompted a review of the anti-proscription policy. The worker in question, a Thomas Davis, had first been found to be suffering from the effects of phosphorus in 1905. At that time, when Dilke had asked a parliamentary question about the case, the home secretary had described it as 'mild'. Moreland were said to have transferred Davis, an inveterate tobacco chewer who had recently lost a tooth, to different work. Accordingly, Dilke was assured that no government interference was required. Eighteen months later Davis was dead. When Dilke resurrected the matter, a different home secretary, Herbert Gladstone, now characterised Davis as a man who had 'long had the seeds of necrosis in his system'. This latest and gravest of a series of cases at the Gloucester firm prompted the Home Office to instruct Cunynghame and Whitelegge to investigate. They found that Davis, a one-legged and therefore comparatively immobile, man, far from being transferred to safe work following his first attack of necrosis, had been given the inappropriate task of removing match splints from dipping paste. Meanwhile, K.W. Goadby, a dental surgeon investigated the working of the special rules while Thorpe analysed the relative merits of various phosphorus and non-phosphorus matches.[114]

Cunynghame and Whitelegge, who reported that Moreland had been quick to adopt the modifications in working practices they had suggested, recommended, as did Goadby, certain changes in the system of special rules. But when they turned to the question of banning white phosphorus they observed that lucifer matches still had advantages over safety matches and also that public demand for them remained buoyant. They also noted that prohibition could throw healthy people, who might have difficulty in finding alternative employment, out of work. Beyond all this was the question of where a policy of prohibition might lead. If white phosphorus were proscribed, why not all the other hazardous materials which were in use in the factories of Britain? On balance, therefore, Whitelegge and Cunynghame concluded that the way forward was through the increased automation of factories and improved ventilation of workrooms.[115]

The government accepted these recommendations. Hence, in April 1907, when it was urged to re-consider its attitude to the Berne Convention, Earl Beauchamp repeated the familiar line that the special rule strategy was working admirably. At this point it had no plans to vary its policy except to ban tobacco chewing.[116] Yet in the following year the same Liberal government introduced a bill to ban the manufacture and import of matches containing white phosphorus. There had been no upsurge in the number of reported necrosis cases, so what prompted this change of heart? The answer is that it represented a response as much to the wishes of the manufacturers as to the needs of endangered workers.

In March 1908 a deputation of match manufacturers, led by Gilbert Bartholomew, the managing director of Bryant and May, met the home secretary, Herbert Gladstone. Bartholomew informed the minister that the availability of efficient substitutes to white phosphorus meant that the trade would prefer a ban on the manufacture and import of white phosphorus matches – 'at the earliest possible date' – in preference to stricter regulation by special rules. The information seems to have taken Gladstone by surprise for he offered no response other than to point out that the suggestion involved international considerations. Even so, in July the home secretary himself brought a prohibition bill before the House. The opposition, in the person of Akers-Douglas, who, previously, had repeatedly denied the need for such a measure, welcomed the move. Gladstone told parliament that the chief reason for the bill's introduction was the necessity 'absolutely to eliminate the necrosis danger'. Without a ban such immunity would be secured only at great trouble and expense. Prohibition, on the other hand, involved no trouble and no expense.[117]

Clearly the government was responding to the demands of the moment, for prohibition suddenly offered an economical and convenient means of satisfying the demands of reformers and manufacturers, meeting demands for international co-operation and offering an escape from a long-running and intractable problem. Less obvious is why the manufacturers suddenly opted for a ban. It was not because a viable alternative to white phosphorus had suddenly become available, for Bartholomew admitted that there had been a suitable substitute since 1900. Neither does it seem likely, given their previous positions, that the manufacturers were moved by a desire to safeguard their workforces. The Earl of Ronaldshay was nearer to the truth when he told parliament that the manufacturers wanted the bill in order to be free of competition from foreign producers of white phosphorus matches. The elimination of Swedish competition, in particular, promised to be of substantial benefit to British producers. The other factor was the prospect of regulations which, unlike those hitherto in force, threatened to impose considerable expense on producers.

The *Factory and Workshop Act, 1901* had greatly reduced the scope for manufacturers to influence the rules by which the health of employees was safeguarded.[118] By removing the old system of special rules, which allowed for independent arbitration, it strengthened the hand of the secretary of state to make regulations for the safety of persons working in dangerous trades. Under the new system there was still provision for objection, including by workers, and for a public inquiry; but the power to modify the rules was left, subject only to parliamentary scrutiny, in the hands of the home secretary, not, as hitherto an arbitrator. Consequently, when, in 1908, the chief inspector of factories speculated about the prospect for regulations covering machinery and ventilation 'entailing large capital outlay', the matchmakers reacted with alarm. Indeed, their deputation to the Home Office spoke of measures 'so stringent in their character as to leave no doubt whatever in the minds of all the Manufacturers, that, if they were to be insisted upon, several Factories would be put out of existence and the rest would be very seriously handicapped'. Faced with a choice of heavy expenditure on remedial measures or a prohibition on the use of white phosphorus which might confer certain competitive advantages on domestic producers, the match manufacturers could realistically reach only one conclusion.[119]

Bryant and May archives further clarify some of these issues by revealing not only the crucial role played by Bryant and May in the move towards prohibition, but also the extent to which business, rather than humanitarian, considerations provided the motive for that move. As Thomas Oliver reported, in July 1898, French inventors appeared to have solved the problem of producing a completely practical match free of white phosphorus. Although Oliver's report did not enter into details, he was almost certainly referring to a new patent process invented by two government scientists, H. Sevène and E.D. Cahen.[120] This used non-toxic sesqui-sulphide of phosphorus as an ingredient of the dipping composition for matchheads. In November 1899 Bryant and May's chairman, Wilberforce Bryant and managing director, Gilbert Bartholomew, visited Paris in order to meet Sevène and Cahen and to negotiate terms for exploiting the patent. The outcome of this visit was that Bryant and May acquired options on the patent for all countries other than France and Russia. After having reported back to their fellow directors Bryant and Bartholomew paid £8000 for the rights to the Sevène-Cahen process. They immediately discontinued all production of white phosphorus matches. This enabled them to close their in-house dental surgery and to cease observing all special rules. As a result, they found it far easier to recruit workers and thereby to increase production and start meeting arrears in orders. Thus, even though Bryant and May were party to the special rule arbitration of March 1900, they had no direct interest in the outcome, except as leading members of the British Matchmakers' Association.[121]

What all this meant was that far from having an interest in safeguarding the right to continue producing white phosphorus matches Bryant and May had a strong pecuniary incentive in seeing the use of phosphorus banned in Britain and elsewhere. If this were to happen it would be in a position to corner as much of the match market as it could handle and, for a fee, to license those companies who wanted a share of that market. This is precisely what happened with British and foreign manufacturers either purchasing licences from Bryant and May or leaving themselves liable to legal action if they used the sesqui-sulphide patent without obtaining such a licence. Thus, Moreland acquired a licence in 1906, agreeing to pay an annual royalty of £350 pa to Bryant and May. Meanwhile, between 1905 and 1909 Bryant and May fought and eventually won, a law suit against a German company deemed to be infringing the patent. By 1908, with Bryant and May paramount in Britain's domestic market – it had amalgamated with the Diamond Match Corporation (a branch of the American Match Trust) in 1901 – the international prohibition of white phosphorus offered an opportunity for the company to 'see off' the international competition.[122]

The *White Phosphorus Matches Prohibition Act* received the Royal Assent on 21 Dec. 1908.[123] Under its terms a ban on manufacture and import was introduced with effect from 1 January 1910. Retail sales were to be allowed for another year in order to give shopkeepers and others the opportunity to shift their stock. The passing of the act enabled Britain to sign the Berne Convention. In order not to disadvantage those domestic manufacturers who had produced only white phosphorus matches and to maintain industry solidarity, the holders of patents for safety matches, that is, Bryant and May, agreed to make their patents available to their few domestic competitors at a modest charge. Hence, as Thomas Oliver observed, the demise of phosphorus match and replacement with non-toxic sesqui-sulphide variety, was 'secured without great cost to the manufacturers, for it has not necessitated any great change of plant and yet what a gain it has been to hundreds of workpeople who have to earn their living in the trade'.[124]

Conclusion

Following implementation of the 1908 act no further necrosis cases were reported to the factory inspectorate. After some seventy years the problem of phosphorus poisoning in match factories had been solved.[125] The main question raised by examination of the history of industrial phosphorus poisoning is: why did the proscription of such a hazardous material take so long. It was not that the dangers of white phosphorus were unknown for, as Charles Dilke pointed out, with little exaggeration, in 1898, 'every fact which is now alleged with regard to that industry was known to Parliament more than 50 years ago and it is a disgrace that no sufficient action has been taken during all those years'.[126] Neither was it a case of the unavailability of alternatives to white phosphorus, for, as we have seen, non-toxic safety matches made with amorphous phosphorus dated from the 1850s. Indeed, Bryant and May's safety matches had won praise at the Paris Exhibition of 1867.[127] Of the various substances used in the manufacture of safety matches sesqui-sulphide of phosphorus, which had been discovered, in France, as long ago as 1864, emerged as the most viable when, in 1898, Sevène and Cahen discovered how it could be used as an ingredient for matchheads. Though a harmless and practical alternative to the dangerous preparations that had dominated the match industry since the 1830s, manufacturers (British and foreign) consistently overlooked its potential, preferring to persist with white phosphorus, even when its perils had become cruelly obvious. As Dixon noted, in 1925, 'it would at the present time appear strange that in spite of the ravages of necrosis, the usefulness of this material was not appreciated until so late a period' as 1898.[128] Dixon believed that conservatism, prejudice and convenience accounted for the lucifer's endurance. In other words public preference dictated the nature of the industry just as, apparently, it dictated that, post-1898, it should change.[129] Yet such an explanation is, at best, incomplete. While consumer preference cannot be ignored – for many years safety matches were slightly more expensive to produce and slightly less reliable in use, at least in certain climates – more fundamental ideological, social and economic factors also need to be taken into account.[130] These factors include considerations of *laissez-faire*, international trade and social class.

Broadly, the perceived economic advantages of continued production of white phosphorus matches were seen to outweigh the health needs of victims who were exclusively drawn from the ranks of 'the lowest of the low and the poorest of the poor'. Hence a ban on the manufacture and import of white phosphorus matches was repeatedly deferred in favour of regulation by special rules, a process which accorded manufacturers, but not (until 1901) workers or their representatives, an important role. As we have seen, regulation by special rules was not unacceptable to industry. For large and successful companies, who were best equipped to negotiate mild rules, it offered an important bonus in that the costs of compliance, which they could easily absorb, could help to eliminate competitors. As a Bryant and May memorandum noted in connection with

German regulations, the effect of the regulations 'has been very good – especially in the way of putting a stop to the small match factories'.[131] Only when special rules threatened to become unacceptably burdensome, in response to the social and political pressures resulting from well-publicised cases of death and disease, was there a change of tack. Meanwhile, civil servants, politicians and others stressed the correlation between lucifer matches and employment and, therefore, the inadvisability of proscribing their manufacture. There was no explanation of why a switch to safety matches should necessarily have destroyed matchworkers' jobs. Indeed, a greater threat to jobs was the move towards automated production which was stimulated by the continued use of white phosphorus. Neither was there any effort either to initiate international talks on proscription or to introduce a unilateral British ban coupled with import restrictions to protect the home industry from foreign competition. Yet such strategies were pursued by overseas match-producing countries. Only belatedly and at the request of financially-threatened manufacturing interests, rather than in response to the needs of imperilled workers, did the British government take action.

Of course, it might be argued that the truth is far simpler; that a ban was never really justified by a disease which, though horrific, was rare; that preventive measures were sufficient to control the small risk which did exist; and that the eventual ban was an emotional reaction unjustified by the facts. Against this it can be said that there is no way of knowing the true incidence of necrosis, let alone of less severe poisoning, even after the introduction of the requirement for statistical returns; that even if the incidence was low, the long-standing emphasis on prevention was not justified given the availability of safe alternatives; and that proscription, far from being an emotional response, was a considered reaction to industrial demand. It is, therefore, hard to avoid the conclusion that in the case of lucifer matches, the state accorded consumers' and manufacturers' interests greater priority than workers' health and that those interests were for many years upheld at the expense of occupational health standards.

Notes

1. *Reports to the Secretary of State for the Home Department on the Use of Phosphorus in the Manufacture of Lucifer matches by Professor T.E. Thorpe, Principal Chemist of the Government Laboratory, Professor Thomas Oliver, Physician to the Royal Infirmary, Newcastle-upon-Tyne*

and George Cunningham, Senior Dental Surgeon to the London Hospital, PP 1899 XII, 549. Recent examinations of historical aspects occupational disease in the match industry include an excellent article by Lowell J. Satre, 'After the Match Girls' Strike: Bryant and May in the 1890s', *Victorian Studies*, 26 (1982), 7–31; Barbara Harrison, 'The Politics of Occupational Health in Late Nineteenth Century Britain', *Sociology of Health and Illness*, 17 (1995), 20–41 and *idem.*, *Not Only the Dangerous Trades. Women's Work and Health in Britain, 1880-1914* (London: Taylor & Francis, 1996). Parts of the present chapter have previously appeared in P.W.J. Bartrip and R.M. Hartwell, 'Profit and Virtue: Economic Theory and the Regulation of Occupational Health in Nineteenth and Twentieth Century Britain' in K.O. Hawkins (ed), *The Human Face of Law. Essays in Honour of Donald Harris* (Oxford: Clarendon Press, 1997), 45–64. For a recent popular history of phosphorus, with sections on matches and poisoning, see John Emsley, *The Shocking History of Phosphorus. A Biography of the Devil's Element* (London: Macmillan, 2000).

2. T.E. Thorpe, *A Dictionary of Applied Chemistry* (London: Longmans, Green, 3 vols. 1893 edn) III, 182; R.E. Threlfall, *The Story of 100 Years of Phosphorus Making, 1851-1951* (Oldbury: Albright and Wilson Ltd., 1951); J.P.W. Hughes *et al*, 'Phosphorus Necrosis of the Jaw: A Present-Day Study', *British Journal of Industrial Medicine*, 19 (1962), 84.
3. See, for example, Robert Hooper, *Lexicon Medicum or Medical Dictionary* (London: Longman, 4th edn, 1820), 679–85; E.A. Kirby, *On the Administration of Phosphorus as a Remedy for Loss of Nerve Power, Neuralgia, Hysteria, Melancholia and other Atonic Conditions of the Cerebro-Spinal System. With the Formulae for its Combination with Iron, Quinine and Nux Vomica* (London: H.K. Lewis, 1875).
4. Thorpe, *op. cit.* (note 2), 194; *Fifth Report of the Medical Officer of the Privy Council (1862)*, PP 1863 XXV, 164–5; 187–8; *First Report of the Children's Employment Commission*, PP 1863 XVIII, 49; *Annual Report of HM Chief Inspector of Factories and Workshops (1879-80)*, PP 1881 XXIII, 115–16; *Reports to the Secretary of State for the Home Department on the Use of Phosphorus in the Manufacture of Lucifer Matches...*, PP 1899 XII, 460.
5. Robert Christison, *A Treatise on Poisons in Relation to Medical Jurisprudence, Physiology and the Practice of Physic* (Edinburgh: Longman, Rees, Orme, Browne and Green, 1829), 134–35.
6. A.S. Taylor, *On Poisons in Relation to Medical Jurisprudence and Medicine* (London: John Churchill, 1848), 295–7. On Taylor see

Noel G. Colley, 'Alfred Swaine Taylor, MD FRS (1806–1880): forensic toxicologist', *Medical History*, 35 (1991), 209–227.

7. T.H.S. Escott, *England. Its People, Polity and Pursuits* (London: Cassell, 2 vols. 1879), I, 256.
8. These figures exclude the one factory, run by the Salvation Army, which produced only phosphorus free safety matches. In 1908 Thomas Oliver indicated that 22 British match firms employed around 4000 workers, 75 per cent of whom were women. See Thomas Oliver, *Diseases of Occupation. From the Legislative, Social and Medical Points of View* (London: Methuen, 1908), 36.
9. Patrick Beaver, *The Match Makers* (London: Henry Melland, 1985), 61.
10. Oliver, *op. cit.* (note 8), 37–41; Michael Heavisides (ed), *The True History of the Invention of the Lucifer Match by John Walker of Stockton-on-Tees in 1827; with an Account of the Ancient Modes of Procuring Light and Fire* (Stockton-on-Tees: Heavisides & Son, 1909); William Hepworth Dixon, *The Match Industry. Its Origin and Development* (London: Pitman, 1925), 14–15, 19–21; Beaver, *op. cit.* (note 9), 18–19; Asa Briggs, *Victorian Things* (London: Batsford, 1988), 188–9; P.A.B. Raffle, W.R. Lee, R.I. McCallum and R. Murray (eds). *Hunter's Diseases of Occupations* (London: Hodder and Stoughton, 1987 edn), 264; *The Times*, 14 Sept. 1842; *Fifth Report of the Medical Officer of the Privy Council*, PP 1863 XXV, 171, 190–2; *First Report of the Children's Employment Commission*, PP 1863 XVIII, 48, 137, 171; *Pharmaceutical Journal* 17 (1858) 410–12; *The Times*, 6 May 1859.
11. In *The Times* the earliest references to lucifer matches dates from 1837. See Palmers Index to *The Times* on CD-ROM.
12. J.E. Archer, *By a Flash and a Scare. Incendiarism, Animal Maiming and Poaching in East Anglia, 1815–1870* (Oxford: Clarendon Press, 1990), 73–4. See also 24 and 251.
13. Quoted in *The Times,* 25 July 1844. See also *The Times,* 11 Sept. 1839, 21 Nov. 1842, 26 Dec. 1843, 5 Dec. 1846.
14. *The Times*, 6 Feb. 25 July 1844; E.P. Thompson, *Whigs and Hunters. The Origins of the Black Act* (London: Allen Lane, 1975), 256; David Jones, *Crime, Protest, Community and Police in Nineteenth-Century Britain* (London, Routledge and Kegan Paul, 1982), esp. chapter 2.
15. William Plomer (ed), *Kilvert's Diary. Selections from the Diary of the Rev. Francis Kilvert* (London: Jonathan Cape, 3 vols. 1980 edn), III, 48.
16. *The Times*, 7 March 1837; 26 Oct. 1837; 14 Sept. 1842; 18 Nov. 1842; 21 Nov. 1842; 4 Jan. 1843; 6 Sept. 1843; 9 Oct. 1843; 26

Dec. 1843; 6 Feb. 1844, 24 Aug. 1844; 5 Dec. 1846; *Metropolitan Buildings Act, 1844* (*7 & 8 Vict. c.84*), s.54.

17. *Provincial Medical Journal and Retrospect of the Medical Sciences*, 24 Dec. 1842, 251; *Lancet*, 30 Dec. 1843, 435–6; *The Times* occasionally carried reports of accidental poisonings from the accidental consumption of lucifer matches. See 2 Aug. 1842 (death of a monkey) and 19 Sept. 1843 (death of a young girl).
18. Dixon, *op. cit.* (note 10), 15–16; Beaver, *op. cit.* (note 9), 21.
19. J.T. Arlidge, *The Hygiene Diseases and Mortality of Occupations* (London: Percival, 1892), 458; Raffle, *et al. op. cit.* (note 10), 264; *First Report of the Children's Employment Commission* PP 1863 XVIII, 137, 179; John Brown, *A Memoir of Robert Blincoe* (Firle: Caliban Books, 1977 edn), 36. Phosphorus matchworkers were also liable to *fragiltas ossium* (brittle bone syndrome). See W.F. Dearden, 'Fragilitas ossium amongst Workers in Lucifer Match Factories', *BMJ*, 29 July 1899, 270–71.
20. *Second Report of the Children's Employment Commission, Appendix to the Commissioners (Trades and Manufacturers) Part I, 'Reports and Evidence from the Sub-Commissioner'*, PP 1843 XII, f253; *First Report of the Children's Employment Commission,* PP 1863 XVIII, 48. On lucifer hawking see Henry Mayhew, *The Morning Chronicle Survey of Labour and the Poor: the Metropolitan Districts* (Horsham: Caliban Books, 6 vols. 1981), II, 38–40. On matchbox making see Margaret Llewellyn Davies (ed), *Life as We Have Known It* (London: Virago, 1977); Raphael Samuel, *East End Underworld. Chapters in the Life of Arthur Harding* (London: Routledge and Kegan Paul, 1981), 21–3, 31, 295.
21. *Second Report of the Children's Employment Commission, Appendix to the Commissioners (Trades and Manufacturers) Part I, 'Reports and Evidence from the Sub-Commissioner', Children's Employment Commission, Appendix*, PP 1843 XII, f253.
22. G.W. Balfour, 'On Necrosis of the Jaw-Bones from the Fumes of Phosphorus', *Northern Journal of Medicine*, iv (1846), 284–7; *Edinburgh Medical and Surgical Journal*, 66 (1846), 254; *Lancet*, 29 Aug. 1846, 248; Curt Proskauer, 'A Civil Ordinance of the Year 1846 to Combat Phosphorus Necrosis', *Bulletin of the History of Medicine*, xi (1942), 561–69; *Fifth Report of the Medical Officer of the Privy Council (1862)*, PP 1863 XXV, 176–80.
23. *British and Foreign Medical and Chirurgical Review*, i (1848), 446–61; *Dublin Quarterly Journal of Medical Science*, xiv (1852), 10–25; *Edinburgh Medical and Surgical Journal*, lxxiv (1853), 123–132.

24. Samuel Wilks, 'Report of the Clinical Society from March 1846 to April 1847: Part ii. Surgical Division', *Guy's Hospital Reports*, 2nd. ser. v (1847), 163.
25. Taylor, *op. cit.* (note 6), 297; Edward Stanley, *A Treatise on the Diseases of Bones* (London: Longman, Brown, Green, & Longmans, 1849), 73–5; see *Lancet*, 30 June 1849, 695–98; 10 Nov. 1849, 498–99; 17 Nov. 1849, 529–30; *Medical Times*, xx (1849), 394.
26. *Lancet*, 12 Jan. 1850, 41–5.
27. *Dublin Quarterly Journal of Medical Science*, xiv (1852), 10–25; *Edinburgh Medical and Surgical Journal*, lxxiv (1853), 123–145; 'One of the Evils of Match-Making', *Household Words*, (1 May 1852), 152–55.
28. *Lancet*, 1 July 1857, 31.
29. *Report on the Laws and Ordnances in Force in France for the Regulation of Noxious Trades and Occupations*, PP 1854–5 XLV, 499–625. On Bristowe see C. Fraser Brockington, *Public Health in the Nineteenth Century* (Edinburgh and London: E & S Livingstone, 1965), 257–59.
30. Arlidge, *op. cit.* (note 19), 456; Hughes, *op. cit.* (note 2), 87.
31. *Dictionary of National Biography. Supplement* (London: Smith Elder, 1909), XXII, 293–94; G.H. Brown (comp.), *Munk's Roll. Lives of Fellows of the Royal College of Physicians of London* (London: RCP, 1955), IV, 92; *BMJ*, 31 Aug. 1895, 563–65; *Lancet*, 31 Aug. 1895, 561–4; Brockington, *op. cit.* (note 29), 257–59.
32. Mixers prepared the hot phosphorus mixture into which the dipper inserted the bundles or clamps of splints which were to become matches. This dipping might be accomplished by hand or by machinery. The dipped matches were then removed to the drying area. Mixers and dippers were usually adults; driers were generally boys.
33. *Fifth Report of the Medical Officer of the Privy Council (1862)*, PP 1863 XXV, 173–74, 181.
34. *Ibid.*, 180–7.
35. Hackney Archives. Bryant and May Mss.D/B/BRY/1/2/571 Papers Concerning 1908 Match Bill...: Ludwig Teleky, 'Die Phosphornekrose' (Vienna, 1907), copied from documents sent by Thomas Legge to Gilbert Bartholomew. Hunter estimated the mortality rate at 20 per cent. Raffle *et al.*, *op. cit.* (note 10), 264.
36. *Fifth Report of the Medical Officer of the Privy Council (1862)*, PP 1863 XXV, 180–87.
37. *Ibid.*, 49.
38. *Ibid.*, 185–6, 188–93.

39. *Ibid.*, 13–16.
40. *First Report of the Children's Employment Commission.* PP 1863 XVIII, 138. See also 48, 54, 141.
41. *Ibid.*, 141–3.
42. *Ibid.*
43. *Ibid.*, 141–3, 154, 159, 161, 171–2.
44. *Ibid.*, 141–3. See also 49.
45. PP 1864 II, 81–90.
46. *Reports of Factory Inspectors, half-year ending 31 Oct. 1864*, PP 1865 XX, 441–6, 449–51; see *Reports of Factory Inspectors, half-year ending 30 April 1866*, PP 1866 XXIV, 427–8.
47. It is not clear when domestic production ceased to be significant. The Commission took evidence suggesting that it remained important, at least in London. At the same time Wilberforce Bryant believed it to have died out in the face of competition from the cheaper, mass produced, article. See *Report of the Commissioners Appointed to Inquire into the Working of the Factories and Workshops Acts with a View to their Consolidation and Amendment, Evidence*, PP 1876 XXIX, 45, 789, 962.
48. 3 *Hansard*, 175 (14 June 1864), 1708–18. More than thirty years later (in 1897) the factory inspector. Rose Squire, noted that matchworkers were 'of the poorest and most down-trodded appearance'. Rose Squire, *Thirty Years in the Public Service. An Industrial Retrospect* (London: Nisbet, 1927), 55. Soon after the *Pall Mall Gazette* (2 June 1898) described them as 'the refuse of the labour market'.
49. Satre, *op. cit.* (note 1), 7–31.
50. Frederick Engels, *The Condition of the Working Class in England* (London: Panther, 1969 edn.), 58; *Half Yearly Report of Inspector Redgrave*, PP 1865 XX, 441–4, 450–1.
51. Satre, *op. cit.* (note 1), 7–31.
52. *Half Yearly Report of Inspector Redgrave*, PP 1865 XX, 441–44, 450–51; Satre, *op. cit*, (note 1), 7–31.
53. Satre, *op. cit*, (note 1), 7–31; *Half Yearly Report of Inspector Redgrave*, PP 1866 XXIV, 269–70; *Half Yearly Report of Inspector Redgrave*, PP 1873 XIX, 71.
54. On the relationship between Baker and Redgrave see P.W.J. Bartrip and P.T. Fenn, 'The Evolution of Regulatory Style in the Nineteenth century British Factory Inspectorate', *Journal of Law and Society*, 10 (1983), 201–22; Public Records Office (PRO) HO 45 OS 8002.
55. *Half Yearly Report of Inspector Baker*, PP 1872 XVI, 123; *Half Yearly Report of Inspector Baker*, PP 1873 XIX, 173–4; *Half Yearly Report of*

Inspector Baker, PP 1874 XIII, 120.

56. *Minutes of Evidence taken before the Commissioners Appointed to Inquire into the Factory and Workshop Acts*, PP 1876 XXX, 789.
57. *Ibid.*, 961.
58. *Ibid.*, 6.
59. On the methods and strategies of the Victorian factory inspectorate see P.W.J. Bartrip and P.T. Fenn, 'The Administration of Safety: the Enforcement Policy of the Early Factory Inspectorate, 1844–1864', *Public Administration*, 58 (1980), 87–102; and *idem.*, *op. cit.* (note 54), 201–22.
60. *Minutes of Evidence taken before the Commissioners Appointed to Inquire into the Factory and Workshop Acts*, PP 1876 XXX, 102, 610.
61. *Ibid.*, 102, 610, 865.
62. Satre, *op. cit.* (note 1), 7–31.
63. *Report of the Commissioners Appointed to Inquire into the Working of the Factory and Workshops Acts with a View to their Consolidation and Amendment*, PP 1876 XXIX, xciv. On this issue see P.W.J. Bartrip, 'State Intervention in Mid-Nineteenth Century Britain: Fact or Fiction', *Journal of British Studies*, xxiii (1983), 63–83.
64. *Minutes of Evidence taken before the Commissioners Appointed to Inquire into the Factory and Workshop Acts*, PP 1876 XXX, 998.
65. *Report of the Commissioners Appointed to Inquire into the Working of the Factory and Workshops Acts with a View to their Consolidation and Amendment*, PP 1876 XXIX, lxxi–lxxii.
66. *Factory and Workshop Act, 1878* (*41 Vict. c.16*) ss.38, 39 and schedules 1 and 2.
67. Arlidge, *op. cit.* (note 19), 456.
68. *Ibid.*, 459–60.
69. *Report on the Laws and Ordnances in Force in France for the Regulation of Noxious Trades and Occupations*, PP 1854–5 XLV, 499–625. On Palmerston as a Home Secretary see David Roberts, 'Lord Palmerston at the Home Office', *The Historian*, xxi (1958), 63–81.
70. PRO HO45 9849 B12393D, Dispatches concerning overseas policies on phosphorus.
71. *Report to the Secretary of State for the Home Department of a Visit of Inspection to French Matchworks at Aubervilliers, Pantin and Marseilles, in June 1898, by Thomas Oliver MD, FRCP*, PP 1898 XIV, 375–84. See PRO HO45 9850 B12393D for letters from inventors of matches free from yellow phosphorus.
72. *Annual Report of HM Chief Inspector of Factories and Workshops (1893)*, PP 1894 XXI, 138–43; *Annual Report of the Chief Inspector*

of Factories and Workshops (1895), PP 1896 XIX, 292–3, 340–2; *Reports to the Secretary of State for the Home Department on the Use of Phosphorus in the Manufacture of Lucifer matches by Professor T.E. Thorpe, Principal Chemist of the Government Laboratory, Professor Thomas Oliver, Physician to the Royal Infirmary, Newcastle-upon-Tyne and George Cunningham, Senior Dental Surgeon to the London Hospital*, PP 1899 XII, 437–730. See PRO HO45 9850 B12393D, reports on match regulations in various countries.

73. *Annual Report of HM Chief Inspector of Factories and Workshops (1891–2)*, PP 1893–4 XVII, 96–8; PRO HO45 9849 B12393D, R.E. Sprague Oram to Godfrey Lushington, 24 May 1892.
74. *Star*, 18, 19, 20, 21, 22, 23, 26 Jan. 1892; Satre, *op. cit.* (note 1), 15–17.
75. *Star*, 27, 29 Jan., 1, 3, 11 Feb. 1892; Satre, *op. cit.* (note 1), 16–17.
76. *BMJ*, 30 Jan. 1892, 238–9.
77. PRO HO 45 9849 B12393D, R.E. Sprague Oram to Godfrey Lushington, 24 May 1892; *Annual Report of the Chief Inspector of Factories and Workshops (1891–2)*, PP 1893–4 XVII, 96–8; Satre, *op. cit.* (note 1), 18–19.
78. *Royal Commission on Labour. Employment of Women. Report by Miss Clara E. Collet (Lady Assistant Commissioner) on the Conditions of Work in London*, PP 1893–4 XXXVII (part 1), 571–4.
79. *Statutory Rules & Orders, 1892* (London: HMSO, 1892), 473.
80. See 4 *Hansard*, 63 (29 July 1898), 474–5.
81. PRO HO45 9849 B12393D, Draft Special Rules for Lucifer Matchmaking.
82. *Star*, 16 March 1893.
83. Satre, *op. cit.* (note 1), 19.
84. PRO HO45 9849 B12393D, letters, petitions and resolutions.
85. PRO HO45 9849 B12393D, Sprague Oram's Memorandum, 6 March 1893; B12393D, James Henderson's letter, 14 April 1893; Inspectors Henderson, Lakeman and Vaughan to Sprague Oram, 14 April 1893; B12393D, Sprague Oram to Lushington, 15 Aug. 1893.
86. PRO HO 45 9849 B12393D, Sprague Oram to Lushington, 15 Aug. 1893. On Abraham and Paterson and the women's inspectorate in general see Mary Drake McFeely, *Lady Inspectors. The Campaign for a Better Workplace, 1893–1921* (Oxford: Basil Blackwell, 1988) and Helen Jones, 'Women Health Workers: The Case of the First Women Factory Inspectors in Britain' *Social History of Medicine*, 1 (1988), 165–82.
87. PRO HO45 9849 B12393D, Sprague Oram to Lushington, 15 Aug. 1893; *Report by the Chemical Works Committee of Inquiry (on Lucifer*

Match Works), PP 1893–4 XVII, 1197–201; *Annual Report of the Chief Inspector of Factories and Workshops (1893)*, PP 1894 XXI, 134–5; Satre, *op. cit.* (note 1), 20–1.

88. PRO HO 45 9850 B12393D, B.A. Whitelegge to Kenelm Digby, 6 July 1898.
89. PRO HO45 9849 B12393D, E. Dixon to Sprague Oram, 15 Jan. 1894; Burrows' memorandum, 19 Feb. 1894; Sprague Oram to Lushington, 24 Feb. 1894; correspondence from match manufacturers; see PRO 9850 B12393D, undated memorandum of Henry Cunynghame (1898); Hackney Archives, Bryant and May Mss. D/B/BRY/1/2/566, Copy of Letter from E.M. Dixon, Managing Director of Bryant and May to Her Majesty's Chief Inspector of Factories, 15 Jan. 1894; *Annual Report of the Chief Inspector of Factories and Workshops (1893)*, PP 1894 XXI, 137–8.
90. PRO HO45 9850 B12393D, undated memorandum of Henry Cunynghame (1898).
91. PRO HO45 9489 B12393D, Sprague Oram's memorandum, 2 March 1895; Satre, *op. cit.* (note 1), 20.
92. *Annual Report of HM Chief Inspector of Factories (1894)*, PP 1895 XIX, 19, 75, 89; *Annual Report of HM Chief Inspector of Factories and Workshops (1895)*, PP 1896 XIX, 137, 251.
93. *Star*, 4, 11, 12, 13 May 1898; *Reynold's Newspaper*, 8 May 1898; *Justice* 14 May 1898; *Daily Chronicle*, 14 May 1898; Satre, *op. cit.* (note 1), 20–1; see Squire, *op. cit.* (note 48), 56–8.
94. PRO HO45 9849 B12393D, W.H. Seal to E. Gould, 5 May 1898; Home Office Memorandum, 10 May 1898; B.A. Whitelegge to Kenelm Digby, 10 May 1898; 4 *Hansard*, 57 (3 May 1898), 171–3; (12 May 1898), 1054–6; (13 May 1898), 1214; *Reports to the Secretary of State for the Home Department on the Use of Phosphorus in the Manufacture of Lucifer matches by Professor T.E. Thorpe, Principal Chemist of the Government Laboratory, Professor Thomas Oliver, Physician to the Royal Infirmary, Newcastle-upon-Tyne and George Cunningham, Senior Dental Surgeon to the London Hospital*, PP 1899 XII, 551.
95. On Troup see Jill Pellew, *The Home Office, 1848–1914. From Clerks to Bureaucrats* (London: Heinemann, 1982), esp. 33–4, 52–3, 71–3, 208; *New DNB* (Oxford: OUP, forthcoming).
96. PRO HO45 9849 B12393D, C.E. Troup's Memorandum, 11 May 1898.
97. *Daily Telegraph*, 3 June 1898; *Westminster Gazette*, 2 June 1898; see *Daily Chronicle*, 2, 3, 8, 9, 13 June 1898; *Pall Mall Gazette* 2 June

1898; *Star* 4 June 1898; *Critic*, 4 June 1898; *St James's Gazette*, 2, 4, 7 June 1898; *Truth,* 9 June 1898; *Daily News*, 4 June 1898; 4 *Hansard*, 63 (29 July 1898), 455, 460.

98. 4 *Hansard*, 58 (7 June 1898), 861–4; *Pall Mall Gazette*, 6 July 1898; *Daily Chronicle*, 12 July 1898; *The Times*, 22 July 1898; for further indications of the pressures on the Home Secretary to act see TUC Library Collections, University of North London. Gertrude Tuckwell Papers, press cuttings, 20e box 4, reel 2.
99. 4 *Hansard*, 59 (14 June 1898), 222; 60 (28 June 1898), 364; 63 (29 July 1898), 460–61; *The Times*, 23 July 1898; *Daily Chronicle*, 14, 23 July 1898.
100. *Annual Report of HM Chief Inspector of Factories and Workshops,* (1898) part 2, PP 1900 XI, 168–70.
101. PRO HO45 9849 B12393D, Report on a Deputation to the Home Office, 21 July 1898; Hackney Archives, Bryant and May Mss. D/B/BRY/1/2/568, Transcription of Notes on Deputation; *The Times*, 12, 22, 25, 27 July 1898.
102. 4 *Hansard*, 63 (29 July 1898), 485; *Reports to the Secretary of State for the Home Department on the Use of Phosphorus in the Manufacture of Lucifer matches by Professor T.E. Thorpe, Principal Chemist of the Government Laboratory, Professor Thomas Oliver, Physician to the Royal Infirmary, Newcastle-upon-Tyne and George Cunningham, Senior Dental Surgeon to the London Hospital,* PP 1899 XII, 474, 552; *Annual Report of the Chief Inspector of Factories and Workshops,* (1898) part 2, PP 1900 XI, 130–1; see PRO HO 45 9850 B12393D, G. Cunningham to B.A. Whitelegge, 12 Oct. 1898 and T.E. Thorpe to T. Legge, 17 March 1899 for reports of an 'astonishing' improvement in conditions at Bryant and May's factory.
103. *Reports to the Secretary of State for the Home Department on the Use of Phosphorus in the Manufacture of Lucifer matches by Professor T.E. Thorpe, Principal Chemist of the Government Laboratory, Professor Thomas Oliver, Physician to the Royal Infirmary, Newcastle-upon-Tyne and George Cunningham, Senior Dental Surgeon to the London Hospital,* PP 1899 XII, 439–46; PRO HO 45 9850 B12393D, file dated Jan. 1899.
104. *Reports to the Secretary of State for the Home Department on the Use of Phosphorus in the Manufacture of Lucifer matches by Professor T.E. Thorpe, Principal Chemist of the Government Laboratory, Professor Thomas Oliver, Physician to the Royal Infirmary, Newcastle-upon-Tyne and George Cunningham, Senior Dental Surgeon to the London Hospital,* PP 1899 XII, 473, 561–2, 699.
105. Hackney Archives, Bryant and May Mss. D/B/BRY/1/2/570

Minutes of Proceedings in the Matter of an Arbitration under the Factory and Workshop Acts between Various Match Companies and Her Majesty's Inspector of Factories; D/B/BRY/1/2/571 Amended Special Rules for Lucifer Match Factories; XP18/1 Directors' Minute Book, 13 Feb., 15 May, 17 July 1899; 4 *Hansard*, 85 (13 July 1900),1383–84.

106. *Annual Report of HM Chief Inspector of Factories and Workshops,* (1900) PP 1901 X, 184, 277, 477; *Annual Report of the Chief Inspector of Factories,* (1901) PP 1902 XII, 206; *Annual Report of Chief Inspector of Factories and Workshops,* (1907) PP 1908 XII, 557; 4 *Hansard*, 170 (11 March 1907), 1224–5.
107. *Annual Report of HM Chief Inspector of Factories and Workshops,* (1899) PP 1900 XI, 259, 613; see PRO LAB14/44 and 14/45 Arbitration on Special Rules in Lucifer Match Factories (1900); *Annual Report of HM Chief Inspector of Factories and Workshops,* (1900) PP 1901 XI, 334, 380, 476–7; 4 *Hansard*, 85 (13 July 1900), 1483–4, 1508–9, 1527–8, 1530–1.
108. *The Times*, 22 July 1898; 4 *Hansard*, 63 (29 July 1898), 470, 473; 85 (13 July 1900), 1527–8.
109. E.P. Hennock, *British Social Reform and German Precedents. The Case of Social Insurance, 1880–1914* (Oxford: Clarendon Press, 1987), 29–32; P.W.J. Bartrip and S.B. Burman, *The Wounded Soldiers of Industry. Industrial Compensation Policy* (Oxford: Clarendon Press, 1983), 215; P.W.J. Bartrip *Mirror of Medicine. A History of the British Medical Journal* (Oxford: BMJ and Clarendon Press, 1990),141–7.
110. *Memorandum on the International Conference on Labour Regulation held at Berne, September 1906, with the Text of the Documents Signed at the Conference*, PP 1906 CXXI, 279–99. The WTUL regretted that the British delegates were denied voting rights. See Trades Union Congress Library Collections, University of North London. Women's Trade Union League. Minutes of Annual Meetings of WTUL, Hanley, 5 Sept. 1905.
111. 4 *Hansard*, 147 (2 June 1905), 569–70; (17 June 1905), 929–30; (20 June 1905), 1098–9; 150 (2 Aug. 1905), 1351–4, 1397–9.
112. *Memorandum on the International Conference on Labour Regulation held at Berne, September 1906 with the Text of the Documents Signed at the Conference*, PP 1906 CXXI, 279–99; *Annual Report of HM Chief Inspector of Factories and Workshops, (1906)* PP 1907 X, 15.
113. 4 *Hansard*, 173 (25 April 1907), 179–85.
114. *Ibid.*, 147 (2 June 1905), 569–70; 169 (26 Feb. 1907), 1414; *Annual Report of HM Chief Inspector of Factories and Workshops,*

(1907) PP 1908 XII, 698–712.

115. *Report to the Secretary of State of the Home Department by H.H.S. Cunynghame, Under Secretary of State and B.A. Whitelegge, HM Chief Inspector of Factories on the Match factory of Messrs Moreland and Sons, Gloucester, with Special Reference to a Recent Fatal Case of Phosphorus Necrosis*, PP 1907 X, 441–7; *The Times*, 6 April 1907.
116. 4 *Hansard*, 173 (25 April 1907), 179–85.
117. *The Times*, 26 March 1908; 4 *Hansard*, 198 (8 Dec. 1908), 206; Hackney Archives, Bryant and May Mss. D/B/BRY/1/2/571 Papers Concerning the 1908 Match Bill...; XP18/1 Directors' Minute Book, 27 March 1908.
118. British Library, Dilke Papers, Add. Mss.43892 ff.259, James of Hereford to Dilke, 10 Dec. 1903.
119. *1 Edw. 7 c.21* ss.79–86; 4 *Hansard*, 197 (3 Dec. 1908), 1746–7; *Annual Report of HM Chief Inspector of Factories,* (1907) PP 1908 XII, 385; *White Phosphorus Matches Prohibition Bill, Memorandum*, PP 1908 V, 951; Hackney Archives, Bryant and May Mss. D/B/BRY/1/2/571 Papers Concerning the 1908 Match Bill....
120. See Oliver, *op. cit.* (note 8), 49. At about this time others were also attempting to develop safe 'strike-anywhere matches. These included Herren S.H. Rosenthal and von Kourocki in Berlin and, in London, a Mr Cordes. See *Daily Chronicle*, 17, 20 Sept. and 6 Dec. 1898.
121. *Report to the Secretary of State for the Home Department of a Visit of Inspection to French Matchworks at Aubervilliers, Pantin and Marseilles, in June 1898, by Thomas Oliver MD, FRCP*, PP 1898 XIV, 375–84; Hackney Archives, Bryant and May Mss. XP18/1 Directors' Minute Book 13 Nov. 11 Dec. 1899, 8 Jan. 26 March, 21 May 18 June 1900.
122. Hackney Archives, Bryant and May Mss. XP18/1 Directors' Minute Book 9 Nov. 1905, 1 Feb. 1906; *Morning Leader*, 1 Jan. 1910. These themes have been explored in P.W.J. Bartrip and R.M. Hartwell, 'Profit and Virtue. Economic Theory and the Regulation of Occupational Health in Nineteenth and Twentieth Century Britain' in Keith Hawkins (ed), *The Human Face of Law. Essays in Honour of Donald Harris* (Oxford: Clarendon Press, 1997), 45–64.
123. *8 Edw.7 c.42.*
124. Oliver, *op. cit.* (note 8), 51.
125. Phosphorus poisoning continued to affect workers in other trades. See Hughes, *op. cit.* (note 2), 83–99.
126. 4 *Hansard*, 63 (29 July 1898), 460.
127. Dixon, *op. cit* (note 10),19–21, 136; Beaver, *op. cit.* (note 9), 24–5, 37–8.

128. Dixon, *op. cit.* (note 10), 19.
129. *Ibid.*, 19–21.
130. On the higher cost of safety matches see *First Report of the Children's Employment Commission. Evidence*, PP 1863 XVIII, 142, 144, 151, 154, 159, 161, 165, 171, 180. *Daily Chronicle*, 14 May 1898; *Westminster Gazette*, 3 June 1898.
131. Hackney Archives, Bryant and May Mss. D/B/BRY/1/2/565 Memorandum concerning German Phosphorus Rules (1893).

7

A Huge Bacterial Bubble: Anthrax in Industry

Origins, incidence and definitions

Anthrax, which has been known by various names including *charbon*, splenic fever and Siberian plague, is an acute infectious disease, mainly of farm animals. It is caused by the bacterium *bacillus anthracis* and can be transmitted to humans by contact with infected animal hair, hides, saliva, urine or faeces. Consequently, anyone who comes into contact with animal parts is potentially at risk. The infective organism can enter the human body, usually as a spore, either by inhalation, ingestion or, most commonly, via a scratch or abrasion. The disease occurs in two forms: pulmonary (or inhalational) anthrax (sometimes known as woolsorters' disease or even *maladie de Bradford*) and cutaneous, in which guise it produces severe ulceration (the so-called 'malignant pustule'). In 1895 the Italian, Achille Sclavo (1861-1930), developed an effective serum and today anthrax can be effectively treated with penicillin or tetracycline.[1] In the nineteenth century the disease was often fatal. It occurred most frequently among dockers, farm labourers, gardeners and workers in trades that used animal products as raw materials. These included the butchery, fur, leather, upholstery, brush and, most notably, the woollen and hair trades.[2]

In a book, which received much attention at the time of its publication in the mid-1980s, a zoologist with a particular interest in rats, Graham Twigg, argued provocatively that the fourteenth century pandemic known as the Black Death was caused not by bubonic plague, as has usually been thought, but by anthrax. In fact most of Twigg's book consists of an argument as to why the bubonic plague explanation is inconsistent with what we know of the epidemiology of the Black Death. Only in his final chapter does Twigg nominate anthrax as a likely alternative candidate.[3] Although one reviewer opined that Twigg made 'a convincing case that the Black Death in Britain was probably not caused by the micro-organism responsible for plague', few reviewers were convinced that Twigg had made a convincing case for anthrax. Indeed, Bill Bynum

TABLE 7.1:
Total Number of Farm Animals Attacked by Anthrax, 1887-1902 (at three year intervals)

Year	Number
1887	636
1890	535
1893	1300
1896	904
1899	986
1902	1032

Source: *Board of Agriculture Returns*

has referred to Twigg's 'rather far-fetched hypothesis'.[4]

The first clinical description of anthrax was provided by Philibert Chabert (1737-1814) in 1780. The bacillus was discovered by Franz Pollender (1800-1879) in 1849, the facts being recorded in a paper published in 1855. In 1850 Pierre Rayer (1793-1867) described how he had inoculated sheep with blood taken from an animal that had died of anthrax. Under the microscope he detected the presence of the bacillus in the inoculated animal. Another anthrax pioneer, Casimir Davaine (1812-1882) later accused Rayer of having pirated his paper. He also became embroiled in a priority dispute with Pollender. Davaine's unambiguous contribution to science was in showing (in 1863) that anthrax could be transmitted to sheep, horses, cattle, guinea pigs and mice. Two years later he demonstrated that a specific disease (anthrax) was caused by a specific micro-organism, thereby doing much to advance the germ theory of disease.[5]

All of these papers, plus the later work of Robert Koch and Louis Pasteur, were written and published on the continent of Europe. French and German researchers predominated, with the British nowhere to be seen. Thus when the Bristol physician and epidemiologist, William Budd, delivered a paper entitled 'Observations on the Occurrence of Malignant Pustule in England: Illustrated by Numerous Fatal Cases' to the British Medical Association's 1862 Annual Meeting, he was able to cite numerous continental authorities on the disease, but only two British practitioners who had produced accounts 'drawn from actual observation'.[6] Why was this so? The explanation might be provided by the higher incidence of the disease on the continent relative to that of the UK. In view of the fact that anthrax attracted much attention in late-nineteenth century Britain, it is possible that, as far as the British were concerned, anthrax was a new disease – a product, perhaps, of industrialisation and the changes it wrought, especially the vast expansion of international trade which led to the spread of the bacillus from areas where it was enzootic. But is this true? Budd felt that there were two reasons why anthrax had been ignored by British researchers. It was a case either that a 'malady which is unlike any other and which, in all respects, is one of the most remarkable to which man is liable, has hitherto escaped general recognition here; or that...malignant pustule (except perhaps as a thing of extremist rarity) is never met with in England'.[7] He opted for the first of these possibilities, for his own experience suggested that anthrax had been rarely written-up by British physicians because it was regularly confused with other maladies. Certainly, Charles Turner Thackrah had noted the ill-health of hair workers without identifying the particular symptoms of anthrax.[8]

Statistics gathered from 1887, when anthrax in farm animals became notifiable (to the Board of Agriculture), enable us to gather some idea, subject to reservations about the accuracy of reporting, of the agricultural incidence of the disease during the late-Victorian and Edwardian periods (see Table 7.1). These figures might suggest that Budd had been right to infer that anthrax had always been more or less prevalent in the UK. But the statistical evidence is inconclusive for it is possible that anthrax became a significant disease on British farms only *after* the practice of importing diseased hides and fleeces had become commonplace. In Bradford, woolsorters' disease, which was later proved to be anthrax, was said to be little known before about 1863 when Van Mohair (produced in the vicinity of Lake Van in Turkey) began to be imported from the Middle East.[9] Waste products from Bradford mills were collected and used in fertilisers that were sold to farmers and gardeners. Since the manufacturing process did not destroy anthrax spores, which are exceptionally durable, it is conceivable that this practice gave what hitherto had been a virtually unknown disease in Great Britain, an established foothold.[10] All that can be said is that while anthrax had 'been known for centuries', in Britain it had been 'almost forgotten' until, in the mid-nineteenth century, its occurrence began to cause concern.[11] In less than 7 years, between 1856 and 1862 Budd had become personally aware of 24 cases, all but one of which resulted in death. He judged that every year there were 'numerous' fatalities in England

and concluded that 'it is high time we should all take serious note of the presence of this disease among us and prepare ourselves to deal with its terrible emergencies'.[12]

From 1863 the Registrar General began to record 'malignant pustule' as a cause of death. Over the next 14 years (1863-76) the official statistics indicate that it was the cause of some three or four deaths a year.[13] Thereafter, under the various categories under which it was recorded, the annual number of fatalities ranged from 3 in 1891 to 21 in 1899. In the six years 1899-1904, 261 cases of anthrax contracted in factories and workshops were reported to the Home Office. Of these, 67 (26%) proved fatal.[14] Statistics of anthrax cases among wool workers in the fifteen-year period, 1899-1913, were collected by a government committee which reported in 1918. These indicated a total of 355 cases, or almost 24 per year, affecting 276 men and 79 among women, among whom there had been 75 deaths (65 men, 10 women).[15]

The accuracy all of these figures is, of course, open to question, not least because diagnosis 'of external anthrax by medical practitioners is sometimes and of internal anthrax is always, difficult' while the obligation to report was, initially at least, not universally known.[16] In 1902 W.H. Hamer, assistant medical officer of health for the City of London, described the official statistics as being 'doubtless...imperfect'. However, he also noted that anthrax was 'of rare occurrence in man'.[17] In the early-twentieth century the number of reported anthrax cases rose slightly, but the average number of fatalities remained below six per year. Hence, the statistics give little indication that anthrax posed a major threat to human life and health. It is therefore difficult to believe that it was the known annual incidence of the disease that prompted statutory intervention in the 1890s. Neither do parliamentary debates provide much of a clue for, at least in the nineteenth century, MPs seldom expressed concern about anthrax as an industrial disease. In 1886, following the death of 21 bullocks, ten sheep and one man in an outbreak at Arnesby, near Leicester, the Anthrax Order, under the terms of the *Contagious Diseases (Animals) Act, 1886*, provided for a ban on the movement of diseased animals, the reporting of all cases to the Board of Agriculture and the destruction of corpses by incineration or chemical means. However, Lord John Manners, the Conservative MP for Melton (Leicestershire) appeared untroubled that 'in many parts of the country' burial was the only available means of carcass disposal.[18] The President of the Local Government Board noted that the danger of anthrax in humans was almost totally confined to those who deal with hides or open bodies of dead animals.[19] Thereafter parliamentary questions about anthrax were occasionally posed, but these dealt, almost exclusively, with anthrax in animals and the prospects of compensation for farmers who lost herds. In other words, in Whitehall and Westminster anthrax was for many years categorised almost exclusively as an agricultural or veterinary, rather than an industrial question.[20] In the early-1900s there was occasional parliamentary discussion about industrial anthrax – usually in connection with the death of an individual worker. This was normally accompanied by suggestions for prevention by statutory regulation.[21] From 1906, perhaps as a result of the influx of Labour MPs into the House in the 1906 General Election, the disease was discussed somewhat more frequently though it cannot be said that the subject fills many columns of *Hansard*.

In fact, the path to regulation of industrial anthrax proceeded less by assiduous statistical evaluation or political controversy, more by way of a series of 'scares' (one might say, 'moral panics') in which anthrax, despite medical uncertainty as to whether the disease was enzootic in Britain, was represented as a mysterious, stealthy and deadly invader from the Czarist empire or elsewhere in the east. The first of the scares occurred in in 1878 when 'a serious outbreak of anthrax' occurred in a Glasgow horsehair factory.[22] On 7 March 1878 the medical officer of health for Glasgow, James Russell, received a letter that drew his attention 'to a report current on the south side of the River Clyde, that several sudden and mysterious deaths had taken place among the workers of the Adelphi Hair Factory (of Messrs John Fraser and Sons), Govan Street, Glasgow'. Investigations revealed that between 1 and 6 March three women workers at the factory had died. Their death certificates recorded three different causes, namely, 'unknown', 'sudden, supposed heart disease' and 'blood poisoning'. Five other women who had experienced symptoms of illness similar to those of the deceased employees had survived. On 1 April Russell was informed of the death of a fourth woman. Her death certificate gave 'malignant vesicle' (anthrax) as the cause of death. Post mortem examination showed that her bodily fluids were teeming with *bacillus anthracis*. Russell attributed all four deaths to anthrax. Although the proprietors of the Adelphi works claimed to have had no similar outbreak of disease in the past, Russell suspected that previous deaths of workers, including three in 1876-7 attributed to pleurisy, bronchitis and *delirium tremens*, had been due to anthrax. He also believed that the deaths of workers in other hair factories had been incorrectly certified. After writing his report Russell's attention was drawn to anthrax cases in other Govan hair works.[23]

What could be done? Russell, who emphasised the importance of prevention, suggested two possibilities. First, prohibiting imports of infected hair, which he recognised would be difficult to enforce since it would require the co-operation of the authorities in the exporting country; or a ban on all Russian hair (on the assumption that Russian hair was particularly hazardous, even though Russell acknowledged that anthrax was epizootic in pastoral regions throughout Europe). Second, disinfection; Russell suggested (erroneously as it later emerged) that the boiling of bales would eliminate all risks in subsequent handling. He also proposed that certain precautionary measures should be taken. These included informing workers of risks, requiring them to wear respirators and close fitting garments, applying carbolic lard to exposed skin (hands and faces), providing washrooms and caustic (for application to suspicious pimples) and banning food and drink in workrooms.[24] There was no immediate move to act upon any of these recommendations.

In 1880 the focus of concern shifted south when 'the attention of the Local Government Board was directed to the occurrence in Bradford and neighbouring districts of an apparently very fatal [sic] malady, locally known as "the Woolsorters' Disease"'.[25] Bradford was, of course, the centre of the British, if not the world's, woollen and worsted industry. Little more than 'an oversized village' in 1801, Bradford grew dramatically in the course of the nineteenth century so much so that, in 1901, its population stood at some 200,000. Although the West Riding of Yorkshire had been a centre of wool production since the middle ages, Bradford's first woollen mill dates from 1801. Hampered by the absence of sufficient water power, the town's manufacturers were quick to see the potential of steam-powered machinery, making use of local iron and coal in the construction and operation of their plant. From around 1830, mechanisation along with a range of production innovations had a profound effect upon the town and its inhabitants. Notwithstanding a number of sharp economic 'downturns', both the number of mills and their average size experienced rapid growth so that, by 1850, Bradford's 128 textile mills employed close to 26,000 hands. This meant that over 50 per cent of inhabitants were directly employed in the woollen industry. The next twenty-five years saw further growth and, in addition, the emergence of the town as an important centre of marketing and finance. The relative importance of wool declined and the industry was badly hit not only by the trade slumps of the 1870s, but also by foreign competition. Even so the 1881 census showed that the industry remained the largest employer of men, women, boys and girls.[26]

Employment in the wool and worsted industry embraced many different occupations. These included spinning, weaving and dyeing, but these processes were all some way down a production line, the first task in which was undertaken by woolsorters. A woolsorter's job was to open the bales of animal wool and hair and to sort their contents into matching piles according to colour, length and quality of fibre. These sorted materials were then washed and combed, though often only after prolonged storage in the sorting room. By the 1870s most of these processes had been mechanised; only in sorting did manual labour remain of primary importance. Woolsorting, which was predominantly a male occupation, could generate clouds of dust and involve contact with dirty and bloody materials. It had acquired a reputation for unhealthiness which, as we have seen, some traced to the introduction of mohair and alpaca fleeces from Asia Minor.[27] Some workers refused to work on certain fleeces; others drew lots to decide who would work on them. But while the sudden death of sorters had aroused serious suspicions that 'something was wrong in the wool', medical practitioners could produce no satisfactory link between the suspect materials and any specific disease. Some suspected a form of septicaemia, while local newspapers speculated on the possibility of bubonic plague. Only with the investigations of John Bell, a local physician and John Spear, a Local Government Board inspector, was it established that woolsorters' or Bradford disease was, in fact, pulmonary anthrax.

J.H. Bell and the Bradford Medico-Chirurgical Society

From 1878, for a period of some four years, the somewhat unlikely setting of Bradford was, at once, a leading edge of medical research and a testing ground for the emergent germ theory of disease. A leading figure in these processes was John Henry Bell, a physician who had first made his name by identifying the disease of miners' nystagmus.[28] On 5 February 1878 Bell read a paper on 'Woolsorters' Disease' to the Bradford Medico-Chirurgical Society (BMCS). According to the society's historian, Bell's paper was the 'most telling' contribution to its sixteenth session.[29] In it Bell discussed the two leading theories of causation: first that the dust and hair that sorters inhaled triggered a respiratory affliction and, second, that sorters contracted an infectious disease from the animals whose fleeces they were handling. He dismissed the respiratory theory on the grounds that sorters were not particularly susceptible to bronchial disorders, that dusty occupations tended to produce chronic rather than acute lung disease, that the introduction of dust-removing fans had had no effect in reducing the frequency of attack and that chemical and microscopical examination revealed no essential difference between dangerous and safe fleeces. But Bell was no more convinced by the theory of cross-infection from animal to man. His main objection to this was that there was no ovine or caprine illness similar to woolsorters' disease. At this point Bell's own theory, which was not based upon microscopical examinations of blood, made no reference to anthrax or invasive micro-organisms. It was that woolsorters' disease was a form of 'septicaemia due to the inhalation of a septic poison produced by the decomposition of animal matter'. Bell's ideas for prevention involved the disinfection or exclusion of suspicious fleeces – though companies that had experimented with washing had given such practices up on grounds of inconvenience.

In the discussion that followed the paper, Bell's ideas attracted considerable support. Although one commentator was reluctant to dismiss the parasitic nature of the disease, another specifically rejected the, still-controversial, germ theory of contagion: 'Mechanical causes and germs should be eliminated from the enquiry. They were not adequate to the production of such sudden effects'. The society's president urged his members to continue investigating the question.[30] In 1879 Bell, having identified the *bacillus anthracis* in the bloodstream of victims, diagnosed the disease as anthrax.[31]

In 1880 five members of the society reported on cases of woolsorters' disease that had come under their care. At the same time Bell delivered a paper which showed the extent to which his views had changed since 1878, probably as a result of Robert Koch and Louis Pasteur's researches on cutaneous anthrax. By 1880 the germ theory of disease was close to gaining acceptance, as was the notion that, as Koch wrote, '*Bacillus anthracis* is the actual cause and contagium of anthrax'.[32] Bell told his audience that he had been wrong to attribute woolsorters' disease to a septic poison attached to the dust and animal matter of fleeces. Instead, the case histories with which he was acquainted 'tended to establish the opinion in his mind that the disease originated in an infective germ-poison, generated in the animal from which certain fleeces were taken'. He had come to the conclusion, he explained, 'that the poison of woolsorters' disease was the same as that inducing splenic fever and anthrax or malignant pustule in animals and that the infective agent was a bacillus called the Bacillus anthracis'.[33]

Although subsequent events proved this analysis to be more or less correct, Bell received little or no support from those BMCS members who heard his paper. One critic, who could not see how the bacillus gained entry to the body, said that 'a more definite pathological knowledge was required before the cause of the mortality could be assigned to such a cause as Dr Bell gave'. Another, David Goyder, who, when writing the Society's history some 18 years later conveniently glossed over his own scepticism whilst deriding that of others, preferred to adhere to the theory of blood poisoning occasioned through the inhalation of decomposing animal matter. A third, the society's president, hedged his bets by suggesting that it was a case of 'two or three diseases mixed up together in one rapid pneumonia'. He proposed that the society should appoint a commission of members to make further investigations. Bell, unabashed, offered to place before the proposed commission all the materials it required and expressed his conviction that his colleagues would sooner or later come to share his views.[34]

Later that year (1880) the society set up a twelve-man Commission on Woolsorters' Diseases (note the plural) 'with a view to the discovery of the nature of the infective poison and for the suggestion of the remedies best calculated to combat and prevent the disease'. The commissioners met thirty times, including to observe various methods of washing, sorting and manufacturing wool and mohair and to conduct experiments on wool dust and animal fluids. They investigated 24 alleged cases of disease, 19 of which involved humans. Of these 19, 9 were agreed by all the commissioners to be woolsorters' disease. An unpublished report, which appeared in 1882, was notable for its differences of opinion, the only point of agreement being that woolsorters' disease involved 'a virulent infective agent'. Otherwise the commissioners were equally divided between the germ theorists and those who adhered to the theory of septicaemia. When it came to the question of remedies the commission had almost nothing to offer beyond speculation that some form of disinfectant, such as carbolic acid, might be of use. The fact is that the disease tended to kill its victims so speedily that the scope for treatment was virtually non-existent. As for prevention, the report had little to suggest beyond the familiar recommendations that the fleeces of 'fallen' animals should not be used and that all other fleeces should be washed before importation. Consequently, in terms of reaching 'a unanimous or almost unanimous conclusion' and producing a 'decisive report', which were the commission's main aims, the inquiry was an almost complete failure.[35]

This failure reflected the deep differences that existed between members of the commission. While these were only hinted at in the report, they received a thorough airing when, in September 1882, the Society met to discuss the findings. On this occasion one of the commissioners, Edward Tibbits, 'charged great inaccuracies on parts of the Report'. In particular, it was far from the case, as the report maintained, that 'a definite conclusion as to the nature of the disease and its prevention', had been reached. He had already, in December 1881, read a paper of his own to the society in which he had dismissed germ theory and emphasised the importance of noxious gases, ingestion of 'excrementitious matter', cold and fatigue. The supposed link between woolsorters' disease and an invasive bacillus was, he maintained, 'a huge bacterial bubble and…it would not be very long before it burst and disappeared'. Bell's response was scathing and, indeed, by this time Tibbits was beginning to look more a fool than a sceptic, for confirmation of Bell's analyses had arrived from other sources.[36]

Spear on tour

In the circumstances of medical uncertainty and public disquiet which prevailed in the Bradford of 1880, John Spear (Local Government Board), accompanied by Professor William Greenfield of the Brown Institution (an animal hospital and experimental centre), visited the borough, in May, to make their own investigations.[37] By means of laboratory analysis combined with examination of case histories, mortality statistics, trading connections and working practices, Spear was able to confirm Bell's claim that woolsorters' disease was indeed anthrax.[38] Like Russell before him, Spear faced the question of what was to be done. A coroner's jury and a committee of Bradford Town Council had already recommended the adoption of preventative measures, a form of which had been agreed by a committee consisting of manufacturers, workers and factory inspectors. Known as the 'Bradford Rules' and dating from 1880, these were essentially forerunners of the special rules that the Home Office began to introduce following the passage of the *Factory and Workshop Act, 1883* and, on a more general basis, the *Factory and Workshop Act, 1891*.[39] They emphasised the washing of dirty fleeces, the maintenance of clean and well-ventilated workshops and the provision of washing and dining facilities for the workforce.[40] Spear, however, questioned whether adoption of these measures would eliminate anthrax. Was it not possible, he speculated, that a warm water soak might actually activate the disease germs? To be sure, anthrax was known to be associated with moist regions such as river valleys, swamps and lake areas. Moreover, Koch's researches in Germany, which had been published in 1877, showed that anthrax spores, which were produced when the bacilli were exposed to air, had remarkable powers of survival: 'Neither years of dryness, nor existence in a putrescent fluid for months, nor repeated drying and moistening, can destroy their power of germination'.[41] Hence, the preventive measures implemented in Bradford promised to effect little improvement – though anecdotal evidence suggests that after 1884, when the rules were implemented, there was a decline in the number of anthrax cases in the Bradford neighbourhood.[42]

Spear recommended action to prevent the wool and hair of dead animals (the so-called 'fallen fleeces') from reaching Britain in bales of uncontaminated material. Separated from the 'probably *innocent*' fleeces they could be disinfected and rendered safe before sorting. One problem with this was that effective means of disinfection which would not ruin the quality of the wool and hair were not available. In any case, as Koch had pointed out, anthrax spores were able to 'withstand the action of most of the chemical disinfectants in ordinary use'.[43] Another difficulty was that of enforcement. Some bales of supposedly uncontaminated wool or hair might contain infected materials. This could be determined, if it could be determined at all, only by examination. If this were to be done, for example by dockside inspectors or customs officers, the risk of contracting anthrax would simply be transferred from factory sorters to bureaucrats.[44] Spear's inquiry therefore led to no significant preventive measures. The 'Bradford Rules' which, following the death of a wool-sorter, Isaac Saville, were revised in 1884, remained for some years the only concrete attempt to deal with occupational anthrax.[45]

Yet anthrax was confined neither to the woollen industry nor to the Bradford region. In 1880 the deaths of two woolsorters in a Leicester factory were attributed to anthrax; in 1882 an outbreak of the disease occurred in the London hide and skin trade. In response to a letter from the London and Southwark coroner concerning the occasional occurrence of malignant pustule among the hide workers and tanners of Bermondsey, the Local Government Board again ordered in Spear. On this occasion he found that most of the 37 cases he investigated originated in wharves and warehouses where the preliminary unpacking and sorting of skins took place. Having traced seven cases, three of which ended fatally, to a Bermondsey tannery in which 'fallen' hides from China were processed, Spear was able to list the countries and ports of origin of the most dangerous consignments. On this occasion he suggested that skins might be rendered safe by immersion in caustic lime.[46] Once again, no action ensued. Why was exposure of these well documented cases not followed legislative or other measures to combat anthrax? The answer would appear to lie in the absence of precedent for statutory intervention to tackle occupational ill health.

A departmental committee

In 1882, when Spear submitted his report, there was still almost no regulation aimed at tackling occupational ill health. Even the factory inspectorate was only just beginning to take cognisance of the problem. In 1880 the inspectorate had investigated the Bradford woollen trade in connection with the outbreak of 'woolsorters' disease'. While it had helped to compile the 'Bradford Rules' it had been obliged to decline requests to help in their enforcement because existing legislation gave it no power to intervene.[47] As we have seen, it was only in the 1890s that occupational ill health and industrial disease began to attract serious and sustained attention. In particular the *Factories and Workshop Act, 1891* focused attention on occupational health by empowering the home secretary to draw up 'special rules' to regulate working conditions wherever life, health or limb were in jeopardy.[48] The 1891-92 report of the chief inspector of factories carried sections on various occupational health risks. In the following year this list was much extended; fully two-thirds of the report proper (excluding a long section on accidents) were devoted to the dangerous trades. In neither of these reports, however, was reference made to anthrax, perhaps reflecting the inspectorate's perception of the limited importance of anthrax as an industrial disease. Only in the 1895 report was it noted that a five-man committee, including two factory inspectors and a future chief inspector, B.A. Whitelegge, who was then medical officer of health for the Yorkshire West Riding, would investigate those industries in which the disease was believed to occur with a view to compiling special rules for the protection of employees. The reasons for the appointment of this committee are obscure but, in general terms, they probably had much to do with the developing interest in occupational health which occurred in the early-1890s. More specifically the spur to action may have been provided by a report from London County Council's assistant medical officer of health,

TABLE 7.2:
Cases of Occupational Anthrax Reported to the Factory Inspectorate, 1896-1919

Year	Cases	Deaths	Year	Cases	Deaths
1896	**17**	**N/A**	**1908**	**45**	**5**
1897	**23**	**N/A**	**1909**	**54**	**10**
1898	**28**	**N/A**	**1910**	**50**	**8**
1899	**55**	**14**	**1911**	**57**	**4**
1900	**36**	**6**	**1912**	**44**	**3**
1901	**39**	**10**	**1913**	**69**	**6**
1902	**37**	**8**	**1914**	**55**	**7**
1903	**47**	**11**	**1915**	**48**	**5**
1904	**49**	**9**	**1916**	**100**	**12**
1905	**52**	**11**	**1917**	**93**	**8**
1906	**62**	**17**	**1918**	**63**	**2**
1907	**57**	**10**	**1919**	**53**	**5**

Source: *Annual Reports of H.M. Chief Inspector of Factories*

published in April 1894, on anthrax in the capital.[49]

The committee visited wool, hair, bone, blanket and other factories throughout the country, concentrating its attention upon premises in Lancashire and Yorkshire. It took evidence from employers, workers, public officials and experts and identified three trades in which anthrax posed a particular threat to human health, namely the wool (including camel and goat hair), hide and skin, and horsehair and bristle industries. For these industries it made certain recommendations, including for the provision of ventilation, use of disinfectants, exclusion of workers with cuts and abrasions, employment on hazardous tasks only of experienced workers and a ban on the taking of meals in workrooms.[50] In the course of this inquiry, following the home secretary's certification of wool sorting (along with the sorting of camel and goat hair) as 'dangerous or injurious to health', special rules for the hide and skin trades and for wool sorting were drawn up.[51] Issued in 1897, they emphasised the importance of hygiene, ventilation and provision of changing and dining rooms. As such, they were broadly similar to the voluntary regulations already observed by many firms in the Bradford area. Disinfection was mentioned only in connection with one material – Persian wool – and then only in the most general terms: 'Persian shall be washed or disinfected as far as possible before being sorted'.[52]

Over the next few years the 1897 special rules for wool sorting were modified, extended and consolidated.[53] However, the one thing these rules, with their emphasis on personal hygiene and cleanliness, could not deliver was effective destruction of anthrax bacilli and spores.[54] Indeed, as was later discovered, ineffectual washing could actually be counter productive in that it could transfer spores from infected to 'clean' materials, thereby increasing the overall quantity of hazardous product.[55] It is not surprising, therefore, that reports of the occurrence of industrial anthrax showed little sign of decreasing (see Table 7.2).

The Anthrax Investigation Board

In July 1905 a joint committee of the Bradford Chamber of Commerce and of local trade unions, meeting in connection with the revision of the woolsorting and woolcombing regulations, decided to set up a specialist standing committee to investigate the anthrax problem. This was the Bradford and District Anthrax Investigation Board (originally known as the Anthrax Committee).[56] Initially set up for a three-year period, it actually lasted for fourteen. Its sphere of activity was the woollen district of West Yorkshire, that is Bradford, Clayton, Shipley, Bingley, Keighley, Queensbury, Halifax and Huddersfield. The Board's funding came partly from the Home Office, which was the single largest contributor, but mainly from small subscriptions, totalling some £250-400 pa. Most of these were contributed by wool and worsted firms located in the Bradford area, subscribing companies being eligible to receive a copy of the Board's annual report. Occasionally individuals, including Thomas Legge, the medical inspector of factories, who had a particular interest in anthrax, and trade unions made donations. Notwithstanding its diverse sources of funding, the Board experienced financial difficulties for, typically, its outgoings exceeded its income by some 25 per cent.[57] The Board was 'established for the purpose of investigating the anthrax question generally and particularly of determining more precisely the classes of wool and hair in connection with which the danger of anthrax arises and to consider further means of prevention'. It did not act as a ginger group for the introduction of legislation. Indeed, in 1906 it firmly opposed Bradford Corporation Health Committee's resolution calling for regulation, including for a ban on the import of dangerous materials. A ban was inappropriate, it argued, 'so long as the Board's operations have not proved unsuccessful'. Probably it was this 'hands off' approach that led some critics to accuse the Board for being either inactive or too solicitous of employers' interests.[58]

For much of its existence the Board consisted of 8 or more local employers from the worsted trade, 2 representatives of operatives, 2 members of Bradford Corporation's Health Committee, a representative of the Chamber of Commerce and a factory inspector – the first incumbent being W.H. Seal. In order to carry out its brief of investigating practical means of sterilising wool, the Board quickly realised that it needed the services of an expert bacteriologist. In October 1905 its chairman, the millowner John Fawcett, discussed the Board's needs with a local physician, Frederick Eurich. Frederick William Eurich (1867-1945) was German by birth and descent, his family having settled in Bradford when he was 8 years of age.[59] After attending Bradford Grammar School the young Eurich studied medicine at Edinburgh University. Following a postgraduate year in Germany he was appointed pathologist to Whittingham County Asylum near Preston. He stayed there for three years, returning to Bradford in 1896 to become a GP. In 1899 he became third assistant physician at the borough's Royal Eye and Ear Hospital and honorary assistant physician at Bradford Royal Infirmary. Soon afterwards he took up an appointment as pathologist and bacteriologist to the Borough of Bradford, thereby resuming the scientific work that had occupied him at Whittingham. Eurich was, therefore, an obvious candidate for the position with the Anthrax Investigation Board (AIB). At its 30 October 1905 meeting he was appointed its bacteriologist. As such he was responsible for investigating anthrax cases, carrying out post-mortem examinations in cases of sudden death, testing wool and hair for the presence of the anthrax bacilli or spores and conducting experiments in washing and disinfection, including with gas, electricity and steam. For these services he received an annual fee of £200. Initially appointed for a twelve month period Eurich's tenure of office actually lasted for the duration of the AIB's existence. From 1907, owing to volume of work, he had the services an assistant, Walter Willey.[60]

Within a few months of taking up his position with the AIB Eurich had established that the immersion of wool in water heated to a temperature of 160 degrees fahrenheit killed anthrax bacilli in 15 to 20 minutes, but left the spores unscathed. In 1908 he reported that to ensure the complete penetration of a disinfectant through all parts of a bale of wool, it would need to be applied under hydraulic pressure. But his 'chief discovery' of that year was that the principal carrier of the anthrax bacillus was not the fleece itself but the traces of blood attached to it.[61] Important as this was in signposting the way towards prevention it was not long before the AIB was receiving criticism from a local MP and two of its own working-class members. Frederick Jowett, the Labour MP for Bradford West criticised the Board for siding with employers.[62] Meanwhile Messrs. Barber and Grundy, AIB members who were, respectively, members of the Bradford Trades and Labour Council and the Woolsorters' Union, complained that after 5 years the Board 'had done little or nothing to eliminate the risk of anthrax'. They suggested that workers' representatives should sever their connections. Although Fawcett expressed his regret and urged the two men to reconsider, they duly resigned their positions. While this was a blow to the Board's representative composition, since it no longer numbered trade unionists among its members, it made little practical difference to its work for it retained the confidence of the Bradford Corporation, the Home Office and local employers. No doubt Barber and Grundy were frustrated by the Board's failure to produce instant solutions to the anthrax problem. After all, its seventh annual report (1911-12) confessed its failure to discover any disinfectant capable of destroying anthrax spore without damaging the fleeces in which they were hidden.[63]

In 1912 a sub-committee of the International Society of Labour Legislation was appointed to investigate and devise regulations for prevention. Yet it was the Anthrax Investigation Board that came up with the breakthrough. Eurich, in collaboration with the factory inspector, Elmhirst Duckering, who had become an AIB member in 1914, devised a means of disinfection that destroyed anthrax bacilli and spores without damaging valuable fibres (the Duckering Process). This involved washing materials such as wool and hair in troughs containing sodium carbonate, sodium hydroxide and formaldehyde. Following the deliberations of a departmental inquiry on *Precautions for Preventing Danger of Infection by Anthrax in the Manipulation of Wool, Goat Hair and Camel Hair*, on which Duckering served as secretary, the *Anthrax Prevention Act, 1919*, gave government the power to prohibit the import of goods infected, or likely to be infected, with anthrax. [64] It also allowed for such goods to be imported only through specified ports in which there was provision for disinfection to be carried out. In 1921 a wool disinfection station was opened in Liverpool with the objective that all hazardous or potentially hazardous wools, hides, fleeces and hairs could be subjected, on one site, to the Duckering

Process. Subsequently, woolsorters' disease, it has been suggested, 'soon became a medical curiosity', the last case of occurring in the 1930s.[65]

Why anthrax?

Medical history has often placed emphasis on the conquest of disease by scientific 'breakthroughs' achieved by dedicated and selfless white-coated workers. The history of industrial anthrax may be viewed in terms of a triumph of medical science and, to a lesser extent, of engineering and bureaucratic expertise over a deadly scourge of humanity. Certainly, the representation of anthrax as a virulent and mysterious disease of man and beast which, having been identified in the laboratory and in the field, was then rendered innocuous makes a compelling tale complete with heroic individuals such as Bell, Koch, Eurich and Duckering. Indeed, this is how the control of anthrax has been presented in at least two studies.[66] But though compelling, the reconstruction is not entirely convincing. In particular, it overlooks the question of why, when anthrax was relatively uncommon – 'rare' according to several authorities – and of localised occurrence it was scheduled as one of the first officially recognised industrial diseases while other, probably commoner, diseases were overlooked? Furthermore, it glosses over the reasons for the long-term twentieth century decline in industrial anthrax while exaggerating the importance of the 1919 act and the establishment of the disinfection centre.

As was the case with all the occupational health problems discussed in this book, official recognition of and action on, anthrax owed something to the growing power and influence of the working class – particularly to competition between the political parties for working-class votes – from around the late-1880s. Following the 1906 General Election, which saw the first arrival of Labour MPs as a significant force, industrial anthrax was raised more frequently as a topic in the House of Commons. Also in common with other occupational diseases, anthrax regulation owed something to the political desire, fuelled by the upsurge of economic and imperial competition to which late-Victorian Britain was being subjected, by Germany in particular, to create a fitter, more efficient workforce.[67] But none of this explains why anthrax in particular was one of the first scheduled industrial diseases. Unlike lead workers, those who worked with hair, wool and hides had no vocal pressure group with friends in parliament – the Women's Trade Union League – or campaigning newspaper – the *Daily Chronicle* or *Star* – to argue their case for protection. When occupational anthrax became subject to regulation there was little appreciation that it was a problem of any significant dimension for the collection of statistics commenced only in 1896. When these were compiled they showed that the number of reported anthrax cases was substantially larger than the number of occupational arsenic or phosphorus poisonings known to the factory inspectorate. At the same time it was much lower than the number of reported lead poisoning cases. The scale of the anthrax problem does not, therefore, explain why this industrial disease was one of the first to be regulated. To appreciate the 'appeal' of anthrax it is necessary to look elsewhere. Should the implications of anthrax as a threat to agricultural prosperity be taken into account?

The first regulatory controls on the disease dealt with agricultural rather than industrial anthrax. Indeed, in some ways animal anthrax was always taken more seriously than anthrax in humans. It was, as we have seen, more often the subject of parliamentary debate. Furthermore, the statistics of animal cases were fuller than those for humans – anthrax in livestock being notifiable, unlike anthrax in humans (except, post-1895, when contracted in a factory or workshop). These statistics show that in late-Victorian Britain some 500-1300 farm animals per year were affected by anthrax (Table 7.1) It is possible, therefore, that efforts to monitor and regulate the industrial workplace originated in anxiety that outbreaks of the disease in Bradford, London or elsewhere might spread to livestock and jeopardise agricultural incomes. Indeed, in 1912 fears were expressed that the use of Bradford mill waste as fertiliser in Kentish hopfields could lead to animal infection.[68] With this exception, however, there is little evidence that farming interests were seriously worried about industrial anthrax as a source of danger to farm animals.

A more convincing explanation for the regulation of industrial anthrax was proffered by an official inquiry that reported in 1960. This suggested that the disease 'became a matter of public concern' in the early-twentieth century not because the number of cases was high, but because of the high fatality rate which prevailed i.e. over 20 per cent in the period 1901-06: 'It was because of the high fatality rate for anthrax that the disease became a matter of public significance and that special legislation was passed'.[69] Because diagnosis was often tardy, surgery impossible and the progress of the disease rapid, contraction of pulmonary anthrax (woolsorters' disease) was virtually a death sentence. As Frederick Jowett, said in 1912: 'even to this day any person who gets anthrax in its pulmonary form, who gets it under such conditions that the surgeon's knife cannot follow it and take it out, is bound to die and no matter what serum is put into him or her, it is fatal'.[70]

Though pulmonary anthrax was a rare form of a rare disease, it exerted an influence far beyond its statistical significance. It encouraged the idea that, whatever form it took, anthrax was, in the words of one MP, an 'extremely fatal disease'.[71] In parliament industrial anthrax was repeatedly referred to as a 'terrible scourge' or 'deadly disease' responsible (somewhat ambiguously) for 'constantly recurring deaths'.[72] Furthermore, Thomas Legge pointed out that the public (mistakenly) 'believes it hardly possible for recovery from anthrax to take place'.[73]

Not only was anthrax represented as particularly horrible, of common occurrence and almost always fatal in its outcome, it was also a slayer of the apparently healthy:

> [He] knew the prevalence of the disease amongst those who worked in wool and also the terrible nature of the disorder. It was a terrible disease and if a man contracted it two days sufficed to kill him. A man went to work perfectly well and came home with a headache and in forty-eight hours he was dead, although previously he was a strong, healthy man. He had seen that happen time after time.[74]

The notion that anthrax was synonymous with death calls to mind Susan Sontag's analyses of late-twentieth century attitudes to cancer and AIDS (see below).[75] Hence, explanation of the public attention devoted towards anthrax in the late-nineteenth and early-twentieth centuries needs to take into account not only mortality rates, but the *mélange* of emotional responses triggered by a disease which has generated its own peculiar mythology.

In the second half of the twentieth century the word 'anthrax' has become associated more with biological warfare than with industrial or agricultural illness.[76] In 1941, as is now well known, the British government explored the possibilities of anthrax as a weapon by exploding bombs containing anthrax spores over the sheep-inhabited island of Gruinard off the west coast of Scotland. Sheep died and subsequent examination revealed much of the island to be contaminated. This contamination with 'viable' spores continued until 1988 when the island was cleaned up and returned by the Ministry of Defence to its original owners.[77] During the 'Gulf War' of 1990 news that 'Deadly anthrax [had been] deployed by Iraq on Saudi border' made front page headlines in the *Sunday Times*.[78] The article, written by the newspaper's Washington correspondent, referred to anthrax as a 'devastating' weapon – 'almost always fatal' – against which standard protective suits were 'no real defence'. It was based on a press briefing provided by 'a senior Pentagon official'. As such, there is reason to view it as having been derived from a partial source interested in making propaganda. It is likely that US intelligence believed that by associating the Iraqi president, Saddam Hussein with what might be considered a dishonourable branch of warfare, the American public (and the public of other western nations) could be more easily persuaded to accept the inevitable sacrifices involved in crushing a tyrant.

The logic that leads biological (or chemical) weaponry to be considered less ethical means of waging war than, for example, high explosive is not altogether clear. In respect of the chemical weapons used by Germany in the First World War Liddell Hart notes persuasively that deployment of chlorine gas 'was undeniably cruel, but no worse than the effect of shell or bayonet and when it was succeeded by improved forms of gas both experience and statistics proved it the least inhumane of modern weapons...it was novel and therefore labelled an atrocity by a world which condones abuses but detests innovations'.[79] Perhaps equally to the point is that allied propaganda saw condemnation of the enemy's use of gas as a useful means of consolidating allied resolve and swinging world opinion against Germany. As the Gruinard experiment indicates, humanitarian or ethical considerations did not deter a later British government from contemplating the development of its own biological weapon. War necessarily involves killing people; the deployment of anthrax, which, if untreated, can lead to a rapid, if relatively painless death, would appear to be no less ethical or humane a way than many of the other methods employed by combatants.[80]

Current attitudes towards biological weapons are perhaps conditioned by the fact that over the last century and a half mankind has battled to minimise or eliminate the ravages of infective micro-organisms. In these circumstances the idea of a part of humanity turning this historical process on its head by systematically deploying bacilli or viruses against its fellows is repugnant. After all, even the viral assault on rabbits, a serious farming 'pest', by means of myxomatosis in the 1950s came to be viewed by many as morally insupportable. Although there are few well documented instances of the use of biological weapons against human adversaries, the association of anthrax and armed conflict does much to explain not only why the disease is now viewed with fear and loathing, but why it has been 'mythologised' so that, for example, it is regarded as having been far more prevalent and more easily transmissable than was ever the case. Thus, in an essay published in the 1950s, which reviewed Bradford's nineteenth century experience of anthrax, Geoffrey Priestman claimed with great exaggeration that 'every week someone died of anthrax'.[81] That such myths were perpetuated, not to say embroidered, thereafter is illustrated by a 1960s article published in a Bradford local paper. This referred to anthrax among wool sorters reaching 'alarming proportions...50 or more years ago'. The disease, it is claimed, though with no evidential basis, 'carried off unrecorded thousands.... Even in 1917 1,200 deaths were noted officially – but a fraction of the unrecorded fatalities of the previous century'.[82] However, while such attitudes may owe something to anthrax's germ warfare associations, the disease's military connexion does not explain Victorian, (that is, pre-biological warfare) attitudes.

At this point it is helpful to turn to Susan Sontag's essays, *Illness as Metaphor* and *Aids and Its Metaphors*. Sontag urges, particularly in relation to cancer and AIDS, against the perception of disease in metaphorical, as against scientific or clinical, terms. To do so, she maintains, leads to the stigmatization of victims, that is, as responsible for their own conditions by virtue of their own unsatisfactory lifestyles or outlooks. But since 'any important disease whose causality is murky and for which treatment is ineffectual, tends to be awash in significance', characterisation in metaphorical terms appears inevitable.[83] For our purposes it is unnecessary to summarise Sontag's argument in full, but it is worth considering those parts that appear to offer insights into our understanding of Victorian and Edwardian responses to anthrax. Sontag maintains that attitudes to disease are culturally rather than scientifically determined. This helps explain why cholera, a 'shock' disease of foreign origins and undignified symptoms, was more feared in the nineteenth century than, say, smallpox or tuberculosis even though, statistically, it was far less significant.[84] It also suggests why tuberculosis, usually a disease of the upper or spiritual body, has been associated, especially in literature, with refinement and sensitivity, whereas cancer, which often attacks the colon, bladder, testicles or rectum has been viewed as evil and ugly. Several aspects of Sontag's analysis are particularly relevant in the anthrax context.

First, the idea that disease 'invariably comes from somewhere else', often somewhere foreign, exotic and primitive. This seems to fulfil a human need to blame serious misfortunes on the failings of others, thereby relieving oneself or one's own society and culture from the burden of responsibility or guilt. Such attitudes have been particularly associated with sexually transmitted diseases; accordingly, some cultures term syphilis the 'French disease' while others dub it the 'German' or 'Chinese' disease. In recent times AIDS has been variously claimed as having originated in Africa and in scientific laboratories in the USA.[85] As far as the Victorians are concerned, dirty foreigners were often perceived to be responsible for infecting a fundamentally healthy and hygienic Britain. By the same token, in 1881, in a report on anthrax submitted to the Veterinary Department of the Privy Council Office, Professor G.T. Brown, the government's chief veterinary officer, maintained that the disease was more virulent and more often fatal in Siberia than it was in Britain.[86] In other words, the British form of the disease was milder, if not, in some sense, benign in comparison with foreign manifestations. As we have seen the British routinely regarded anthrax, like cholera, the mantle of which seems to have been, at least partly, assumed by anthrax, following the last European cholera epidemic of 1866-77, as an alien invader from the primitive, insanitary and exotic east.

Second, the most terrible diseases are seen as de-humanising. Sontag cites rabies – a disease of animals communicable to humans – and leprosy – a disease connected with mutation and animality.[87] Historically the number of cases of rabies in Britain has always been very small; as has been the threat it poses to humans – 79 deaths in 1877 'by far the worst year on record'.[88] It has, nevertheless, given rise to periodic 'panics'. Leprosy, though seldom fatal and not highly contagious, has been perceived as plague-like. Anthrax, because it is primarily a disease of lower animals, has clear parallels with both these diseases, particularly with rabies which has also been seen as another 'shock' disease, brought to Britain from outside and as a 'socially loaded affliction', contraction of which meant certain death.[89]

Third, the application of military metaphors to disease. Cancer has been described as 'a ruthless, secret invasion' by alien cells and as 'an evil, invincible predator'.[90] The military metaphor was encouraged by acceptance of the germ theory of causation, for microscopic organisms could actually be seen as 'an invasion of alien organisms'. As we have seen, anthrax researchers were among the first to establish germ theory.

In summary, the symbolism of anthrax – 'that foreign disease' as the home secretary called it in 1912 – involves its conceptualisation in terms of unclean, almost sub-human, aliens colonising and defiling the inhabitants of a pure, unsullied Great Britain.[91] It is, therefore, instructive to note that public anxiety about anthrax coincided with rising public antipathy towards immigrants and immigration. Hence, while Sontag notes that epidemic disease often prompts demands to prohibit the entry of aliens, a historian of British immigration refers to evidence of concern, in 1901, about an 'alien immigration plague'.[92] Hostility centred upon those coming from the Czarist Empire, many of whom were Jews. They were seen not only as offering a competitive threat in the areas of housing and unemployment, but also as an attraction to British women. Their numbers were small, though they tended to be concentrated in certain areas e.g. Jews in London's East End and Lithuanians in Scotland. There were, of course, no restrictions on the admittance of foreigners to Britain until the passing of the *Aliens Act, 1905*.[93] As this account suggests, there are parallels between the geography, psychology and chronology of immigration and anthrax scares. In these circumstances, it is peculiarly fitting that the measure that has conventionally been seen as leading directly to the 'conquest' of *bacillus anthracis*, the 1919 *Anthrax Prevention Act*, was evolved in the course of a struggle with and the eventual defeat of a real military enemy. As Britain triumphed over the 'Hun' and helped to prepare a 'world fit for heroes' at Versailles, so the bacteriological equivalent of the aggressive and aggrandising foreigner also appeared to have been sanitised, thereby also rendering the world a safer place in which to live.

In passing, it might also be noted that fearful crimes also tended to evoke the 'round up all foreigners' response. Most notoriously, the 1888 'Ripper' murders in Whitechapel, for which, of course, no arrest was ever made, were, in some minds, linked with Russians and Jews. As William Fishman notes, 'it was in accord with current belief in British pride and moral superiority, that no Christian Englishmen could have perpetrated such abominations; therefore it *must* have been a foreigner. Easiest to pinpoint were the Russians, settled locally.... It was inevitable [too] that suspicion would fall on the old scapegoat, the foreign Jew'.[94] There are echoes of such ideas not only in the Revd. Francis Kilvert's notion – which seems a curious one for a man who represented a religion founded in the middle east – that '[a]ll evil things have always come from the East, the plague, cholera and man', but also in the *British Medical Journal*'s (much later) criticism of 'Britain's highly promiscuous infected male homosexuals, who are mainly of European stock'.[95]

Finally, though strictly the question lies beyond the chronological limits of this study, it is worth asking whether the 1919 act was responsible for the elimination of industrial anthrax. In the first place, it is not true that the disease did disappear following establishment of the government disinfecting centre. The total of recorded cases of external industrial anthrax in the period 1900-56 was 2145, of which 261 were fatal. Of the total number of cases, 987, about 46 per cent occurred between 1921 and 1956 inclusive. In the case of internal anthrax, only 75 cases were recorded in the period 1900-56 (of which 74 were fatal); 26 (about 35 per cent) of these occurred in or after 1921. External anthrax was reported at a rate of about 58 cases per year in the period 1900-20 and at about 27 cases per year between 1921 and 1956; in other words, after the passing of the *Anthrax Prevention Act, 1919* cases of human anthrax occurred at rather less than 50 per cent of the previous rate. These statistics show that from being a rare disease at the beginning of the twentieth century, anthrax became extremely rare, though not completely extinct. As the Ministry of Labour's Committee on Anthrax reported in 1960:

> The incidence of death from anthrax of both types, internal and external, is now so slight – an average of under one a year in cases reported under the Factory Acts since the end of the War – that it cannot be said that any serious public problem is now presented by the disease.

Yet the committee did not attribute the decline of anthrax to the measures taken in 1919 and implemented in 1921: 'We wish to emphasise at this point that at most only a small part of this fall in the incidence of anthrax can be ascribed to the working of the Government Wool Disinfecting Station'.[96] This was because the materials scheduled in 1921 – East India goat hair and Egyptian/Sudanese wool and hair – had been responsible for a maximum of 7 per cent of the anthrax cases in the period 1900-20. The materials responsible for all other cases were not scheduled, yet the incidence of anthrax contracted from these other materials fell in line with cases arising from scheduled materials. The committee identified six factors as being potentially responsible for the overall decline of industrial anthrax. These were: improved animal hygiene in exporting countries, improved hygiene in woollen mills, improved hygiene on the part of workers, substitution of machinery for manual labour, a smaller number of employees in the woollen trade (down by about one-third in the period 1921-48), and the use of antibiotics (since 1945) which cured anthrax before it was even diagnosed.[97] In other words, neither advances in medical science nor the introduction of 1919 regulations were especially significant in bringing occupational anthrax under control. It would seem, therefore, that, to some extent at least, the history of anthrax in Britain lends support to what might broadly be termed the McKeownesque model of why health standards improved and life expectancy advanced in nineteenth and twentieth century Britain.

In summary, the late Thomas McKeown, who for many years was Professor of Social Medicine at the University of Birmingham, argued that increased life expectancy in modern Britain owed little to public health measures and even less to improvements in medical science. Far more important was a higher standard of living which, in particular, facilitated developments in the quality and quantity of food intake and, hence, the better state of nutrition which means greater resistance to infectious disease. In this view longer life expectancy would have occurred whether or nor scientific medicine had advanced or public health acts had been passed. Although McKeown's views, which were presented in numerous papers and books over a protracted period, came to be widely accepted, they have been questioned in recent years.[98] In particular, Simon Szreter has strongly argued the case for public health exerting a powerful influence on life expectancy.[99] While anthrax developments do not directly pertain to this debate, it can be argued that the decline in occupational anthrax owed little either to medical advances in prevention or treatment or to the regulatory measures introduced in late-nineteenth and twentieth century Britain. Although improved industrial hygiene was a factor in the decline of occupational anthrax, it is probable that the disease would have all but disappeared even if the entire paraphernalia of inquiry, legislation and inspection never been.

Notes

1. *Concise Medical Dictionary* (Oxford, OUP, 1987); Leslie T. Morton, *A Medical Bibliography* (Garrison and Morton). *An Annotated Check-List of Texts Illustrating the History of Medicine* (Aldershot: Gower, 4th edn, 1983), 687–8; *BMJ*, 22 July 1905, 207. If the organism is ingested (eg through drinking infected milk) anthrax may develop gastro-intestinally. Although common in herbivores which graze on infected pastures, this form of the disease is rare in humans.
2. In 1881 a government scientist dismissed the likelihood of anthrax being contracted via contact with infected manure but farmworkers

top Hunter's list of occupations most commonly affected by anthrax. See P.A.B. Raffle, W.R. Lee, R.I. McCallum, R. Murray (eds), *Hunter's Diseases of Occupations* (London: Hodder and Stoughton, 1987), 718; *Report of Professor Brown on Anthrax or Woolsorters' Disease*, PP 1881 LXXV, 413–14; Annual Report of the Medical Officer of the Local Government Board, 1880, *PP 1881 XLVI*, Appendix A no.8, 804–5.

3. Graham Twigg, *The Black Death: a Biological Reappraisal* (London: Batsford, 1984).
4. See reviews by Ann Carmichael and William Tigertt in *Journal of the History of Medicine,* 41 (1986), 485–9 and by Lise Wilkinson in *Medical History*, 29 (1985), 326–8; W.F. Bynum, '"C'est un Malade": Animal Models and Concepts of Human Diseases', *Journal of the History of Medicine and Allied Sciences,* 45 (1990), 397–43.
5. Morton, *op. cit.* (note 1), 687–8; John Theodorides, 'Casimir Davaine (1812-1882): a precursor of Pasteur', *Medical History,* 10 (1966), 155–65; K. Codell Carter, 'The Koch-Pasteur Dispute on Establishing the Cause of Anthrax', *Bulletin of the History of Medicine,* 62 (1988), 42–57; see J.E. Schmidt, *Medical Discoveries. Who and When* (Springfield, Illinois: Thomas, 1959), 26–7. On developments in anthrax research before 1870 see Lise Wilkinson, *Animals and Disease: an Introduction to the History of Comparative Medicine* (Cambridge: Cambridge University Press, 1992) esp. 123–30.
6. *BMJ*, 24 Jan. 1863, 85–7.
7. *Ibid.*, 87.
8. C.T. Thackrah, *The Effect of Arts, Trades and Professions and of Civic States and Habits of Living, on Health and Longevity: with Suggestions for the Removal of Many of the Agents which Produce Disease and Shorten the Duration of Life* (London: Longman, Rees, Orme, Brown, Green and Longman, 2nd edn, 1832), 69; J.T. Arlidge, *The Hygiene Diseases and Mortality of Occupations* (London: Percival, 1892), 417.
9. In Britain little was published about anthrax as an animal disease before the early-1860s. See *Sixth Report of the Medical Officer of the Privy Council,* 1863, PP 1864 XXVIII, Appendix 17, *Report by Mr. Robert Ceely on an Outbreak of Cattle Disease* (Anthrax Fever) at Swineshead, 769–78.
10. By 1905, when Thomas Legge took 'Industrial Anthrax' as the subject of his Milroy Lectures, it was also established that viable anthrax spores could be carried by wind or running water to areas

remote from woollen or other factories. *Lancet*, 18 March 1905, 695.

11. *Annual Report of the Medical Officer of the Local Government Board, 1880*, PP 1881 XLVI, Appendix A no.8, 788.
12. *Lancet*, 18 March 1905, 695; see 31 Jan. 1863, 110–3; 14 Feb. 1863, 159–61; 7 March 1863, 237–41; 28 March 1863, 316–18; 30 May 1863, 557–8; *Report of the Departmental Committee Appointed to Inquire into the Conditions of Work in Wool-Sorting and other Kindred Trades*, PP 1897 XVII, 5. The committee obviously did not read Budd's paper. Probably it consulted a later report which stated that Budd had found no evidence of the existence of anthrax in the English hair trade. When compiling its report the Committee omitted this important qualification. See *Annual Report of the Medical Officer of the Local Government Board,1878*, PP 1878-9 XXIX, Appendix 7, R*eport by James B. Russell, Medical Officer of Health for Glasgow, on Certain Cases of Sickness and Death Occurring among the Workers in Adelphi Horsehair Factory, Glasgow in March and April 1878, with Remarks upon the Communication of Animal Poisons by means of Horsehair*, 321–46.
13. Thomas Oliver (ed.), *Dangerous Trades. The Historical, Social and Legal Aspects of Industrial Occupations as Affecting Health, by a Number of Experts* (London: John Murray, 1902), 623.
14. The figures are taken from the annual reports of the chief inspector of factories. See also Thomas Oliver, *Diseases of Occupation From the Legislative, Social and Medical Points of View* (London: Methuen, 1908), 335; Thomas Legge, 'The Milroy Lectures on Industrial Anthrax', *British Medical Journal*, 11 March 1905, 529–31; 18 March 1905, 589–93; 25 March 1905, 641–3.
15. *Report of the Departmental Committee Appointed to Inquire as to Precautions for Preventing Danger of Infection by Anthrax in the Manipulation of Wool, Goat Hair and Camel Hair*, PP 1918 VI, Appendix 1 and 2, 267.
16. Ibid., 117; see *Annual Report of HM Chief Inspector of Factories and Workshops*, (1896) PP 1897 XVII, 247; *Lancet*, 18 March 1905, 689.
17. W.H. Hamer. 'Anthrax' in Oliver, *op. cit.* (note 13), 621, 623.
18. The decomposition of animals dead from anthrax can lead to the entry of anthrax spores into the soil, thereby creating contaminated pasture. However, the formation of spores follows exposure of bacilli to the atmosphere. Burial of a recently deceased, unopened, animal will result in the rapid destruction of the bacilli and therby precluding spore formation. See *Ministry of Labour. Report of the*

Committee of Inquiry on Anthrax, PP 1959-60 VIII, 1001.

19. 3 *Hansard,* 308 (7 Sept. 1886), 1467–8; 312 (25 March 1887), 1468–9.
20. In the 1890s *Hansard* index entries for anthrax direct the reader to 'Agriculture'; the Parliamentary Papers index advises: 'see Cattle'. Compensation to farmers whose animals died of anthrax was not paid. It was available only to those required to slaughter herds. Compulsory slaughter was seldom necessary in anthrax cases because the progress of the disease was so rapid.
21. See eg 4 *Hansard,* 131 (17 March 1904), 1384; 139 (1 Aug. 1904), 260; 139 (4 Aug. 1904), 1008, 1013, 1028.
22. *Report of the Departmental Committee Appointed to Inquire into the Conditions of Work in Wool-Sorting and other Kindred Trades,* PP 1897 XVII, 5.
23. A*nnual Report of the Medical Officer of the Local Government Board,1878,* PP 1878-9 XXIX, Appendix 7, Report by James B. Russell, 321–5, 336–7, 345–6.
24. *Ibid.*
25. *Annual Report of the Medical Officer of the Local Government Board,* 1880, PP 1881 XLVI, Appendix A no.8, 788.
26. See Karl Ittmann, *Work, Gender and Family in Victorian England* (Basingstoke: Macmillan, 1995), particularly chapter 1. Notwithstanding its title, Bradford supplies this book's exclusive focus. See also Jack Reynolds, *The Great Paternalist. Titus Salt and the Growth of Nineteenth Century Bradford* (London: St Martin's Press, 1983).
27. *Annual Report of the Medical Officer of the Local Government Board, 1880,* PP 1881 XLVI, Appendix A no.8, 804–5.
28. Margaret Bligh, *Dr Eurich of Bradford* (London: James Clarke, 1960), 83.
29. West Yorkshire Archives Bradford (WYAB), 40D89/1, Bradford Medico-Chirurgical Society, 1874-1934, *History, Rules and Reports; David Goyder, History of the First Twenty-Five Years of the Bradford Medico-Chirurgical Society* (Bradford: Toothill, 1898), 29–30.
30. WYAB, 40D89/2, Bradford Medico-Chirurgical Society, 1874-1934, Minutes, 1874-84.
31. *Lancet*, 20 Dec. 1879, 920; see A.H. Japp, *Industrial Curiosities. Glances Here and There in the World of Labour* (London: Marshall Japp & Co., 1882), 68–73.
32. Quoted in Carter, *op. cit.* (note 5), 48.
33. WYAB, 40D89/2, Bradford Medico-Chirurgical Society, 1874-1934,

Minutes, 1874-84.

34. *Ibid.*
35. *Ibid.*; Bradford Central Library Local Collection, Bradford Medico-Chirurgical Society. *Report of the Commission on Woolsorters' Disease* (Bradford: Toothill, 1882).
36. WYAB, 40D89/2, Bradford Medico-Chirurgical Society, 1874-1934, Minutes, 1874-84.
37. *Annual Report of the Medical Officer of the Local Government Board, 1880,* PP 1881 XLVI, vi-vii, Appendix A no.8, 788–857. On the Brown Institution and Professor Greenfield see Wilkinson, *op. cit.* (note 3), chapter 10; Sir Graham Wilson, 'The Brown Animal Sanitary Institution', *Journal of Hygiene*, 82 (1979), 155–76, 337–52, 501–21 and 83 (1979) 171–97; W.D. Tigertt, 'Anthrax. William Smith Greenfield, MD FRCP, Professor Superintendent the Brown Animal Sanctuary Institution (1878-1881) Concerning the Priority Due to him for the Production of the First Vaccine against Anthrax', *Journal of Hygiene*, 85 (1980), 415–20.
38. *Annual Report of the Medical Officer of the Local Government Board, 1880*, PP 1881 XLVI, Appendix A no.8, 788.
39. *46 & 47 Vict. c.53*; *54 & 55 Vict. c.75*. As stated above, regulation by special rules dates back to the *Mines Act, 1855* (*18 & 19 Vict. c.108*).
40. *Annual Report of HM Chief Inspector of Factories and Workshops, (1879-80*) PP 1881 XXIII, 129–40.
41. F. Marc Laforce, 'Woolsorters' Disease in England', *Bulletin of the New York Academy of Medicine*, 54 (1978), 956–63; *Ministry of Labour. Report of the Committee of Inquiry on Anthrax*, PP 1959-60 VIII, 1001.
42. See e.g. F.W. Eurich, 'Anthrax in the Woollen Industry, with Special Reference to Bradford', *Proceedings of the Royal Society of Medicine*, VI (1912-13), 219.
43. *Annual Report of the Medical Officer of theLocal Government Board, (1880)* PP 1881 XLVI, Appendix A no.8, 'Report by Mr. J. Spear on the so-called "Woolsorters' Disease," as Observed in Bradford and in Neighbouring Districts in the West Riding of Yorkshire', 830–5; see *Report of the Committee on Dangerous Trades (Anthrax), P*P 1897 XVII, 7–9.
44. See *Report of Professor Brown on Anthrax or Woolsorters' Disease,* PP 1881 LXXV, 414.
45. In an amended form the 'Bradford Rules' were adopted by the Borough of Keighley.

46. *Annual Report of the Medical Officer of theLocal Government Board, 1882*, PP 1883 XXVIII, viii and Appendix 13, *Report by John Spear on the Occurrence of Anthrax amongst Persons Engaged in the London Hide and Skin Trades*, 746–81.
47. *Annual Report of HM Chief Inspector of Factories and Workshops* (1895), PP 1896 XIX, 120–22.
48. 54 & 55 Vict. c.75 ss.8–12.
49. *Report of the Departmental Committee Appointed to Inquire into the Conditions of Work in Wool-Sorting and other Kindred Trades,* PP 1897 XVII, 7.
50. *Ibid.*, 12.
51. *Statutory Rules & Orders*, 1896 no. 646 (London: HMSO, 1896), 110–1.
52. *Report of the Departmental Committee Appointed to Inquire into the Conditions of Work in Wool-Sorting and other Kindred Trades,* PP 1897 XVII, Appendix iv; *Annual Report of HM Chief Inspector of Factories and Workshops.* (1897) PP 1898 XIV, 63–4; *Statutory Rules & Orders 1896* (note 51).
53. *Statutory Rules & Orders,* 1898 no. 278 (London: HMSO, 1898), 358; *Statutory Rules & Orders, 1899* no. 841 (London: HMSO, 1899), 603–4; *Statutory Rules & Orders, 1905* no. 1293 (London: HMSO, 1905), 90–6.
54. *Report of the Departmental Committee Appointed to Inquire into the Conditions of Work in Wool-Sorting and other Kindred Trades,* PP 1897 XVII, 9; see 4 *Hansard,* 162 (1 Aug. 1906), 1105–6 where Jowett suggested that pressurised steam heated to 230 degrees fahrenheit would remove danger while Herbert Gladstone pointed out that the search for effective disinfection continued.
55. Public Record Office (PRO) LAB 46/10, Seventh Annual Report of the Anthrax Investigation Board (AIB).
56. PRO LAB 46/4, Summary of Evidence Contained in the Annual Reports of the AIB.
57. WYAB, Anthrax Investigation Board, (AIB), 71D80/1/66, Minutes, 1905-19. On AIB finances see PRO LAB 46/1-16, *Annual Reports of the AIB*, 1906–18; Lancet, 18 March 1905, 689–96; 25 March, 765–6; 1 April, 841–6. See PRO LAB 46/3, T.M. Legge, *Report on the Incidence of Anthrax in the Manipulation of Horsehair and Bristles* (London: HMSO, 1906); Thomas Legge, *Industrial Maladies* (London: OUP, 1934), 36–44. A colleague, Rose Squire, called Legge 'the expert on the subject'. Rose E. Squire, *Thirty Years in the Public Service. An Industrial Retrospect* (London: Nisbet & Co.,

1927), 59.

58. WYAB, 39D84/1, Anthrax Investigation Board (AIB) Correspondence; Bradford Central Library (BCL), AIB Annual Reports; WYAB, 71D80/1/66AIB, AIB Minutes, 1905-19. Meetings of 23 April, 2 May, 9 Oct. 1906, 27 Dec. 1910, 12 Jan. 1911, 9 Feb. 1912; PRO LAB 46/4, Summary of Evidence Contained in the Annual Reports of the AIB.
59. Prior to the First World War Bradford had a thriving German community. See J.B. Priestley, *English Journey* (London: BCA, 1984 edn), 124-25.
60. WYAB, 71D80/1/66, AIB Minutes, 1905-19. Meetings of 30 Oct. 1905, 14 Aug. 1907; PRO LAB 46/5, First Annual Report of the AIB. PRO LAB 46/6, Second Annual Report of the AIB; Bligh, *op. cit.* (note 28), esp. chapters I and X.
61. PRO LAB 46/7, Third Annual Report of the AIB.
62. PRO LAB 46/4, Summary of Evidence Contained in the Annual Reports of the AIB. Jowett had personal experience of working conditions in Bradford mills both as an operative worker and in management. Born in 1864 he became a child worker at the age of eight. He ultimately became a mill manager. See Dod's *Parliamentary Companion, 1910* (London: Whittaker, 1910).
63. WYAB, 71D80/1/66, AIB Minutes, 1905-19. Meetings of 27 Dec. 1910, 30 March 1911, 9 Feb. 1912; BCL, AIB 7th Annual Report (1911-12), 19; PRO LAB 46/4, Summary of Evidence Contained in the Annual Reports of the AIB; PRO LAB 46/10, Seventh Annual Report of the AIB. See also *Yorkshire Observer*, 1 Dec. 1913.
64. PP 1918 VI; 9 & 10 Geo. V c.23.
65. Laforce, *op. cit.* (note 41), 962.
66. *Ibid.*, and Raffle *et al.*, *op. cit.* (note 2), 718–25.
67. Bernard Semmel, *Imperialism and Social Reform. English Social-Imperial Thought, 1895-1914* (London: George Allen & Unwin, 1960); B.B. Gilbert, *The Evolution of National Insurance in Great Britain. The Origins of the Welfare State* (London: Michael Joseph, 1966); G.R. Searle, *The Quest for National Efficiency. A Study in British Politics and Political Thought, 1899-1914* (Oxford: Basil Blackwell, 1971); J.R. Hay, *The Origins of the Liberal Welfare Reforms, 1906-1914* (London and Basingstoke: Macmillan, 1975); Tony Novak, *Poverty and the State. An Historical Sociology* (Milton Keynes: Open University Press, 1988); Geoffrey Finlayson, *Citizen, State and Social Welfare in Britain, 1830-1990* (Oxford: OUP, 1994).
68. 5 *Hansard*, 44 (2 Dec. 1912), 1860-61; see *Lancet*, 18 March 1905,

695.

69. *Ministry of Labour. Report of the Committee of Inquiry on Anthrax*, PP 1959-60 VIII, 1003. The committee stated (1061) that: 'If anthrax were not liable to kill it would not be a disease of any particular significance in this country, where few people contract it'. See 4 *Hansard*, 74 (7 July 1899), 235 where a Bradford MP claimed that around 50 per cent of industrial anthrax cases were fatal. In 1905 Legge estimated the mortality rate to be 'at least 25 per cent'. See also *Lancet*, 25 March 1905, 765.
70. 5 *Hansard*, 41 (17 July 1912) 464. Between 1900 and 1956 inclusive seventy-five cases of internal anthrax were recorded. Of these, seventy-four terminated fatally. *Ministry of Labour. Report of the Committee of Inquiry on Anthrax*, PP 1959-60 VIII, 1104.
71. 5 *Hansard*, 40 (26 June 1912), 338.
72. See eg 4 *Hansard*, 162 (1 Aug. 1906), 1094, 1097, 1105; 5 *Hansard*, 18 (20 June 1910), 49; 41 (17 July 1912), 466.
73. *Lancet*, 18 March 1905, 689–90.
74. 4 *Hansard*, 162 (1 Aug. 1906), 1097. Said by William Byles, a Bradford man who was MP for Salford North. He had been a journalist and chief proprietor of the *Bradford Observer* which had been founded by Byles's father. See Dod's *Parliamentary Companion 1906* (London: Whittaker, 1906).
75. S. Sontag, *Illness as Metaphor* (London: Allen Lane: 1979); *idem.*, *Aids and Its Metaphors* (London: Allen Lane, 1989).
76. See Robert Harris and Jeremy Paxman, *A Higher Form of Killing. The Secret Story of Gas and Germ Warfare* (London: Chatto & Windus, 1983).
77. R.J. Manchee *et al.*, 'Bacillus Anthracis on Gruinard Island' *Nature*, 19 Nov. 1981, 254–5.
78. 2 Sept. 1990. Use of anthrax as a biological weapon made front page headlines following the 11 September 2001 attacks on the Pentagon and World Trade Centre. See *The Times*, 9 Oct. 2001.
79. B.H. Liddell Hart, *History of the First World War* (London: Cassell, 1970 edn), 195–6.
80. On the ethics of bombing urban targets in the Second World War see Stephen A. Garrett, *Ethics and Air Power in World War II: the British Bombing of German Cities* (New York: St. Martin's Press, 1997).
81. Geoffrey Priestman, 'Frederick William Eurich and Anthrax – the Woolsorters' Disease', *Journal of the Bradford Textile Society*, (1956-7), 107–10.

82. *Bradford Telegraph and Argus*, 2 June 1967.
83. Sontag, *op. cit.* (note 75), *Aids and its Metaphors, op. cit.* (note 75), 58.
84. R.J. Morris, *Cholera 1832 The Social Response to an Epidemic* (London: Croom Helm, 1976); Charles Rosenberg, *The Cholera Years. The United States in 1832, 1849 and 1866* (Chicago: University of Chicago Press, 1962); F.B. Smith, *The Retreat of Tuberculosis, 1850-1950* (Beckenham: Croom Helm, 1988); Linda Bryder, *Below the Magic Mountain. A Social History of Tuberculosis in Twentieth Century Britain* (Oxford: Clarendon Press, 1988).
85. Sontag, *op. cit.* (note 75), *Aids and Its Metaphors, op. cit.* (note 75), 47–8, 50–4.
86. *Report of Professor Brown on Anthrax or Woolsorters' Disease,* PP 1881 LXXV, 413. On Brown see *Dictionary of National Biography. Second Supplement, 1901-11* (London: Smith Elder, 1912), I, 236–7.
87. Sontag, *op. cit.* (note 75), *Aids and Its Metaphors, op. cit.* (note 75), 38–9, 41, 44.
88. Harriet Ritvo, *The Animal Estate The English and Other Creatures in the Victoria Age* (Cambridge Mass.: Harvard University Press, 1987), 169.
89. *Ibid.,* chapter 4; Sontag, *op. cit.* (note 75), *Aids and Its Metaphors, op. cit.* (note 75), 44.
90. Sontag, *op. cit.* (note 75), *Illness as Metaphor,* 5–7, 14.
91. 5 *Hansard,* 41 (17 July 1912), 482; see 4 *Hansard,* 162 (1 Aug. 1906), 1094; 187 (31 March 1908), 315.
92. Sontag, *op. cit.* (note 75), *Aids and its Metaphors, op. cit.* (note 75), 62; Colin Holmes, *John Bull's Island. Immigration and British Society, 1871-1971* (Basingstoke: Macmillan, 1988), 297.
93. *Ibid.*, 25–9, 295–307.
94. William J. Fishman, *East End 1888. A Year in a London Borough Amomg the Labouring Poor* (London: Duckworth, 1988), 217; Judith R. Walkowitz, *City of Dreadful Delight. Narratives of Sexual Danger in Late Victorian London* (London: Virago, 1992).
95. William Plomer (ed.), *Kilvert's Diary. Selections from the Diary of the Rev. Francis Kilvert,* (London: Jonathan Cape, 3 vols. 1980 edn), I, 238; *BMJ*, 23 June 1962, 1752.
96. *Ministry of Labour. Report of the Committee of Inquiry on Anthrax*, PP 1959–60 VIII, 1006.
97. *Ibid.*, 1028–9.
98. McKeown's views are succinctly presented in *The Modern Rise of Population* (London: Edward Arnold, 1976).

99. Simon Szreter, 'The Importance of Social Intervention in Britain's Mortality Decline c.1850-1914: a Re-interpretation of the Role of Public Health', *Social History of Medicine*, I (1988), 1–38.

8

Conclusion

Costs, benefits and bans

In many respects, not least in that it witnessed tremendous strides in the application of science and technology to manufacturing industry, communications and to medicine and surgery, the Victorian era may be characterised as an 'heroic age'. It is certainly possible to exaggerate the speed and scope of change – the application of steam power in industry and agriculture was far from universal even when electricity and the internal combustion engine appeared on the scene towards the end of the nineteenth century.[1] Furthermore the horse remained of vital importance in relation to agriculture and the carriage of goods deep into the inter-war period, if not beyond. Indeed, the armies of the First World War, for all their participation in a military-industrial conflict which saw the emergence of aerial combat, the tank and gas warfare, were to a large extent, horse-drawn hosts.[2] Even so, wherever one looked in Victorian Britain, science and technology were extending their reach. This was true of transport where railways and metallic steamships came to rival and in many contexts replace, the horse, the coach, the canal boat and wooden-hulled sailing vessels. It was equally true of manufacturing industry which was producing a constant stream of new products while introducing refinements to old.[3]

In all of this there were huge financial gains for individuals (not all of whom were captains of industry) and institutions; there were also great consumer benefits.[4] A combination of swift transport links and refrigeration meant that well before the end of the century the British people were able to eat bread baked from wheat grown on the North American prairies and dine on meat raised on the South American pampas or Australasian grasslands. Undoubtedly, 'the rich got richer' but overall standards of living among the population at large also showed substantial gains (notwithstanding the continued existence of – sometimes dire – poverty). It was, after all, the economic vitality of the 'workshop of the world' which sustained Britain's huge population growth (from some 10.5m in 1801 to around 40.8m in 1911), her position as a European 'power' and, to a large extent, her imperial status. Of course, there were also costs.

Sometimes these were a consequence of exploitation (for example, the vast fortunes gained by patent medicine men such as Thomas Holloway were acquired by duping a gullible public); sometimes they were the product of ignorance, folly, or carelessness (for example, the use of public water courses as open sewers). In the context of this study gains included the capacity to kindle flame instantly and easily; the provision of cheap dyes for home furnishings, ornaments and clothing; and brilliantly coloured and glazed china and earthenware. The costs were visited on a workforce, some of whom experienced sickness and death because their labour brought them into contact with deadly poisons or germs. Were sick and dead workers the victims of ignorance, carelessness, or exploitation?

There is no simple answer to this question. At certain junctures, Bryant and May, some pottery manufacturers and other industrialists do seem, calculatedly, to have placed their own commercial interests a long way ahead of the health of their workers. Aware though they were that certain materials used in their workplaces were responsible for serious illness and even death, they did their utmost both to suppress knowledge of the true conditions that pertained in their factories and uphold their freedom to use such raw materials and manufacturing processes as they saw fit, regardless of the hazards they posed. Only prosecution, the full weight of state intervention, or the potential loss of markets and customers could persuade them to do things differently. However, Bryant and May and their ilk were, so far as can be ascertained, not necessarily typical of industrialists within the so-called 'dangerous trades'. When the Home Office and factory inspectorate issued special rules for the protection of workers, most manufacturers accepted them without demur. As for anthrax in the woollen industry, the failure to regulate this disease into oblivion by 1914 owed more to scientific ignorance than culpability and neglect. In the first place the cause of woolsorters' disease was obscure until the 1880s. In the second, knowledge that the disease was pulmonary anthrax and that it was caused by the inhalation of the spores of a living organism was of no avail in terms of devising a solution. That solution, in the form of the 'Duckering Process' (of disinfection) was not available until the end of the period covered by this study. Prior to this both the woollen industry itself (through the Bradford Rules of 1880) and the state (through special rules first compiled in 1897) sought to modify working conditions with a view to protecting workers. The success of these initiatives was limited because they did not tackle the root cause of the anthrax problem – namely the destruction of bacilli and spores. But this is not to categorise those endeavours as insincere. Only the eradication of the woollen industry itself could have guaranteed the elimination of anthrax among woolsorters. Yet costs and benefits surely had to be considered. Given the incidence of anthrax, the destruction of an important industry was, surely, not a price worth paying.

In the twentieth century similar dilemmas have been thrown up in relation to the benefits of motor transport (including widely affordable, door-to-door, personal mobility) *versus* its costs. In the UK alone the annual cost includes some 3000-4000 accidental deaths and the far larger toll of personal injury from road accidents, thousands more premature deaths resulting from atmospheric pollution created by the car, and environmental destruction in both town and country. Even when seen purely in relation to personal injury and death, the carnage wrought on the roads has sometimes been worse than that inflicted by warfare.[5] Yet the response of successive governments has been to regulate safety either by such means as licensing of drivers and vehicles, establishing speed limits and traffic control systems or, more recently, using the price mechanism to deter car use. Few, if any, politicians of national standing have ever advocated the banning of motorised transport. Implicitly, such a 'solution' to the problem of ill health and injury caused by motor vehicles has been and is seen as unacceptable both to governments and the voters who elect them. To put it another way, the British people and the politicians who represent them are willing to see 3000-4000 people per year die in road accidents (not to mention all the other 'downsides' of a 'car culture') in return for the perceived benefits of motoring. Curiously, however, when a relatively small number of people die in a rail accident (as at Southall in 1987 or Ladbroke Grove in 1999 or Hatfield in 2000) there is an all but universal cry for the investment of huge sums of money which, perhaps, will transform a comparatively safe form of transport into an absolutely safe one.[6]

Similar considerations applied in the Victorian period in relation to lead glazed pottery, lucifer matches, exotic wools and a wide variety of popular consumer goods, the benefits of which were not to be lightly discarded. But the choices span wider issues than, for example, cars *versus* safety or matches *versus* health. To ban the motor car or restrict its use either through draconian regulations or massive tax 'hikes' would have incalculable economic implications, including loss of livelihood not only for those directly employed in the motor industry, whether in its manufacturing, retailing, or maintenance sectors, but also for those whose employment is possible only because cars exist. In Victorian industry any move to ban lead, phosphorus, arsenic, or wools and hair would, in the absence of suitable alternatives, have meant unemployment. As we have seen, the regulation of occupational health was often seen explicitly, by workers, trade unionists, employers, civil servants and politicians in terms of jobs versus health. While some, such as Herbert Burrows of the Matchmakers' Union, thought that possible illness was a risk worth running for the reality of a job, others were less certain. As John Burns told the House of Commons in 1898 in respect of lead poisoning in the Potteries, if the cost of safeguarding British workers was the export of jobs to the continent, then so be it: 'If an industry can only be carried on by the destruction of the health of the potential mothers of many of our working classes, well, then, I say Germany can have that industry'.[7]

If such analyses suggest that choices were simple, albeit Hobsonian, this was far from being the case, for the commercial impact of occupational health regulation in the Victorian and Edwardian periods was assessed differently by different groups and individuals. Thus, in the pottery industry to which Burns referred, scientists (Thorpe and Oliver) believed that safe glazes would do little or nothing to disadvantage businesses. It followed, therefore, that their compulsory introduction would neither reduce profitability nor lead to job losses. Pottery manufacturers, on the other hand, who not unreasonably maintained that they knew their businesses best, thought otherwise. In this particular conflict between business and science, business triumphed, for manufacturers were not obliged to conform to the standards suggested by the two professors. The same was also true in respect of safety matches. As early as 1863 the scientist, Henry Letheby, believed that there existed suitable alternatives to the phosphorus match (see above 186–7), but such an analysis failed to carry the day then or indeed, for decades afterwards. When it did, it had much to do with the fact that Bryant and May, who had acquired domination of the British match market, saw commercial advantages in the proscription of phosphorus. Outside our period, in the 1920s, we find another example of how scientific analysis could be downgraded relative to other priorities. In 1922 the senior medical inspector of factories, as he then was, Thomas Legge, attended an international conference in Geneva at which it was agreed that the use of lead paint in buildings should be banned from 1926. When 1926 arrived the British Government declined to implement the agreement on the grounds that it was no longer necessary owing to the decline in lead poisoning from paint in the years since the conference convened. Instead, it introduced the *Lead Paint (Protection Against Poisoning) Act, 1926* which, *inter alia*, restricted the employment of women and minors and required that instances of poisoning be reported to the factory inspectorate.[8] Legge disagreed with such an approach and resigned in protest, thereby bringing to an end a distinguished career in the factory inspectorate that had lasted some twenty-eight years. The recently-knighted Legge's gesture was to no avail since the government had no second thoughts about banning lead paint. Once again scientific opinion was far from being the decisive factor in deciding policy on hazardous materials.

A question raised by Legge's resignation is whether the inspector was correct to resign on a point of principle if the statistics of poisoning were falling. He felt that a treaty commitment was a binding obligation, but if circumstances had changed, was it not reasonable that government policy should also change? A notable example of acceptance of this second alternative is provided by the attitude of Gertrude Tuckwell. As a leading light of the Women's Trade Union League (WTUL), Tuckwell was, in the Edwardian era, a fierce advocate for a ban on the use of lead glazes. By the 1920s, however, she took the view that inspection and regulation had achieved so much that proscription was no longer necessary.[9] In her unpublished *Reminiscences* she contrasted the fourteen cases of lead poisoning that occurred in the pottery and earthenware industry in 1929 with the 'hundreds' that had been an annual occurrence in the 1890s. She went on to explain this decline in the following terms:

> ...the end of the dangerous trades...did not come about by the abolition of all poisons as I had thought.... Good results were being obtained under the Home Office rules, increased inspection...that is to say by the perfected administration and not by the abolition of the dangerous ingredient [i.e. lead] that we had asked for.[10]

Two distinguished lady inspectors of factories, Adelaide Anderson and Hilda Martindale, held similar opinions – and not merely in respect of lead poisoning in the pottery and earthenware industry. Martindale wrote:

> Gradually, under the Chief Inspector of Factories, Sir Arthur Whitelegge and the Medical Inspector, Dr. Legge, knowledge of causes and precautions grew and Dame Adelaide Anderson was undoubtedly right when she said: 'The early years of the twentieth century saw what was unquestionably the most remarkable

> development that had ever yet been attempted in any age or country in applying scientific knowledge and care to the protection of workers from industrial disease and injury.' One by one, these injurious or dangerous trades or processes were brought under special regulations and the risks of working in them greatly lessened, if not eliminated.[11]

In other words, regulation was successful in mitigating hazard.

Women and networks

Not that it was regulation alone that came to the aid of workers; consumer choice also played its part. Importantly, this was an area where women, who were often the purchasers of products that contained toxic ingredients, could play a part in reducing the hazards, including those faced by women workers (who always formed a significant presence) in the dangerous trades. The WTUL recognised that its predominantly middle-class supporters, by insisting on pottery and earthenware free of lead glaze, might persuade manufacturers to alter their practices. Others believed that match manufacturers might be forced to produce only safety matches if they were subject to sufficient consumer pressure presumably, in this instance, mainly from men. The influence of the consumer in these two areas is insufficiently documented for us to reach conclusions about impact. In relation to arsenical colours, however, particularly in respect of wallpapers, there can be little doubt that consumer demand, driven in large part, no doubt, by the desire for self-preservation, was a major factor in the introduction of 'safe' dyes. Here again, women, not least as members of the Ladies' Sanitary Association had an important role to play.[12]

To be sure, women were prominent in the occupational health context in a number of contexts, including as 'victims'. Concern about women's health (especially that of young women) and the health of their unborn children was a factor – often a major one – in encouraging regulation. Indeed, in several cases, for example, those of Alice Skeeles (an artificial flower-maker) and Matilda Scheurer (a matchmaker), their ill-health or death triggered a regulatory response. At a slightly later date a further example of 'one woman who made a difference' is provided by Nellie Kershaw. Mrs Kershaw, who died in 1924, has the 'distinction' of being the first identifiable victim of an asbestos-related disease. Her death prompted a coroner's inquest and Dr William Cooke's pathological investigation of her lungs. Cooke's findings, first published in the *British Medical Journal* in 1924 stimulated further investigations into asbestos and occupational health, including by the factory inspectorate. The outcome of this process was the enactment of the Asbestos Industry Regulations, 1931, which sought to tackle the disease of asbestosis among workers in the asbestos industry.[13]

Aside from their roles as consumers and victims, women were also prominent as occupational health reformers. Most notable in this respect were women factory inspectors. First appointed in 1893 to enforce the factory acts as they related to women workers, the lady inspectors (as they were known) took a keen interest in occupational health issues and were important in accelerating the process of government intervention. Neither were women factory inspectors the only female officials concerned with such issues. Before they were even appointed the lady assistant commissioners on the Royal Commission on Labour were investigating problems of health in industry. Beyond the government service the WTUL was an influential 'ginger group' on occupational health. As I have argued elsewhere, the league, far from being an obscure feminist organisation functioning on the fringes of the labour movement, operated not only by mobilising workers but by exploiting, mainly *via* the extensive personal connections of Gertrude Tuckwell and the league's president, Lady Emilia Dilke, a complex network of reformers.

Lady Dilke was, of course, the wife of Sir Charles Dilke who, prior to the Crawford divorce scandal in 1885-6, which wrecked his political ambitions, was widely expected to be a future Liberal prime minister. After Charles' death in 1911 Tuckwell co-wrote his biography and 'weeded' his papers of potentially embarrassing material. Tuckwell, who idolised the Dilkes, was Emilia's niece. She became her secretary when her close friend, May Abraham, who had held that position (as well as the treasurership of the Women's Provident and Protective League), was appointed the first lady inspector of factories. In 1895, in her capacity as chief lady inspector of factories Abraham was appointed a member of the Dangerous Trades Committee chaired by H.J (Jack) Tennant MP. A year later she resigned her official positions when she and Tennant married. Tennant had previously served as secretary to the 1893 Departmental Committee on the Lead Industries. Along with Dilke, he was the chief parliamentary advocate for occupational health regulation. He was also private secretary to Asquith who, as home secretary between 1892 and 1895 took a number of important initiatives concerning the dangerous trades. Towards the end of the 1890s, when Asquith was in opposition, he became a supporter of tougher regulations for the control of lead poisoning. He was drawn closer to the regulationists when, in 1894, he married Tennant's sister, Margot, who was another WTUL activist. By the early-twentieth century Asquith was in favour of abandoning the 'moral suasion' approach in dealing with hazardous industries for a more forceful style of regulation.[14]

During the period when Tuckwell and Abraham lived together in Chelsea they had become friendly with the journalist Vaughan Nash (1861-1932) who, with his wife, Rosalind, went on to serve on the committee of the WTUL. Nash, who was an expert on labour questions wrote an important article, 'The Home Office and the Deadly Trades', for the *Fortnightly Review*. He also wrote articles on occupational disease for the *Daily Chronicle*.[15] Until his resignation in November 1899, Nash was the labour correspondent of the *Daily Chronicle*, the 'most radical' London newspaper which, in the 1890s, including under H.W. Massingham's editorship, not only achieved the highest circulation of any metropolitan newspaper, but, with the *Star*, was the principal organ for exposure of occupational disease scandals.[16] When Asquith was prime minister Nash served as his private secretary (1908-12), having previously held the same position for Campbell-Bannerman (1905-8).[17] The *Chronicle* devoted many column inches to occupational health issues and was the organ in which the WTUL chose to launch its public appeal on behalf of lead-poisoned pottery workers. Home Office files indicate that civil servants paid close attention to what the newspaper had to say about industrial disease. Massingham was a friend of Herbert Burrows of the Matchmakers Union. Indeed, during the match girls' strike of 1888 Massingham had helped to raise money for the strikers.[18] As for Burrows, he too was a leading member of the WTUL.

Neither does this web of personal and professional linkages indicate the full extent of the reformers' connections. Charles Dilke once boasted that he had 'known everyone worth knowing' between 1850 and his death.[19] Either through him or their own circles of acquaintances, his wife and Gertrude Tuckwell had the ears of a vast range of powerful people, including industrialists, aristocrats, lawyers, politicians, civil servants and churchmen. There are many indications of this in Tuckwell's unpublished autobiography. One example must suffice here to illustrate the point. Tuckwell's father, the so-called 'radical parson',

> had been Lord James' 'right hand man' in the old days when he [Lord James] was a Liberal candidate and then member for Taunton. He was a friend of my uncles and talked to me a good deal of old days when he dined at Sloane Sq. As children we used to support him by driving each other about with yellow reins and listening to all the items of information we could pick up. There was a petition of bribery against him and when he triumphantly cleared himself, he came to my home with Sergeant Ballantyne, his counsel. I ran out from our schoolroom to see what he looked like, as he had just been promoted.[20]

Since Lord James (1828-1911) was first elected MP for Taunton in 1869 it would appear that Tuckwell's acquaintance with him stretched back as far as the 1860s (she was born in 1861). Lord James was also connected to the reform movement by virtue of the fact that he was Charles Dilke's lawyer and personal friend. In 1901, Lord James was 'umpire' in the pottery arbitration. While undertaking this task he stayed with the Duchess of Sutherland. Given that she was a prominent WTUL supporter who was antipathetic towards the use of lead in pottery glazes, this alone raises questions as to whether his independence was compromised. It threatened to be more so when Tuckwell, having heard about the arbitration 'privately', gained an audience with her old friend and 'in my utter ignorance of procedure, tried to brief him on the sufferings of the women'.[21]

In 1902-03 James was in regular, and somewhat conspiratorial, correspondence with Dilke about the pottery arbitration. During this period the arbitration was in a state of suspension pending, *inter alia*, establishment of a compensation scheme for lead poisoning victims. James assured his client and friend that he would 'with pleasure see anybody you suggest in relation to the Pottery scheme'.[22] He also showed Dilke copies of correspondence he had with A.P. Llewellyn (the arbitrator nominated by the pottery manufacturers), took advice from Dilke in drafting replies to Llewellyn, and confidentially made his sympathies with the WTUL very clear.[23] In August 1903, at which point the arbitration was about to resume, James informed Dilke of his belief that the employers 'are acting very unreasonably'. With a view to accounting 'for the delay in issuing my award…so as to let him account for my non-action' he drafted a question for Dilke to put to the home secretary.[24] That James was aware of the extreme sensitivity of these dealings in the highly charged atmosphere of the time was made clear in a letter in which he enjoined Dilke to 'consider this letter written to yourself alone'.[25]

Responsibilities

To return to the question of why occupational disease existed in Victorian and Edwardian Britain. Although it is tempting to focus on exploiters and victims – not least because of some well-documented instances in which such a characterisation clearly holds good – the truth is rather more complex. This complexity lies partly in the behaviour of manufacturers intent on maximising profits, but also in the attitudes and actions of shareholders who did not hold companies to account, of trade unions that placed little emphasis on the health of members, of governments that were in some degree, at least, antipathetic towards intervening in the workplace, of a factory inspectorate that lacked both resources and medical expertise within its ranks and, indeed, a 'mindset' (shared by some workers and some government ministers) that questioned the value of regulations that threatened to destroy industries, export jobs and benefit overseas competitors.

At the time, workers were often criticised for not complying with regulations by, for example, not making use of washing facilities, or failing to wear the respirators and protective clothing specified in special rules. Such accusations of worker indifference or bravado ring true (for who has not, in our own day, seen construction workers cutting stone amid a cloud of dust while not wearing a mask or visor, or operating a pneumatic drill without using ear protectors?), but for several reasons blaming workers for their own occupational ill health does not take us far. Workers in the dangerous trades were poorly (if at all) educated and seldom in a position to understand, much less assess, the risks they ran. Those who worked within the dangerous trades were also, by virtue of their position at the base of the employment ladder, often desperate for work of any sort; as such, they could not afford to be selective in their choice of work. So although workforces were often criticised for lack of personal hygiene, the reality is that their health was being undermined not by lack of personal cleanliness (over which they might have been able to exert some control – subject to the provision of properly maintained washing facilities and the like) but by an atmosphere suffused with dust or fume over which they could exert no control. Thomas Legge recognised that workers ought to be expected to do their bit to safeguard their own health, but he also recognised, in the first of his famous 'axioms', that the primary responsibility rested with employer or others who controlled the workplace. As such, it was invidious to place blame (as Alexander

Redgrave frequently had) on workers who failed to wash their hands:

> 1. Unless and until the employer has done everything, the workman can do next to nothing to protect himself.[26]

In other words a healthy workplace, like so much else in the sphere of industrial relations was about power and control.

The question of responsibility for occupational ill health and its containment, leads to the related point of those factors that led to the state to regulate workplace disease and, indeed, why certain diseases were chosen for regulation in preference to others, notably, dust diseases. Clare Holdsworth has pondered this question, not in relation to all four diseases considered on this book but in respect of occupational health regulation in the pottery industry. She emphasises the 'political expediency of rules to control lead exposure, compared with those introduced to control dust within workshops' and proceeds to identify four specific points in support of this observation. First, the existence of a 'practical alternative' to 'raw' lead glazes in the form of leadless or low solubility glazes and technical difficulties of improving ventilation, especially in small pot-banks which lacked steam or electrical power. Second, the 'pattern of susceptibility' whereby women and young persons were deemed to be those most at risk from lead. This allowed the authorities to introduce protective regulation without interfering with the contractual freedom between adult workers and their employers. Such legislation, she points out, accorded not only with the long-established traditions of the factory acts, but with the late-Victorian and Edwardian obsession with restricting the employment of wives and mothers. Third, doctors could diagnose lead poisoning (or believed they could), whereas their knowledge of occupational dust disease was strictly limited. Fourth the popular campaign involving involving newspapers such as the *Daily Chronicle*. This was critical because it awakened public sympathy over an emotional issue.[27]

Holdsworth's analysis, though compelling, is not completely convincing. The present author agrees with those explanations that emphasise the importance of popular campaigning and the strengths and weaknesses of medical expertise, but, for several reasons, is less convinced by the others. In particular, Holdsworth's references to the 'practicality' and 'political expediency' of regulating some health hazards rather than others, raise difficulties. While political expediency did play a part in determining the nature and severity of the regulations established – particularly in terms of the compilation of rules that would not undermine industrial competitiveness and employment opportunities – neither expediency nor considerations of practicality explain why regulators ignored dust (if they did) and targeted lead. The practicality of alternatives to dangerous materials such as raw lead in pottery glaze or white phosphorus in matches, far from being a matter of consensus was actually a question of fierce dispute. As Holdsworth acknowledges, only 'a small minority of manufacturers' during the period in question accepted that either fritted or leadless glazes were practical. Consequently, as Holdsworth also acknowledges, efforts to restrict the use of lead in pottery and earthenware glazes 'were as strongly contested' as regulatory efforts relating to ventilation. As a result, it is hard to agree that lead was somehow seen as an 'acceptable' area of regulation while dust diseases were not. In fact efforts to control dust emissions in factories dating, as they do, from 1864, long pre-date any attempt to regulate the use of lead (or other hazardous raw materials). Equally, they long pre-date any attempt to tackle any specific occupational diseases among factory workers. Whitelegge recognised that china and earthenware production was hazardous because of the presence of lead *and* dust. Not only was 'the unhealthiness of the industry as a whole...beyond question' but '[p]ractically all the "processes" are dangerous either from lead or from dust'.[28] It was presumably for this reason that in the 1890s some clauses in codes of special rules did focus specifically on dust. For example, rule 3 of the 1894 special rules for the pottery industry required the 'use of fans or other mechanical means for the removal of dust'. In any case, the idea that dust diseases and lead poisoning are sharply differentiated is debatable for, as Thomas Legge observed: 'Practically all industrial lead poisoning is due to the inhalation of dust and fumes; and if you stop their inhalation you will stop the poisoning'.[29]

The fact is that the regulation of occupational health in the late-nineteenth and early twentieth centuries focused on particular *diseases*, rather than workplace environments. As such it contrasted with earlier legislation, such as the *Factory Acts Extension Act, 1864*, clause four of which required that factories should be kept clean and be ventilated in such a way as to render harmless 'so far as is practicable' any gases, dust and impurities that posed a threat to health.[30] The new emphasis that emerged in the 1880s and especially from the 1890s, reflected the inadequacy of the earlier, rather generalised, approach. In these circumstances the diseases that were selected for attention by doctors, campaigners and the state were what might be termed 'gross' diseases – that is, those with obvious and horrible symptoms, or those which were quick to develop, had high fatality rates, or awakened some sort of emotional aversion. Dust diseases fell into none of these categories. They were relatively under-researched, hard to diagnose, usually slow and insidious in their development and not easily distinguished from respiratory diseases, particularly tuberculosis, that were not occupationally related. These factors meant that the regulation of and compensation for dust diseases were primarily developments of the inter-war period and after. Silicosis was regulated in 1918, asbestosis in the asbestos industry in 1931 and byssinosis as late as the 1940s. In terms of industrial disease the decades after the First World War have rightly been termed, 'the age of dust'. In the 1960s the chief inspector of factories observed that: 'In the early part of this century industrial health made great and rapid strides at comparatively little cost. Today we are left with only the difficult problems; the easy ones have been solved'.[31] Lead, arsenic and phosphorus poisoning, along with anthrax, were not necessarily 'easy' problems, but they were obvious ones.

Another aspect of Holdsworth's analysis that gives rise to doubt is her suggestion that lead poisoning in potteries became a subject of regulation because women and young persons were at risk. In identifying links between age, gender and occupational health regulation Holdsworth is not alone. Carolyn Malone, for example, has emphasised that public concern about unhealthy conditions in the dangerous trades had much to do with a desire to protect women workers and, thereby, wives, mothers, their children and even the concept of femininity and the future of the race by imposing restrictions on the liberty of women to work where and when they wished. However, by the 1890s the notion that the state had no right to intervene between employer and adult male employee, with a view to safeguarding the latter, was effectively moribund. As early as the 1840s industrial safety legislation had sought, at least to a degree, to protect males and females, young and old.[32] Hence, to characterise the occupational health regulation of the 1890s and after simply (or especially) in terms of protecting women and young persons is erroneous. For various reasons, as indicated in the present study, women occupy a prominent place in the history of occupational health regulation in the Victorian and Edwardian periods. Nevertheless, their significance should not be exaggerated, for the regulation of the late-nineteenth and early-twentieth centuries went beyond a desire to protect women (for whatever motive).

Malone makes far-reaching claims about the centrality of women in the regulation of the dangerous trades. She argues not only that the medical profession, press and the public singled out women as being in need of protection, but also that between 1891 and 1914 they were removed from the best paid jobs in the name of 'protective legislation'.[33] If the latter were the case it would lend support to the notion that protective legislation really served the interests of men and/or the state. However, both her points are contestable. First, most workers in the dangerous trades, regardless of gender and regardless of whether they were employed in white lead manufacture, artificial flower production or matchmaking, far from being prominent in the best paid jobs, were actually engaged in the worst paid. As Redgrave observed as early as 1875, '[t]he people employed in these [white lead] works...the women especially are of the very poorest class.[34] This point was endorsed by Mrs Charles Mallet nearly twenty years later:

> It is mostly women of the very poorest and roughest class who offer themselves to work in the White Lead Factory. 'The widow who has a family to support, the wife of a drunken husband, the girl whose character will not bear scrutiny' – these are the applicants for employment. Poor and of impaired vitality, badly nourished and careless of personal cleanliness, their constitutions are ill-fitted to cope with the poison and they readily succumb to it. This industry represents for women very much what the Dockers' industry is to men.[35]

Although there is some evidence of danger money and wage premiums being paid to workers in the dangerous trades, it was more usual, as Mallet indicates, that those who worked with poisonous substances simply occupied the jobs that others would not do.

If women were not in the best paid jobs, what of the suggestion that the object of the dangerous trades legislation was their removal from the workplace? Again, this is an unconvincing hypothesis. First, in the dangerous trades context, protective legislation usually meant not removal from employment but the establishment of regulations (albeit often misconceived), such as provision of protective clothing and washing facilities, to mitigate hazards. Second, while the press certainly did highlight the 'problem' of women in the dangerous trades, it did not do this to the exclusion of their male counterparts. By the same token, neither bureaucrats nor the legislature focused exclusively on removing women from the dangerous trades or on introducing protective measures for their benefit. Indeed, this was far from being the case. The main objective of the factory acts from the passing of the *Health and Morals of Apprentices Act, 1802* and for much of the nineteenth century was the protection not of women but of children and young persons. Insofar as they did apply to adults they were not exclusively concerned with women. To quote Redgrave again: 'I do not think it is sufficient for an employer to say that the operatives who come to him accept the work with its consequences. Is he justified in placing *men and women* [author's emphasis] in jeopardy without providing and insisting upon the adoption of some sufficient precautions?'[36]

With one exception (that baths should be provided for women workers) the white lead sections in the *Factory and Workshop Act, 1883* applied to men and women equally. Barbara Harrison is mistaken in claiming that overalls, head coverings, and respirators had to be provided for women alone.[37] Neither this act nor the 1892 rules for arsenic or the white lead rules of, 1892 or 1894 banned the employment of women. Similarly, none of the three codes of special rules for matchmaking (1892, 1894, 1899) included any gender-specific rules. In the special rules for the pottery industry, issued in 1894, only one of the eleven clauses – that which referred to the provision of overalls and head coverings – applied to women alone. Since this rule did not seek to exclude women from any work process it is hard to see it as being exclusionist as well as protective in intent. By 1900 the Home Office was persuaded of the need for medical inspection of all pottery workers, including adult males, who encountered lead. The 1904 pottery rules introduced routine medical inspection for males. While women were excluded from certain dangerous occupations, this was not the main thrust of dangerous trades regulation. Certainly, to see the 'elimination of women from the most dangerous, and highest paying, parts of the lead trade' as 'a prime example of social policy making in England in the two decades before World War I' is to go too far. Malone herself recognises in another context, lead work in pottery manufacture, that the government consistently rejected the prohibition of women workers. As Barbara Harrison points out, the 'prohibition or the exclusion of women was not accepted as a legislative remedy'. Furthermore, in those few instances where an exclusionary approach was adopted 'the actual impact on women's participation in paid work seems to have been minimal'.[38]

Malone, citing John Tosh, notwithstanding that his recently-published book places little emphasis on the relation between bodily power and male identity, maintains that the masculine ideology of the Victorian period stressed the virtue of physical strength.[39] From this observation she concludes (though with no evidential basis beyond a quotation from a male potter that 'we take our risk on ourself; we know the risk when we go working), that 'working men accepted personal risk and danger as a natural part of their worklives'. However, if men were passive and resigned in their approach to occupational risk, it is hard to see why the trade unions to which they belonged and, in particular, the Trades Union Congress, wanted to see reform in employers' liability law, including the abolition of the common law concept of *volenti non fit injuria* which held that in accepting a job a worker implicitly and voluntarily accepted all the risks that went with it.[40] It is more plausible that male workers, far from being cavalier in their attitudes to safety, recognised, as the trade unionist Herbert Burrows pointed out (see above 203–4), that employment in a hazardous occupation was preferable to unemployment. In so doing they reached a conclusion that was shared by many women.

Insofar as dangerous trades regulation did target women, for example through the white lead rules issued in 1896 and 1899, this reflected the state of medical and scientific knowledge about the cause, prevention and impact of specific diseases. Lead poisoning was thought to be to some extent a woman's problem. The lead trades also happened to be occupations in which women formed a large proportion of the labour force. Accordingly some special regulations in those industries were devised to protect women, including by removing them from places of risk. Other diseases either were not seen to pose a particular threat to women (phosphorus poisoning, arsenic poisoning and anthrax) or affected workforces that were predominantly male (notably, anthrax among woolsorters). Since protective regulations were introduced in all of these areas, it is difficult to see the regulation of the dangerous trades exclusively, or even mainly, in gender specific terms. Consequently, suggestions that 'the gendered vision of Victorian and Edwardian England blinded social policy makers and allowed them to neglect the health in trades where few or no women worked' cannot be substantiated.[41]

Finally, if it is implied that the exclusion of women from certain occupations was some sort of male conspiracy to remove women from the 'public sphere' (the workplace) and confine them to their own 'separate sphere' (the home), it is well to bear in mind that the WTUL, which was run by women for women, was at the forefront of those who demanded the exclusion of women from the dangerous trades – notably employment in lead processes in the pottery industry.[42] It is also well to remember that the league was an advocate of further recruitment of women by the factory inspectorate and, as such sought to promote women's employment. But, leaving this point on one side, in opposing the employment of women in lead processes in pottery and earthenware manufacture the WTUL was following the best medical advice as it stood in the 1890s and early-1900s. During this period, the two leading experts on occupational health, Thomas Arlidge and Thomas Oliver, agreed that lead poisoning was, particularly, a 'woman's problem'. In this assessment they may have been mistaken but at the time such a view was the received medical opinion of the day. It is hard to see that Arlidge, Legge, Oliver, the Dilkes or Tuckwell *et al* had any motive in favouring the removal of women from the workplace (or certain areas thereof) beyond reducing the toll of pain, suffering, ill health and death which they believed was the lot of women who worked with hazardous substance.

A matter of timing

From a late-twentieth century vantage point it is tempting to ask why occupational health regulation came so 'late', that is, mainly from the 1890s, when industrial disease was clearly neither a new phenomenon in this decade nor an insignificant problem hitherto. Why did overwork, education, the employment of juveniles and factory accidents all take precedence? This question has already been addressed in the introduction to this study where attention was directed towards the unspectacular and insidious nature of much occupational disease. Beyond this, however, lies the problem of hindsight, for it is mainly with the benefit of hindsight that one is led to ask why something did not occur earlier than it did. Why, an undergraduate once asked, did the government not establish a National Health Service in 1911-13 rather than the much more limited national health insurance scheme that was then introduced? The real answer to this profoundly 'unhistorical' question is that history is a matter of process, that (albeit not inevitably) one thing leads to another and that the National Health Service was introduced in 1948 partly because the inadequacies of national health insurance had by then become clear for most to see. Whether the NHS would have been established if the Second World War had not occurred is a difficult question. But what seems probable is that the experience of war, the precedent of the wartime Emergency Medical Service, the importance of maintaining civilian morale by prioritising post-war 'reconstruction' even at the height of the conflict were all factors in the emergence of the new regime of 'nationalised' health care.

How does all of this relate to occupational disease in the nineteenth century? Early-nineteenth century observers saw for themselves that cotton mills were horribly dusty and noisy places. Some, workers among them, believed, furthermore, that the inhalation of dust was a health hazard (even though others, including medical practitioners, regarded cotton dust as harmless). It hardly needs to be said that there was no suggestion that the cotton industry should be destroyed because it brought about ill health and loss of life. Neither were there any proposals for mitigating the health hazards of the textile industry. How could there have been when there was then no medical consensus on the existence of a hazard and no scientific or clinical understanding either of the dangers posed by cotton dust? Neither was there a precedent for occupational health regulation; in no quarter was there any recognition that the state had a role to play in terms of ensuring that the atmosphere of the cotton mill held little or no dust. Even if there had been the technology for removing dust from the atmosphere had not then progressed beyond the stage of opening windows – a solution which, given the physical location of the British cotton industry, was seldom compatible with the maintenance of optimum spinning conditions (warmth and humidity).

The point has been made in relation to asbestos and occupational health that regulation came 'late', that is, as much as thirty years after the hazard had been recognised and that this tardiness reflected an outlook that was heedless of workers' suffering and, therefore, worthy of condemnation by historians.[43] An alternative perspective, however, is that for formal regulations to be introduced there had to be understanding both that a process or material did give rise to significant harm, that the technology existed to mitigate such harm and that in removing this harm fresh harms (e.g. unemployment, the introduction of unsafe alternatives, or the destruction of a vital industry) were not created in its place. This is not to say that occupational health reform gained a place on the political and administrative agenda from the 1880s because the time was then 'ripe' for regulation (which is a meaningless tautology). Neither is it to say that there was anything inevitable about the enactment of occupational health regulation in the 1880s, 1890s and after; neither should we dismiss as unimportant the role of the people involved in its enactment. The question of why was there a surge of interest in the occupational health in this period is not easily answered, not least because of the difficulties of disentangling causes from consequences. For example, did legislative change such as the *Factory and Workshop Act, 1895*, which provided for the collection of occupational disease data, reflect or stimulate a burgeoning of interest? Probably it did both, but the relative importance of stimulus and response is not easily gauged. Hence, any explanation for the late-Victorian expansion of interest in industrial disease must take account of a multiplicity of factors that operated at different levels.

Reference has been made to the impact of individual victims such as Skeeles and Scheurer. By the same token, 'moral entrepreneurs' such as Thomas Burt, Henry Broadhust, John Burns; Gertrude Tuckwell, the Dilkes (Charles and Emilia), and the Duchess of Sutherland played key roles in placing occupational health reform on the political agenda and mobilising support for it.[44] In August 1903, at the height of the lead poisoning controversy in the Potteries, Dilke observed that the 'the H.O. will…be kept up to the mark' in the task of protecting workers, by 'the fear of what [John] Burns and others might afterwards say in the House of Commons'.[45] Medical experts such as Arlidge and Oliver were also to the fore. Changes of personnel in the factory inspectorate and at the Home Office, notably the retirement of the highly conservative Alexander Redgrave as chief inspector of factories and workshops, in 1891 and appointment of the progressive Asquith as home secretary, in 1892, certainly helped prioritise workers' health. Redgrave's departure was followed by a considerable 'shake-up' in the factory department. The inspectorate was expanded, including by the appointment (in 1893) of the first women inspectors (who took a particular interest in occupational health); at the same time the number of prosecutions for breach of safety regulations multiplied; most importantly, occupational health regulations were introduced. In the latter connection the passing of the *Factory and Workshop Act, 1891*, was important. This act empowered the home secretary to certify particular industries and processes as dangerous to health and to make special rules for their conduct. This was an important extension of a principle first established, though seemingly never invoked, in the *Factory Acts Extension Act, 1864*. Although the reform achieved limited impact, owing to the safeguard of an arbitration procedure which effectively accorded employers a power of veto over the rule-making process, it helped to put occupational health 'on the map'. Thus, for the first time ever the inspectorate's 1891-92 report contained a section on 'dangerous and unhealthy processes'.[46]

Organisations such as the Ladies' Sanitary Association, the WTUL and, more broadly elements of the press need to be emphasised. Also important in awakening public interest in occupational diseases were the reports of the factory inspectorate and Labour Commission. Numbers were not particularly significant, not least because nobody had even a vague idea of the toll exerted by occupational disease. Well-publicised individual cases, on the other hand were important – especially when exploited by the skilled reporters of the 'new journalism' – which brings us back to Skeeles and Scheurer. We come back also to questions of 'history as process'. Occupational health regulation was part of a process of factory regulation that dated from 1802. In many ways this process fits the model proposed by Oliver MacDonagh in his famous 1958 article on the 'Nineteenth Century Revolution in Government' and developed subsequently. MacDonagh argued that government intervened to remedy abuses when it was obliged to do so by intolerable circumstances. He suggested that the initial intervention was insufficient to remove the abuse and that as this registered so further intervention was essayed usually, at some point, including the appointment of executive officers (inspectors) to oversee and enforce regulations. These officials than came to play a part in extending the intervention for they identified deficiencies in the statute and also acted as proponents of further intervention. The possibility of solving a problem through a once-and-for-all act of parliament comes to be recognised as misguided. Hence MacDonagh's model sees subsequent legislation as a dynamic process whereby loopholes are constantly being identified and closed and the reach of regulations and the regulators steadily extended.[47] Although MacDonagh's stress on intolerability has been justifiably criticised, in many respects occupational health regulation in Victorian and Edwardian Britain can be said to fit this broad model of social reform and administrative growth.

In addition, occupational health reform fits neatly into a 'national efficiency' model of reform. Some years historians have explained the Liberal Welfare Reforms of 1906-14, in part at least, as a response to broad concerns about national decline. This decline related to the spread of Darwinist ideas, particularly within the contexts of Britain's 'poor' military performance in the Anglo-Boer War; alarm about the physical status of the British people, as evidenced by a high rate of rejection of men volunteering for military service during the Boer War; and anxiety about Britain's technological and economic decline relative to international competitors, especially Germany and the

USA. Investment in the health and fitness of the people, including, though not exclusively, in mothers, possible future mothers and the young would, some thought, help to reverse such trends.[48]

In his book, *Dangerous Trades*, Thomas Oliver suggests that lack of emphasis on health and safety was a factor in Britain's relative industrial decline. He accused the leaders of British industry of being set in their ways, lethargic and insular, of being technologically and scientifically ignorant – relative to their continental counterparts – and wedded to old-fashioned methods. He foresaw that heightened international competition in the field of manufacturing would lead to increased speed of production and the imposition of extra strain upon workers. He went on to speculate that such developments, along with, for example, urban overcrowding, could damage workers' physiques. Rural depopulation – a recurrent theme among those who feared physical deterioration among the British people – would produce a less robust population: 'There is something in the air of such factories (textile), it may be the excessive heat and moisture, or the animal products given off during perspiration and breathing, that interferes with the nutrition of the body and checks its growth'. For Oliver, therefore, improved health and safety opened the way to greater national efficiency and an opportunity to reverse trends that were inimical to the physical status of the great mass of the people. Since a fit workforce was the key to national survival, power and prosperity, the regulation of the dangerous trades ought to be welcomed by manufacturers and the nation at large rather than feared. Indeed, Oliver saw factory legislation as something that 'has not paralysed but has improved trade as well as the conditions of labour'. In his view further emphasis upon a healthy workplace was a natural legislative development. If Oliver's analysis was correct and his argument is compelling, it suggests that occupational health regulation in the late-nineteenth and twentieth centuries deserves to be seen not only in terms of an extension of humanitarian concern or the triumph of scientific and medical 'progress', as it sometimes has been, especially by the occupational health specialists who have hitherto dominated the field of occupational health history, but also in relation to wider objectives in public policy.[49]

Looking to the future

What of the post-Edwardian period, as Britain emerged from the heroic age of industrialisation; was it the case that occupational illness diminished and, perhaps, became a thing of the past? Although Gertrude Tuckwell referred, in 1929, to 'the end of the dangerous trades', the answer to this question is in the negative. [50] It is true that the diseases discussed in this volume were brought under some degree of control (there were only 23 cases of occupational arsenic poisoning during the the whole of the 1930s) and even eradicated (as in the case of phosphorus necrosis among matchmakers), but some hazards remained significant for many years.[51] Thus, in the inter-war period (1919-39 inclusive) almost 5000 cases of lead poisoning were reported to the factory inspectorate under the terms of the *Factory and Workshop Act, 1901* (s.73) and (from 1927) the *Lead Paint (Protection Against Poisoning Act), 1926* (s.3). This figure excluded the, sometimes substantial, number of house painters and plumbers (56 in 1922) whose poisoning was not required to be reported, either at all or, in the case of painters, until 1927. Among those whose sickness was reportable were 497 workers who died as a result of occupational lead poisoning.

Neither are the numbers for other diseases insignificant; for example, the inter-war period saw 827 case of occupational anthrax, (including over 100 fatalities). Furthermore, beginning with mercury poisoning (as early as 1898) new hazards and diseases were identified and made reportable.[52] These included toxic jaundice or TNT poisoning (with effect from 1916), epitheliomatous ulceration and chrome ulceration (both effective from 1920), carbon bisulphide, aniline and chronic benzene poisoning (all with effect from 1925) and two more diseases (compressed air illness and manganese poisoning) in the 1930s. Toxic jaundice was particularly a disease of First World War munitions workers exposed to TNT (trinitrotoluene);[53] epitheliomatous ulceration, known as 'mule spinners' cancer' when it affected cotton workers, could affect those whose work brought them into contact with tar, soot, mineral oil or pitch;[54] chrome ulceration affected a number of occupations but was a particular hazard of the chromium plating and dyeing industries. There was a statutory obligation on all medical practitioners to notify the factory inspectorate of cases of these diseases whenever they had reason to believe them to have been contracted in a factory or workshop. Some of the diseases that became reportable after those originally scheduled in the 1895 act, notably carbon bisulphide and chronic benzene poisoning affected very few workers. Toxic jaundice was, initially widespread, with over 400 cases between 1916 and 1918, inclusive. However, with the end of the First World War the numbers declined steeply. Other diseases took a more consistent toll – there were 146 cases of aniline poisoning in the thirties (with 1 death). The greatest number of occupational cases in inter-war factories involved epitheliomatous and chrome ulceration. Between 1920 and 1939 (inclusive) there were 2772 case of the former (including 645 fatalities) and 1666 of the latter (though no deaths). So it is clear that in the inter-war period thousands suffered and hundreds died from industrial diseases reported to the factory inspectorate. The toll would be higher if diseases that were either not notifiable or reportable under different codes of regulation (eg. silicosis, asbestosis, or fatigue) were included.

Precisely what should be made of these figures is unclear. Since we do not have data for the working population exposed to the risk of, say, lead poisoning, it is not possible to reach any conclusions about rising, falling, or static levels of incidence in the inter-war period. Neither is it the intention at this point to explore this issue. The continued existence of occupational health hazards after 1914 has led Barbara Harrison to conclude that late-Victorian and Edwardian regulation 'failed' in terms of having 'a major influence on disease prevention and thence the improvement of workers' health'.[55] But how should 'success' be judged?. Diseases such as occupational lead poisoning or anthrax were not 'solved' in terms of being eliminated. But this should not prompt us to minimise the achievements of the late-nineteenth and early-twentieth centuries when grave problems were identified and tackled with at least some measure of success. Indeed, occupational phosphorus poisoning was eradicated. Occupational illness is the almost inevitable consequence of work. As work evolves so new hazards emerge. Even in a 'post-industrial society' in which coal mines, for example, have become more a feature of the heritage industry than a vital source of domestic and industrial fuel, and in which most workers are employed in service industries rather than in manufacturing, occupational illness continues to be reported at high levels. The classic poisonings and infections may be largely things of the past, but they have been replaced by such disorders as repetitive strain injury, vdu radiation and, that ubiquitous condition of the modern workplace, stress.[56]

Notes

1. See G.N. von Tunzelmann, *Steam Power and British Industrialisation to 1860* (Oxford: Clarendon Press, 1978).
2. See *Horses in European Economic History. A Preliminary Canter* (Reading: British Agricultural History Society, 1983); F.M.L. Thompson, 'Nineteenth Century Horse Sense', *Economic History Review*, 29 (1976), 60–81.

3. Asa Briggs, *Victorian Things* (London: Batsford, 1988).
4. Some lawyers made fortunes out of their services to the emergent railway companies. See R.W. Kostal, *Law and English Railway Capitalism, 1825-1875* (Oxford: Clarendon Press, 1994).
5. See Bill Luckin, 'War on the Roads: Traffic Accidents and Social Tension in Britain, 1939-45' in Roger Cooter and Bill Luckin (eds), *Accidents in History: Injuries, Fatalities and Social Relations* (Amsterdam and Atlanta: Rodopi, 1997), 234–54; Sean O'Connell, *The Car in British Society. Class, Gender and Motoring, 1896-1939* (Manchester and New York: Manchester University Press, 1998). O'Connell marvels, surely with good reason, that road traffic deaths and injuries have been accepted with so little protest.
6. See Simon Jenkins, 'Risking our Sanity', *The Times*, 20 Oct. 1999.
7. 4 *Hansard*, 63 (29 July 1898), 504–5. John Elliot Burns (1858-1943) was elected to the Commons, in 1892, as one of the first Independent Labour MPs. In 1905 he became 'the first artisan' to enter the cabinet. *Dictionary of National Biography, 1941-1950* (London: OUP, 1959), 121–4.
8. (*16 & 17 Geo.V c. 37*). See this author's entry on Legge in the *New Dictionary of National Biography* (Oxford: OUP, forthcoming).
9. See*Report of the Departmental Committee Appointed to inquire into the Dangers attendant on the Use of Lead and the Danger or Injury to Health arising from Dust and other Causes in the Manufacture of Earthenware and China and in the Processes incidental thereto including the Making of Lithographic Transfers*, PP 1910 XXIX, Memorandum by Miss Tuckwell, 223–4; Peter Bartrip, '"Petticoat Pestering": the Women's Trade Union League and Lead Poisoning in the Staffordshire Potteries, 1890-1914', *Historical Studies in Industrial Relations*, 2 (1996), 3–26.
10. TUC Library Collections. North London University Library. Gertrude Tuckwell Papers. Unpublished Reminiscences of Gertrude Tuckwell, 190–1.
11. Hilda Martindale, *From one Generation to Another, 1839-1944. A Book of Memoirs* (London: George Allen & Uniwin, 1944), 152; Adelaide Mary Anderson, *Women in the Factory. An Administrative Adventure* (London: John Murray, 1922), 97.
12. See P.W.J. Bartrip, 'How Green was My Valance: Environmental Arsenic Poisoning and the Myth of Victorian Domesticity', *English Historical Review*, cix (1994), 891-913; *idem., op. cit.* (note 9), 3–26.
13. On the Kershaw case see Peter Bartrip, 'Nellie Kershaw, Turner and Newall, and Asbestos-Related Disease in 1920s Britain', *Historical*

Studies in Industrial Relations Historical Studies in Industrial Relation, 9 (June 2000), 101–16; *idem., The Way from Dusty Death. Turner & Newall and the Regulation of the British Asbestos Industry, 1890-1970* (London: Athlone, 2001); Irving J. Selikoff and Morris Greenberg, 'A Landmark Case in Asbestosis', *JAMA*, 265 (20 Feb. 1991), 898. David J. Jeremy, 'Corporate Responses to the Emergent Recognition of a Health Hazard in the UK Asbestos Industry: The Case of Turner & Newall, 1920-1960', *Business and Economic History*, 24 (1995), 254–65.

14. 4 *Hansard*, 139 (4 Aug. 1904), 1028.
15. *Fortnightly Review*, 59 (1893), 169–83; Rosalind Nash also wrote on the dangerous trades. See Carolyn Malone, 'Sensational Stories, Endangered Bodies: Women's Work and the New Journalism in England in the 1890s' *Albion*, 31 (1999), 68–9.
16. Before moving to the *Chronicle*, which he edited from 1895-1899, Massingham had briefly edited the *Star* (1890-91). See Alan J. Lee, *The Origins of the Popular Press in England* (London: Croom Helm, 1976), 164–5; Alfred H. Havighurst, *Radical Journalist: H.W. Massingham (1860-1924)* (London: Cambridge University Press, 1974), esp. chapter 2, 103, 108.
17. *Who Was Who, 1929-1940* (London: Adam & Charles Black, 1947).
18. Havighurst, *op. cit.* (note 16), 16, 20.
19. Roy Jenkins, *Dilke. A Victorian Tragedy* (London: Collins, 1965), 20.
20. TUC Library Collections, University of North London. Gertrude Tuckwell Papers. Unpublished Reminiscences of Gertrude Tuckwell, 188–89.
21. *Ibid.*; *Dictionary of National Biography, 1901-1911* (Oxford: OUP, 1920), 359–61.
22. British Library, Dilke Papers, Add. Mss.43892 ff.259, James of Hereford to Dilke, 29 July 1902.
23. *Ibid.*, 1, 5, 6, Aug. 1902.
24. *Ibid.*, 8 Aug. 1903. The question to Akers-Douglas (home secretary) asked: 'If he is in a position to state when the final award in respect of the Lead Poisoning Rules will be published'. See copy of letter from Dilke to James, 9 Aug. 1903 in which he agrees to pose the question.
25. *Ibid.*, 7 Aug. 1902. See also James to Dilke, 5 Nov. 1903.
26. Sir Thomas Morrison Legge, *Thirty Years' Experience of Industrial Maladies* (London: Royal Society of Arts, 1929), 4.
27. Clare Holdsworth, 'Potters' Rot and Plumbism: Occupational Health in the North Staffordshire Pottery Industry', Liverpool

University Ph.D. thesis (1995), 28 *et seq* and 192. On the role of the press see Malone, *op. cit.* (note 15), 49–71.

28. PRO HO 45/9852/B12393E. B.A. Whitelegge to Kenelm Digby, 28 April 1898.
29. *Annual Report of HM Chief Inspector of Factories and Workshops,* (1894) PP 1895 XIX, 94; Thomas Legge, *Industrial Maladies* (London: OUP, 1934), 3.
30. *27 & 28 Vict. c.48* s.4.
31. *Annual Report of HM Chief Inspector of Factories on Industrial Health,* (1966) PP 1967 XXXI (Cmnd.3359), 525.
32. *Factory Act* (*7&8 Vict. c.15*). Although section 21 of the act stipulated that certain machinery should be fenced, applied only in respect of equipment on which children and young persons were employed or were 'liable to pass', the clause was bound also to confer protection upon adults. Clauses 22 and 23, which provided for the notification and investigation of accidents, applied to all workers, regardless of age or gender. Similarly, clauses 24 and 25, which allowed for the compensation of accident victims were also applicable to the workforce as a whole.
33. Malone, *op. cit.* (note 15), 50; *idem.*, 'Gendered Discourses and the Making of Protective Labor Legislation in England, 1830-1914', *Journal of British Studies*, 37 (1998), 185; *idem.*, 'The Gendering of Dangerous Trades: Government Regulation of Women's Work in the White Lead Trade in England, 1892-1898', *Journal of Women's History*, 8 (1996), 15; *idem.*, 'Sex in Industry: Protective Labor Legislation in Engand, 1891-1914', University of Rochester Ph.D. (1991), 4–6 and chapter V.
34. *Report of Inspector Redgrave for the Half-Year Ending 31 October 1875*, PP 1876 XVI, 34–5. See *Report upon the Precautions which can be Enforced under the Factory Act and as to the need of further powers for the Protection of Persons employed in White Lead Works*, PP 1882 XVIII, 960.
35. C. Mallet, *Dangerous Trades for Women* (London: William Reeves, 1893), 8.
36. *Report of Inspector Redgrave for the Half-Year Ending 31 October 1875*, PP 1876 XVI, 34–5. *Report upon the Precautions which can be Enforced under the Factory Act and as to the need of further powers for the Protection of Persons employed in White Lead Works*, PP 1882 XVIII, 960.
37. Barbara Harrison, *Not Only the 'Dangerous Trades'. Women's Work and Health in Britain, 1880-1914* (London: Taylor & Francis, 1996), 61.

38. *Ibid.*, 229 and 230; Malone, *op. cit.* (note 33), 'Sex in Industry', 152–53.
39. Malone, *op. cit.* (note 15), 68; John Tosh, *A Man's Place. Masculinity and the Middle Class Home in Victorian England* (New Haven and London: Yale University Press, 1999).
40. See P.W.J. Bartrip and S.B. Burman, *The Wounded Soldiers of Industry. Industrial Compensation Policy, 1830-1897* (Oxford: OUP, 1983), 123–2, 137, 184 and 191.
41. Malone, *op. cit.* (note 33), 'Sex in Industry', 80.
42. In its early years, the Women's Provident and Protective League (the forerunner of the WTUL) opposed the imposition of restrictions on women's labour. See e.g. G. Boone, *The Women's Trade Union Leagues in Great Britain and the United States of America* (New York: Columbia University Press, 1942); C. Bolt, *The Women's Movements in the United States and Britain from the 1790s to the 1920s* (London: Harvester Wheatsheaf, 1993); H. Goldman, *Emma Paterson* (London: Lawrence & Wishart, 1974).
43. See, in particular, Morris Greenberg, 'Knowledge of the Health Hazard of Asbestos Pior to the Merewether and Price Report of 1930', *Social History of Medicine*, 7 (1994), 493–516.
44. P.W.J. Bartrip and R.M. Hartwell, 'Profit and Virtue. Economic Theory and the Regulation of Occupational Health in Nineteenth and Twentieth Century Britain' in Keith Hawkins (ed.), *The Human Face of Law. Essays in Honour of Donald Harris* (Oxford: Clarendon Press, 1997), 47.
45. British Library, Dilke Papers, Add. Mss.43892 ff.259, copy of letter from Dilke to James, 10 Aug. 1903.
46. *Annual Report of HM Chief Inspector of Factories*, (1891-2) PP 1893-4 XVII, 87–90; *Royal Commission on Labour. The Employment of Women*, PP 1893-4 XXVII pt.1, 600–703; 4 *Hansard*, 63 (29 July 1898), 471, 475–6, 520; H.J. Tennant, 'Dangerous Trades. A Case for Legislation', *Fortnightly Review*, 71 (Feb. 1899), 317; Adelaide Mary Anderson, *Women in the Factory* (London: John Murray, 1922), 10–11; Jill Pellew, *The Home Office, 1848-1914: from Clerks to Bureaucrats* (London: Heinemann, 1982), 151; P.W.J. Bartrip and P.T. Fenn, 'The Measurement of Safety: Factory Accident Statistics in Victorian and Edwardian Britian', *Historical Research*, 63 (1990), 58–72; Mary Drake McFeely, *Lady Inspectors. The Campaign for a Better Workplace, 1893-1921* (Oxford: Blackwell, 1988); Helen Jones, 'Women Health Workers: the Case of the First Women Factory Inspectors in Britain', *Social History of Medicine*, I (1988),

165–82; S. Koss, *Asquith* (New York: Columbia University Press, 1976); Roy Jenkins, *Asquith* (London: Collins, 1964). Gertrude Tuckwell, secretary and, later, president of the WTUL attributed the appointment of women factory inspectors to 'the wisdom of Mr Asquith'. See TUC Library Collections, University of North London. Gertrude Tuckwell Papers. Unpublished Reminiscences of Gertrude Tuckwell, 107.

47. O. MacDonagh, ' The Nineteenth Century Revolution in Government: a Re-appraisal', *Historical Journal*, I (1958), 52–67; *idem., A Pattern of Government Growth, 1800-60: the Passenger Acts and their Enforcement* (London: MacGibbon & Key, 1961).
48. See Bernard Semmel, *Imperialism and Social Reform. English Social-Imperial Thought, 1895-1914* (London: George Allen & Unwin, 1960); B.B. Gilbert, *The Evolution of National Insurance in Great Britain. The Origins of the Welfare State* (London: Michael Joseph, 1966); G.R. Searle, *The Quest for National Efficiency. A Study in British Politics and Political Thought, 1899-1914* (Oxford: Basil Blackwell, 1971); J.R. Hay, *The Origins of the Liberal Welfare Reforms, 1906-1914* (London and Basingstoke: Macmillan, 1975); Tony Novak, *Poverty and the State. An Historical Sociology* (Milton Keynes: Open University Press, 1988); Geoffrey Finlayson, *Citizen, State and Social Welfare in Britain, 1830-1990* (Oxford: OUP, 1994).
49. Thomas Oliver (ed), *Dangerous Trades: The Historical, Social and Legal Aspects of Industrial Occupations as Affecting Health by a Number of Experts* (London: John Murray, 1902), 5–7.
50. TUC Library Collections, University of North London. Gertrude Tuckwell Papers. Unpublished Reminiscences of Gertrude Tuckwell, 190–91.
51. With the exception of 1919, when one case of industrial phosphorus poisoning was reported to the factory inspectorate, there were no reports of phosphorus-related disease among British workers in the inter-war period. See *Annual Reports of HM Chief Inspector of Factories and Workshops*. It is important to stress that even where problems were 'solved' the question arose of whether the alternatives were entirely safe. Thus, in 1900 Thomas Legge reported that non-poisonous substitutes for white phosphorus were causing 'severe conjuntivitis', oedema of eyelids and eczema. See *Annual Report of HM Chief Inspector of Factories and Workshops,* (1900) PP 1901 X, 477.
52. See W.R. Lee, 'The History of Mercury Poisoning in Great Britain', *British Journal of Industrial Medicine*, 25 (1968), 52–62.

53. See Antonia Ineson and Deborah Thom, 'T.N.T. Poisoning and the Employment of Women Workers in the First World War' in Paul Wendling (ed), *The Social History of Occupational Health* (London: Croom Helm, 1985), 89–107.
54. See Alan Fowler and T.J. Wyke (eds), *The Barefoot Aristocrats: A History of the Amalgamated Association of Operative Cotton Spinners* (Littleborough: George Kelsall, 1987), chap. 10.
55. Harrison, *op. cit.* (note 37), 229.
56. *The Times*, 14 July 1999.

Works Cited

Archive Sources

Public Record Office. Files HO 45, LAB 14, 46

Bodliean Library. Ms. Asquith

Bradford Central Library, Anthrax Investigation Board Annual Reports

British Library, Dilke Papers, Add. Mss.43892

Hackney Archives. Bryant and May Mss.

TUC Library Collections. North London University Library. Gertrude Tuckwell Papers. Unpublished Reminiscences of Gertrude Tuckwell

TUC Library Collections, University of North London. Women's Trade Union League Minutes

TUC Library Collections, University of North London. WTUL Ledger on Health and Work in the Potteries District

West Yorkshire Archives Bradford, 39D84/1, Anthrax Investigation Board (AIB) Correspondence

West Yorkshire Archives Bradford, Bradford Medico-Chirurgical Society, 1874-1934, 40D89/1, History, Rules and Reports

West Yorkshire Archives Bradford, Bradford Medico-Chirurgical Society, 1874-1934, 40D89/2, Minutes, 1874-84

West Yorkshire Archives Bradford, 71D80/1/66, Anthrax Investigation Board Minutes, 1905-19

Acts of Parliament

Anthrax Prevention Act, 1919 (9 & 10 Geo. V c.23)

Aliens Act, 1844 (7&8 Vict. c.66)

Aliens Act, 1905 (5 Edw.7 c.13)

Arsenic Act, 1851 (14 & 15 Vict. c.13)

Bleaching Works Act, 1860 (23 & 24 Vict. c.78)

Coal Mines Regulation Act, 1872 (35 & 36 Vict. c.76)

Contagious Diseases (Animals) Act, 1886 (41 & 42 Vict. c.74)

Factory Act, 1833 (3&4 Will.4 c.103)

Employer's Liability Act, 1880 (43 & 44 Vict. c.42)

Factory Act, 1844 (7 & 8 Vict. c.15)

Factory Act, 1856 (19 & 20 Vict. c.38)

Factory Acts Extension Act, 1864 (*27 & 28 Vict. c.48*)
Factory Acts Extension Act, 1867 (*30 & 31 Vict. c.46*)
Factory and Workshop Act, 1871 (*34 & 35 Vict. c.104*)
Factory and Workshop Act, 1878 (41 Vict. c.16)
Factory and Workshop Act, 1883 (*46 & 47 Vict. c.53*)
Factory and Workshop Act, 1891 (*54 & 55 Vict. c.75*)
Factory and Workshop Act, 1895 (*58 & 59 Vict. c.37*)
Factory and Workshop Act, 1901 (*1 Edw.7 c.22*)
Health and Morals of Apprentices Act, 1802 (*42 Geo.3 c.73*)
Health and Safety at Work Act, 1974 (*22&23 Eliz. 2 c 37*)
Lead Paint (Protection Against Poisoning) Act, 1926 (*16 & 17 Geo.V c. 37*)
Medical Act, 1858 (*21 & 22 Vict. c.90*)
Metropolitan Buildings Act,1844 (*7 & 8 Vict. c.84*)
Metropolitan Police Act, 1829 (*3&4 Will.4 c.89*)
Mines Act, 1842 (*5&6 Vict. c.99*)
Mines Act, 1855 (*18 & 19 Vict. c.108*)
Poor Law Amendment Act, 1834 (4 & 5 Will.4 c.76)
Print Works Act, 1845, (*8 & 9 Vict. c.29*)
Prisons Act, 1823 (*4 Geo.4 c.64*)
White Phosphorus Matches Prohibition Act (*8 Edw.7 c.42*)
Workmen's Compensation Act, 1897 (*60 & 61 Vict. c.37*)
Workmen's Compensation Act, 1906 (*6 Edw.7 c.58*)
Workshop Regulation Act, 1867 (*30 & 31 Vict. c.146*)

Official Publications

Annual Report of the Medical Officer of the Local Government Board,1878, PP 1878-9 XXIX
Annual Report of the Medical Officer of the Local Government Board, 1880, PP 1881 XLVI
Annual Report of the Medical Officer of theLocal Government Board, 1882, PP 1883 XXVIII
Appendix to the Second Report of the Children's Employment Commission. Trades and Manufactures, part 1. Reports and Evidence from the Sub-Commissioners, Reports by Samuel Scriven, PP 1843 XV, 216
Bill to Amend the Law Relating to the Liability of Employers for Injuries to their Workmen, PP 1893-4 III
Board of Agriculture Returns
Census of England and Wales. 1901. Summary Tables, PP 1903 LXXXIV
Civil Service Estimates
Communications Addressed to the Secretary of State on the Subject of White Lead Poisoning, with Report by the Chief Inspector of Factories upon the Same Subject, PP 1883 XVIII

Departmental Committee Appointed to Inquire into and Report upon Certain Miscellaneous Dangerous Trades, Interim Report, PP 1896 XXXIII
Dod's Parliamentary Companion
Employers' Liability Amendment Bill, PP 1894 IV
Factory Acts Extension Bill, PP 1864 II
Factory & Workshops Bill, PP 1895 III
Fifth Report of the Children's Employment Commission, PP 1866 XXIV
Fifth Report of the Medical Officer of the Privy Council, PP 1863 XXV
Final Report on the First Census of Production of the United Kingdom (1907), PP 1912-13 CIX
First Report of the Central Board of His Majesty's Commissioners for Inquiry into the Employment of Children in Factories; with Minutes of Evidence and Reports by Medical Commissioners, PP 1833 XX
First Report of the Children's Employment Commission, PP 1863 XVIII
Fourth Report of the Children's Employment Commission. PP 1865 XX
Fourth Report of the Medical Officer of the Privy Council, PP 1862 XXII
Hansard's Parliamentary Debates
Interim Report of the Departmental Committee Appointed to Inquire into and Report upon Certain Miscellaneous Dangerous Trades, PP 1896 XXXIII
Irish University Press Reprints of British Parliamentary Papers (Industrial Revolution Children's Employment 9). Second Report of the Commissioners on Trades and Manufactures
Memorandum on the International Conference on Labour Regulation held at Berne, September 1906, with the Text of the Documents Signed at the Conference, PP 1906 CXXI
Ministry of Labour. Report of the Committee of Inquiry on Anthrax, PP 1959-60 VIII
Minutes of Evidence taken before the Commissioners Appointed to Inquire into the Factory and Workshop Acts, PP 1876 XXX
Minutes of Evidence Taken before the Select Committee on the State of the Children Employed in the Manufactories of the United Kingdom, PP 1816 III
On the State of the Public Health. The Annual Report of the Chief Medical Officer of the Department of Health for the Year 1994 (London: HMSO, 1995)
Report by the Chemical Works Committee of Inquiry (on Lucifer Match Works), PP 1893-4 XVII
Report from the Departmental Committee on the Various Lead Industries, PP 1893-4 XVII
Report from the Select Committee on the 'Bill to Regulate the Labour of Children in the Mills and Factories of the United Kingdom'; with the Minutes of Evidence, Appendix and Index, PP XV 1831-2

Report of Professor Brown on Anthrax or Woolsorters' Disease, PP 1881 LXXV
Report of the Commissioners Appointed to Inquire into the Working of the Factory and Workshops Acts with a View to their Consolidation and Amendment, PP 1876 XXIX
Report of the Committee on Dangerous Trades (Anthrax), PP 1897 XVII
Report of the Departmental Committee Appointed to Inquire into the Conditions of Work in Wool-Sorting and other Kindred Trades, PP 1897 XVII
Report of the Departmental Committee Appointed to Inquire as to Precautions for Preventing Danger of Infection by Anthrax in the Manipulation of Wool, Goat Hair and Camel Hair, PP 1918 VI
Report of the Departmental Committee Appointed to inquire into the Dangers attendant on the Use of Lead and the Danger or Injury to Health arising from Dust and other Causes in the Manufacture of Earthenware and China and in the Processes incidental thereto including the Making of Lithographic Transfers, PP 1910 XXIX
Report on the Conditions of Labour in Potteries, the Injurious Effects upon the Health of the Workpeople and the Proposed Remedies, PP 1893-4 XVII
Report on the Employment of Compounds of Lead in the Manufacture of Pottery, PP 1899 XII
Report on the Laws and Ordnances in Force in France for the Regulation of Noxious Trades and Occupations, PP 1854-5 XLV
Reports of Factory Inspectors
Report to the Secretary of State of the Home Department by H.H.S. Cunynghame, Under Secretary of State and B.A. Whitelegge, HM Chief Inspector of Factories on the Match factory of Messrs Moreland and Sons, Gloucester, with Special Reference to a Recent Fatal Case of Phosphorus Necrosis, PP 1907 X
Report to the Secretary of State for the Home Department of a Visit of Inspection to French Matchworks at Aubervilliers, Pantin and Marseilles, in June 1898, by Thomas Oliver MD, FRCP, PP 1898 XIV
Reports to the Secretary of State for the Home Department on the Use of Phosphorus in the Manufacture of Lucifer matches by Professor T.E. Thorpe, Principal Chemist of the Government Laboratory, Professor Thomas Oliver, Physician to the Royal Infirmary, Newcastle-upon-Tyne and George Cunningham, Senior Dental Surgeon to the London Hospital, PP 1899 XII
Report upon the Precautions which can be Enforced under the Factory Act and as to the need of further powers for the Protection of Persons employed in White Lead Works, PP 1882 XVIII
Royal Commission on Labour. The Employment of Women. Report of May Abraham on the White Lead Trade, PP 1893-4 XXXVII

Royal Commission on Labour. The Employment of Women. Report of Clara Collet on the Staffordshire Potteries, PP 1893-4 XXXVII (pt1)
Royal Commission on Labour. Employment of Women. Report by Miss Clara E. Collet (Lady Assistant Commissioner) on the Conditions of Work in London, PP 1893-4 XXXVII (pt1)
Royal Commission on the State of Large Towns and Populous Districts, PP 1844 XVII, Second Report of the Central Board of His Majesty's Commissioners for Inquiry into the Employment of Children in Factories; with Minutes of Evidence and Reports by Medical Commissioners. Dr James Mitchell's Report, PP 1833 XXI
Select Committee of the House of Lords on the Sale of Poisons etc. Bill (H.L.), PP 1857(2) XII
Sixth Report of the Medical Officer of the Privy Council. Appendix by George Whitley, PP 1864 XXVIII
Statutory Rules & Orders
Supplementary Report of the Central Board of His Majesty's Commissioners for Inquiry into the Employment of Children in Factories; with Minutes of Evidence and Reports by Medical Commissioners. Dr Bisset Hawkins's Reports on Lancashire, Derbyshire and Cheshire, D3, PP 1834 XIX
Third Interim Report of the Departmental Committee on Dangerous Trades, PP 1899 XII
White Phosphorus Matches Prohibition Bill, Memorandum, PP 1908 V

Books and Pamphlets

Aikin, J. *A Description of the Country from Thirty to Forty Miles Round Manchester* (London: John Stockdale, 1795)
Alfred (Samuel H.G. Kydd), *The History of the Factory Movement from the Year 1802, to the Enactment of the Ten Hours' Bill in 1847* (London: Simpkin, Marshall and Co., 1857)
Anderson, A.M. *Women in the Factory. An Administrative Adventure* (London: John Murray, 1922)
Archer, J.E. *By a Flash and a Scare. Incendiarism, Animal Maiming and Poaching in East Anglia, 1815-1870* (Oxford: Clarendon Press, 1990)
Arlidge, J.T. *On the Mortality of Stoke-upon-Trent and its Causes, with Especial Reference to Children and Potters*, (Newcastle-under-Lyme: np, 1864)
Arlidge, J.T. *On the Diseases Prevalent Among Potters* (London: np, 1872)
Arlidge, J.T. *Hygiene, Diseases and Mortality of Occupations* (London: Percival, 1892)
Ashford, N. A. *Crisis in the Workplace: Occupational Diseases and Injury* (Cambridge, Mass.: MIT Press, 1976)

Asquith, Earl of Oxford and *Fifty Years of Parliament* (London: Cassell, 1926)

Baines, E. *History of the Cotton Manufacture of Great Britain* (London: Frank Cass, 1966 edn)

Bartrip, P.W.J. *Workmen's Compensation in Twentieth Century Britain* (Aldershot: Gower, 1987)

Bartrip P.W.J. *Mirror of Medicine. A History of the British Medical Journal* (Oxford: BMJ and Clarendon Press, 1990)

Bartrip, P.W.J. *The Way from Dusty Death. Turner & Newall and the Regulation of Asbestos-Related Disease in Britain, 1890s-1970s* (London: Athlone, 2001)

Bartrip P.W.J. and Burman, S.B. *The Wounded Soldiers of Industry. Industrial Compensation Policy, 1833-1897* (Oxford: Clarendon Press, 1983)

Bayer R. (ed) *The Health and Safety of Workers. Case Studies in the Politicsd of Professional Responsibility* (New York: Oxford University Press, 1988)

Beaver, P. *The Match Makers* (London: Henry Melland, 1985)

Berman, D. *Death on the Job. Occupational Health and Safety Struggles in the United States* (New York: Monthly Review Press, 1979)

Bligh, M. *Dr Eurich of Bradford* (London: James Clarke, 1960)

Bolt, C. *The Women's Movements in the United States and Britain from the 1790s to the 1920s* (London: Harvester Wheatsheaf, 1993)

Boone, G. *The Women's Trade Union Leagues in Great Britain and the United States of America* (New York: Columbia University Press, 1942)

Booth C. *Life and Labour of the People in London* (London: Macmillan, 10 vols, 1892-97)

Booth, General W. *In Darkest England and the Way Out* (London: Charles Knight, 1970 edn)

Boston, S. *Women Workers and the Trade Union Movement* (London: Davis-Poynter, 1980)

Boucherett J. and Blackburn H. *The Condition of Working Women and the Factory Acts* (London: Elliot Stock, 1896)

Bradford Central Library Local Collection, *Bradford Medico-Chirurgical Society. Report of the Commission on Woolsorters' Disease* (Bradford: Toothill, 1882)

Briggs, A. *Victorian Things* (London: Batsford, 1988)

Bristow, E.J. *Vice and Vigilance. Purity Movements in Britain Since 1900* (Dublin: Gill & Macmillan, 1977)

Brockington, C.F. *Public Health in the Nineteenth Century* (Edinburgh & London: E.S. Livingstone, 1965)

Brown G.H. (comp) *Munk's Roll. Lives of the Fellows of the Royal College of Physicians of London, 1826-1925* IV (London: RCP, 1955)

Brown, J. *A Memoir of Robert Blincoe, an Orphan Boy; Sent from the Workhouse of St. Pancras, London, at Seven years of Age, to Endure the Cotton-Mill, through His Infancy and Youth, with a Minute Detail of his Sufferings, being the First Memoir of the Kind Published* (Firle: Caliban Books, 1977)

Brown, L. *Victorian News and Newspapers* (New York, Oxford University Press, 1985)

Bryder, L. *Below the Magic Mountain. A Social History of Tuberculosis in Twentieth Century Britain* (Oxford: Clarendon Press, 1988)

Buck, A. *Victorian Costume and Costume Accessories* (Carlton, Bedford: Ruth Bean, 1984 edn)

Burchill F. and Ross, R. *A History of the Potters' Union* (Stoke-on-Trent: CATU, 1977)

Byrde, P. *Nineteenth Century Fashion* (London: Batsford, 1992)

Carr, H. *Our Domestic Poisons; or, the Poisonous Effects of Certain Dyes and Colours Used in Domestic Fabrics* (London: William Clowes, 1879)

Chapman, S.D. *The Early Factory Masters* (Newton Abbot: David & Charles, 1967)

Christison, R. *A Treatise on Poisons in Relation to Medical Jurisprudence, Physiology and the Practice of Physic* (Edinburgh: Longman, Rees, Orme, Browne and Green, 1829)

Clarke, A. *The Effects of the Factory System* (Littleborough: George Kelsall, 1989)

Clegg H.A., Fox Alan and Thompson A.F. *A History of British Trade Unions since 1889* (Oxford: Clarendon Press, 1964-94)

Corn, J.K. *Response to Occupational Health Hazards. A Historical Perspective* (New York: Van Nostrand Reinhold, 1992)

Cullen, M.J. *The Statistical Movement in Early Victorian Britain* (Brighton: Harvester Press, 1975)

Cunnington, C.W. *English Women's Clothing in the Nineteenth Century* (London: Faber & Faber, 1937)

Davies M.L. (ed) *Life as We Have Known It* (London: Virago, 1977)

Dawson, A. *Bernard Moore. Master Potter, 1850-1935* (Richard Dennis: London, 1982)

Derickson, A. *Workers' Health, Workers' Democracy. The Western Miners' Struggle for Health and Safety, 1891-1925* (Ithaca: Cornell University Press, 1988)

Derickson, A. *Black Lung. Anatomy of a Public Health Disaster* (Ithaca and London: Cornell University Press, 1998)

Dickens, C. *The Uncommercial Traveller* (London: Everyman edn, 1911)

Dictionary of National Biography

Digby, A. *Making a Medical Living. Doctors and Patients in the English Market for Medicine, 1720-1911* (Cambridge: CUP, 1994)

Digby, A. *The Evolution of British General Practice, 1850-1948* (Oxford: Oxford University Press, 1999)

Dixon, W.H. *The Match Industry. Its Origin and Development* (London: Pitman, 1925)

Driver, C. *Tory Radical. The Life of Richard Oastler* (New York: Oxford University Press, 1946)

Duckham, H. and B. *Great Pit Disasters: Great Britain 1700 to the Present Day* (Newton Abbot: David & Charles, 1970)

Dupree, M.W. *Family Structure in the Staffordshire Potteries* (Oxford: Clarendon Press, 1995)

Emsley, J. *The Shocking History of Phosphorus. A Biography of the Devil's Element* (London: Macmillan, 2000)

Engels, F. *The Condition of the Working Class in England* (London: Panther, 1969 edn)

Escott, T.H.S. *England. Its People, Polity and Pursuits* (London: Cassell, 2 vols, 1879)

Eyler, J. *Victorian Social Medicine. The Ideas and Methods of William Farr* (Baltimore: Johns Hopkins University Press, 1979)

Finlayson, G. *The Seventh Earl of Shaftesbury, 1801-1885* (London: Eyre Methuen, 1981)

Finlayson, G. *Citizen, State and Social Welfare in Britain, 1830-1990* (Oxford: Oxford University Press, 1994)

Fishman, W. J. *East End 1888. A Year in a London Borough Amomg the Labouring Poor* (London: Duckworth, 1988)

Forbes, J. Tweedie A. and Conolly, J. *Cyclopaedia of Practical Medicine* (London: Sherwood, Gilbert and Piper and Baldwin and Cradock, 1833)

Fowler Alan and Wyke T.J. (eds), *The Barefoot Aristocrats: A History of the Amalgamated Association of Operative Cotton Spinners* (Littleborough: George Kelsall, 1987)

Furnival, W. *Researches on Leadless Glazes* (Stone: W.J. Furnival, 1898)

Garfield, S. *Mauve. How one Man Invented a Colour that Changed the World* (London: Faber and Faber, 2000)

Garrett, S.A. *Ethics and Air Power in World War II: the British Bombing of German Cities* (New York: St. Martin's Press, 1997)

Gaskell, P. *Artisans and Machinery: the Moral and Physical Condition of the Manufacturing Population considered with Reference to Mechanical Substitutes for Human Labour* (London: Frank Cass, 1968)

General View of the Agriculture and Minerals of Derbyshire (London: Board of Agriculture, 3 vols, 1811-17)

Gersuny, C. *Work Hazards and Industrial Conflict* (Hanover NH: University Press of New England, 1981)

Gilbert, B.B. *The Evolution of National Insurance in Great Britain. The Origins of the Welfare State* (London: Michael Joseph, 1966)

Gilfillan, S. Colum *Rome's Ruin by Lead Poison* (Long Beach: Wenzel Press, 1990)

Gloag, J. *Victorian Comfort. A Social History of Design from 1830 to 1900* (Newton Abbot: David & Charles, 1973 edn)

Goldman, H. *Emma Paterson* (London: Lawrence and Wishart, 1974)

Goyder, D. *History of the First Twenty-Five Years of the Bradford Medico-Chirurgical Society* (Bradford: Toothill, 1898)

Gray, R. *The Factory Question and Industrial England, 1830-1860* (Cambridge, CUP, 1996)

Hammond P.W. and Egan, H. *Weighed in the Balance. A History of the Laboratory of the Government Chemist* (London: HMSO, 1992)

Harris R. and Paxman, J. *A Higher Form of Killing. The Secret Story of Gas and Germ Warfare* (London: Chatto & Windus, 1983)

Harrison, B. *Not Only the 'Dangerous Trades'. Women's Work and Health in Britain, 1880-1914* (London: Taylor & Francis, 1996)

Hastings, C. *A Treatise on the Inflammation of the Mucous Membrane of the Lungs* (London: Thomas & George Underwood, 1820)

Hastings, C. *Illustrations of the Natural History of Worcestershire* (London & Worcester: Sherwood, Gilbert & Piper, 1834)

Havighurst, A.H. *Radical Journalist: H.W. Massingham (1860-1924)* (London: Cambridge University Press, 1974)

Hay, J.R. *The Origins of the Liberal Welfare Reforms, 1906-1914* (London and Basingstoke: Macmillan, 1975)

Heavisides M. (ed) *The True History of the Invention of the Lucifer Match by John Walker of Stockton-on-Tees in 1827; with an Account of the Ancient Modes of Procuring Light and Fire* (Stockton-on-Tees: Heavisides & Son, 1909)

Hennock, E.P. *British Social Reform and German Precedents. The Case of Social Insurance, 1880-1914* (Oxford: Clarendon Press, 1987)

Henriques, U.R.Q. *Before the Welfare State. Social Administration in Early Industrial Britain* (London: Longman, 1979)

Hodder, E. *The Life and Work of the Seventh Earl of Shaftesbury K.G.* (London: Cassell, 1893)

Holland, G.C. *Diseases of the Lungs from Mechanical Causes; and Inquiries into the Condition of Artisans Exposed to the Inhalation of Dust* (London: John Churchill, 1843)

Holmes, C. *John Bull's Island. Immigration and British Society, 1871-1971* (Basingstoke: Macmillan, 1988)

Hooper, R. *Lexicon Medicum or Medical Dictionary* (London: Longman, 4th edn 1820)

Hopkins, E. *Childhood Transformed. Working Class Children in Nineteenth Century England* (Manchester: Manchester University Press, 1994)

Hunter, D. *The Diseases of Occupations* (London: English Universities Press, 1955)

Hutchins B.L.and Harrison, A. *A History of Factory Legislation* (London: P.S. King, 1926 edn)

Hyam E. (trans) *Taine's Notes on England* (London: Thames and Hudson, 1957 edn)

Isaacson, E. *The Forgotten Physician* (no publishing details)

Ittmann, K. *Work, Gender and Family in Victorian England* (Basingstoke: Macmillan, 1995)

Japp, A.H. *Industrial Curiosities. Glances Here and There in the World of Labour* (London: Marshall Japp & Co., 1882)

Jenkins, R. *Asquith* (London: Collins, 1964)

Jenkins, R. *Dilke. A Victorian Tragedy* (London: Collins, 1965)

Jones, D. *Crime, Protest, Community and Police in Nineteenth-Century Britain* (London, Routledge and Kegan Paul, 1982)

Jones, H. *Health and Society in Twentieth Century Britain* (London: Longman, 1994)

Judkins, B. M. *We Offer Ourselves. Towards Workers' Control of Occupational Health* (Westport: Greenwood Press, 1986);

Kay, J.P. *The Moral and Physical Condition of the Working Classes Employed in the Cotton Manufacture in Manchester* (London: Ridgway, 1832)

Kinnersly, P. *The Hazards of Work. How to Fight Them* (London: Pluto Press, 1973)

Kirby, E.A. *On the Administration of Phosphorus as a Remedy for Loss of Nerve Power, Neuralgia, Hysteria, Melancholia and other Atonic Conditions of the Cerebro-Spinal System. With the Formulae for its Combination with Iron, Quinine and Nux Vomica* (London: H.K. Lewis, 1875)

Koss, S. *Asquith* (New York: Columbia University Press, 1976)

Kostal, R.W. *Law and Englsih Railway Capitalism, 1825-1875* (Oxford: Clarendon Press, 1994)

Lambert, R. J. *Sir John Simon and English Social Administration* (London: MacGibbon & Key, 1963)

Lee, A.J. *The Origins of the Popular Press in England, 1855-1914* (London: Croom Helm, 1976)

Legge, T.M. *Report on the Incidence of Anthrax in the Manipulation of Horsehair and Bristles* (London: HMSO, 1906)

Legge, Sir T.M. *Thirty Years' Experience of Industrial Maladies* (London: Royal Society of Arts, 1929)

Legge, Sir T.M. *Industrial Maladies* (London: Oxford University Press, 1934)

Legge T.M. and Goadby, K.W. *Lead Poisoning and Lead Absorption* (London: Edward Arnold, 1912)

Lewenhak, S. *Women and Trade Unions* (London: Benn, 1977)

Lewis, J. *The Politics of Motherhood. Child and Maternal Welfare in England, 1900-1939* (London: Croom Helm, 1980)

Luson T. and Hyde, R. *The Diseases of Workmen* (London: Butterworth, 1908)

MacDonagh, O. *A Pattern of Government Growth, 1800-60: the Passenger Acts and their Enforcement* (London: MacGibbon & Key, 1961)

MacKenzie, D. *Statistics in Britain, 1865-1930: the Social Construction of Scientific Knowledge* (Edinburgh: Edinburgh University Press, 1981)

Major, R.H. *A History of Medicine* (Oxford: Blackwell, 1954)

Mallet, Mrs C. *Dangerous Trades for Women* (London: William Reeves, 1893)

Martindale, H. *From one Generation to Another, 1839-1944. A Book of Memoirs* (London: George Allen & Uniwin, 1944)

Mayhew, H. *The Morning Chronicle Survey of Labour and the Poor: the Metropolitan Districts* (Horsham: Caliban Books, 1981)

McFeely, M.D. *Lady Inspectors. The Campaign for a Better Workplace, 1893-1921* (Oxford: Blackwell, 1988)

McIvor, A.J. *A History of Work in Britain*, 1880-1950 (Basingstoke: Palgrave, 2001)

McKeown, T. *The Modern Rise of Population* (London: Edward Arnold, 1976)

McMenemy, W. H. *The Life and Times of Sir Charles Hastings. Founder of the British Medical Association* (Edinburgh and London: Livingstone, 1959)

Meiklejohn, A. *The Life Work and Times of Charles Turner Thackrah, Surgeon and Apothecary of Leeds (1795-1833* (Edinburgh and London: E&P Livingstone, 1957)

Mess, H.A. *Factory Legislation and its Administration, 1891-1924* (London: P.S. King, 1926)

Morris, R.J. *Cholera 1832 The Social Response to an Epidemic* (London: Croom Helm, 1976)

Munk's Roll. Lives of Fellows of the Royal College of Physicians IV (London: RCP, 1955)

Neild, P. *Byssinosis—'The Lancashire Disease'* (London: Chartered Insurance Insurance Institute, 1982)

Neff, W. F. *Victorian Working Women. An Historical and Literary Study of Women in British Industries and Professions, 1832-1850* (London: Frank Cass, 1966 edn)

New Dictionary of National Biography (forthcoming)

Newsam, Sir F. *The Home Office* (London: George Allen & Unwin, 1954)

Nichols, T. *The Sociology of Industrial Injury* (London: Mansell, 1997)

Nicholls, D. *The Lost Prime Minister. A Life of Sir Charles Dilke* (London: Hambledon Press, 1995)

Norman J.M. (ed) *Morton's Medical Bibliography. An Annotated Check-list of Texts Illustrating the History of Medicine (Garrison and Morton)* (Aldershot: Scolar Press, 1991 edn)

Novak, T. *Poverty and the State. An Historical Sociology* (Milton Keynes: Open University Press, 1988)

Nriagu, J.O. *Lead and Lead Poisoning in Antiquity* (New York: Wiley, 1983)

O'Connell, S. *The Car in British Society. Class, Gender and Motoring, 1896-1939* (Manchester and New York: Manchester University Press, 1998)

Oliver, T. (ed) *Dangerous Trades: The Historical, Social and Legal Aspects of Industrial Occupations as Affecting Health by a Number of Experts* (London: John Murray, 1902)

Oliver, T. *Diseases of Occupation. From the Legislative, Social and Medical Points of View* (London: Methuen, 1908)

Owen, R.D. *Threading My Way. Twenty Seven Years of Autobiography* (London: Trubner, 1874)

Page J.A. and O'Brien, M.-W. *Bitter Wages: Ralph Nader's Study Group Report on Disease and Injury on the Job* (New York: Grossman, 1973)

Papers and Discussions on Public Health: Being the Transactions of the Fourth Department of the National Association for the Promotion of Social Science (London: Emily Faithful, 1862)

Paulus, I. *The Search for Pure Food: a Sociology of Legislation in Great Britain* (London: Martin Robertson, 1974)

Pellew, J. *The Home Office, 1848-1914. From Clerks to Bureaucrats* (London: Heinemann Educational Books, 1982)

Percival, T. *Observations and Experiments on the Poison of Lead* (London: Johnson, 1774)

Perkin, H. *The Origins of Modern English Society, 1780-1880* (London: Routledge & Kegan Paul, 1969)

Pinchbeck, I. *Women Workers and the Industrial Revolution, 1750-1850* (London: Frank Cass, 1969 edn)

Plomer W. (ed) *Kilvert's Diary. Selections from the Diary of the Rev. Francis Kilvert* (London: Jonathan Cape, 3 vols, 1980 edn),

Prendergast, W.D. *The Potter and Lead Poisoning* (Stoke-on-Trent: n.p., 1898)

Priestley, J.B. *English Journey* (London: BCA, 1984 edn)

Prochaska, F.K. *Women and Philanthropy in Nineteenth Century England* (Oxford: Clarendon Press, 1980)

Raffle, P.A.B. Lee, W.R. McCallum, R.I. Murray R. (eds) *Hunter's Diseases of Occupations* (London: Hodder and Stoughton, 1987)

Reeves, M.P. *Round About a Pound a Week* (London: Virago, 1979 edn)

Reynolds, J. *The Great Paternalist. Titus Salt and the Growth of Nineteenth Century Bradford* (London: St Martin's Press, 1983)

Ritvo, H. *The Animal Estate The English and Other Creatures in the Victoria Age* (Cambridge Mass.: Harvard University Press, 1987)

Roberts, E. *Women's Work, 1840-1940* (Basingstoke: Macmillan, 1995)

Rose, S. *Limited Livelihoods. Gender and Class in Nineteenth Century England* (Berkeley: University of California Press, 1992)

Rosen, G. *The History of Miners' Diseases: a Medical and Social Interpretation* (New York: Schuman's, 1943)

Rosenberg, C. *The Cholera Years. The United States in 1832, 1849 and 1866* (Chicago: University of Chicago Press, 1962)

Rosner D. and Markowitz G. (eds) *Dying for Work. Workers' Safety and Health in Twentieth-Century America* (Bloomington: Indiana University Press, 1987)

Rosner D. and Markowitz, G. *Deadly Dust: Silicosis and the Politics of Occupational Disease in Twentieth Century America* (Princeton: Princeton University Press, 1991)

Rowe, D.J. *Lead Manufacturing in Great Britain. A History* (Beckenham: Croom Helm, 1983)

Rule, J. *The Experience of Labour in Eighteenth Century Industry* (London: Croom Helm, 1981)

Sadler, T. (ed) *Diary, Reminiscences and Correspondence of Henry Crabb Robinson, Barrister-at-Law* (London: Macmillan, 3 vols, 1869)

Samuel, R. *East End Underworld. Chapters in the Life of Arthur Harding* (London: Routledge and Kegan Paul, 1981)

Sarsby J. *Missuses & Mouldrunners. An Oral History of Women Pottery Workers at Work and at Home* (Milton Keynes: Open University Press,1988)

Schilling, R. *A Challenging Life. Sixty Years in Occupational Health* (London: Canning Press, 1998)

Schmidt, J.E. *Medical Discoveries. Who and When* (Springfield, Illinois: Thomas, 1959)

Searle, G.R. *The Quest for National Efficiency. A Study in British Politics and Political Thought, 1899-1914* (Oxford: Basil Blackwell, 1971)

Sellers, Christopher C. *Hazards of the Job. From Industrial Disease to Environmental Health Science* (Chapel Hill and London: University of North Carolina Press, 1997)

Semmel, Bernard *Imperialism and Social Reform. English Social-Imperial Thought, 1895-1914* (London: George Allen & Unwin, 1960)

Shaw, Charles *When I Was a Child* (Firle: Caliban Books, 1980)

Sherard, R.H. *The White Slaves of England. Being True Pictures of Certain Social Conditions in the Kingdom of England in the Year 1897* (London: James Bowden, 1897)

Simon, Sir John *English Sanitary Institutions* (London: John Murray, 1897)

Smith, A. *The Wealth of Nations* (London: Everyman edn, 2 vols, 1970)

Smith, B.E. *Digging our Own Graves: Coal Miners and the Struggle over Black Lung Disease* (Philadelphia: Temple University Press, 1987)

Smith, F.B. *The Retreat of Tuberculosis, 1850-1950* (Beckenham: Croom Helm, 1988)

Smith, P. *Disraelian Conservatism and Social Reform.* (London: Routledge & Kegan Paul, 1967)

Sontag, S. *Illness as Metaphor* (London: Allen Lane: 1979)

Sontag, S. *Aids and Its Metaphors* (London: Allen Lane, 1989)

Spanton W.D. (ed. E.E. Young) *The Story of My Life* (London: The Connoisseur, 1920)

Squire, R. *Thirty Years in the Public Service. An Industrial Retrospect* (London: Nisbet, 1927)

Stanley, E. *A Treatise on the Diseases of Bones* (London: Longman, Brown, Green, & Longmans, 1849)

Stigler, S.M. *The History of Statistics. The Measurement of Uncertainty before 1900* (Cambridge, Mass. and London: Belknap Press, 1986)

Stuart, D. *Millicent Duchess of Sutherland, 1867-1955* (London: Gollancz, 1982)

Taylor, A.S. *On Poisons in Relation to Medical Jurisprudence and Medicine* (London: John Churchill, 1848)

Taylor, W. C. *Notes of a Tour in the Manufacturing Districts of Lancashire* (London: Frank Cass, 1968)

Teleky, L. *History of Factory and Mine Hygiene* (New York: Columbia University Press, 1948)

Thackrah, C.T. *The Effect of Arts, Trades and Professions and of Civic States and Habits of Living, on Health and Longevity: with Suggestions for the Removal of Many of the Agents which Produce Disease and Shorten the Duration of Life* (London: Longman, Rees, Orme, Brown, Green and Longman, 2nd edn, 1832)

Thomis, M. I. *The Town Labourer and the Industrial Revolution* (London: Batsford, 1974)

Thomis, M. I. *Responses to Industrialisation. The British Experience, 1780-1850* (Newton Abbot: David & Charles, 1976)

Thompson, E.P. *Whigs and Hunters. The Origins of the Black Act* (London: Allen Lane, 1975)

Thompson F.M.L. *Horses in European Economic History. A Preliminary Canter* (Reading: British Agricultural History Society, 1983)

Thompson F.M.L. (ed), *The Cambridge Social History of Britain, 1750-1950. vol.3 Social Agencies and Institutions* (Cambridge: CUP, 1990)

Thorpe, T.E. *A Dictionary of Applied Chemistry* (London: Longmans, Green, 3 vols, 1893 edn)

Threlfall, R.E. *The Story of 100 Years of Phosphorus Making, 1851-1951* (Oldbury: Albright and Wilson Ltd., 1951)

Tosh, J. *A Man's Place. Masculinity and the Middle Class Home in Victorian England* (New Haven and London: Yale University Press, 1999)

Troup, C.E. *The Home Office* (London and New York: G.P. Putnam's Sons Ltd., 1925)

Tunzelmann, G.N. von *Steam Power and British Industrialisation to 1860* (Oxford: Clarendon Press, 1978)

Tweedale, G. *From Magic Mineral to Killer Dust. Turner & Newall and the Asbestos Hazard* (Oxford: Oxford University Press, 2000)

Twigg, G. *The Black Death: a Biological Reappraisal* (London: Batsford, 1984)

Ure, A. *The Philosophy of Manufactures: or, an Exposition of the Social, Moral and Commercial Economy of the Factory System of Great Britain* (London: Charles Knight, 1835)

Walby, S. *Patriarchy at Work. Patriarchal and Capitalist Relations in Employment* (Cambridge: Polity, 1986)

Walkowitz, J. R. *City of Dreadful Delight. Narratives of Sexual Danger in Late Victorian London* (London: Virago, 1992)

Warren, C. *Brush with Death. A Social History of Lead Poisoning* (Baltimore and London: The Johns Hopkins University Press, 2000)

Weatherill, L. *The Pottery Trade and North Staffordshire, 1660-1760* (Manchester: Manchester University Press, 1971)

Weindling P.(ed) *The Social History of Occupational Health* (London: Croom Helm, 1985)

Weiner J. H. (ed) *Papers for the Millions, the New Journalism in Britain, 1850s to 1914* (London and New York: London ,1988)

Whipp, R. *Patterns of Labour. Work and Social Change in the Pottery Industry* (London: Routledge, 1990)

Who Was Who

Wikeley, N.J. *Compensation for Industrial Disease* (Aldershot: Dartmouth, 1993)

Wilkinson, L. *Animals and Disease: an Introduction to the History of Comparative Medicine* (Cambridge: Cambridge University Press, 1992)
Wohl, A. S. *Endangered Lives. Public Health in Victorian Britain* (London: Methuen, 1984)
Wright, M. *Treasury Control of the Civil Service, 1854-1874* (Oxford: Clarendon Press, 1969)
Wright, W.C. *De Morbis Artificum. Bernardini Ramazzini. Diatriba. Diseases of Workers. The Latin Text of 1713 Revised with Translation and Notes* (Chicago: University of Chicago Press, 1940)
Yarwood, D. *The English Home* (London: Batsford, 1979)

Journal Articles and Chapters in Edited Books

Allison, W.P. 'Observations on the Pathology of Scrofulous Diseases with a View to their Prevention', *Transactions of the Medico-Chirurgical Society of Edinburgh*, I (1824)
Anderson, A. 'Historical Sketch of the development of Legislation for Injuries and Dangerous Industries in England', in Thomas Oliver, (ed.), *Dangerous Trades: The Historical, Social and Legal Aspects of Industrial Occupations as Affecting Health by a Number of Experts* (London: John Murray, 1902)
Arlidge, J.T. 'Diseases Incident to the Manufacture of Pottery', *BMJ*, 26 Aug. 1876
Baines, M.A. 'The Ladies' National Association for the Diffusion of Sanitary Knowledge', in Hastings G.W. (ed.) *Transactions of the National Association for the Promotion of Social Science* (London: John Parker, 1859)
Balfour, G.W. 'On Necrosis of the Jaw-Bones from the Fumes of Phosphorus', *Northern Journal of Medicine*, iv (1846)
Bartrip, P.W.J. 'British Government Inspection, 1832-1875. Some Observations', *Historical Journal*, 25 (1982)
Bartrip, P.W.J. 'State Intervention in mid-Nineteenth Century Britain: Fact or Fiction?', *Journal of British Studies*, xxxiii (1983)
Bartrip, P.W.J. 'Expertise and the Dangerous Trades, 1875-1900' in R.M. MacLeod (ed.), *Government and Expertise. Specialist, Administrators and Professionals, 1860-1919* (Cambridge: Cambridge University Press, 1988)
Bartrip, P.W.J. 'Accidents and Ill-Health: The Hidden Wages of the Workplace', *Social History of Medicine*, 3 (1990)
Bartrip, P.W.J.'A "Pennurth of Arsenic for Rat Poison": the Arsenic Act, 1851 and the Prevention of Secret Poisoning', *Medical History*, 36 (1992)

Bartrip, P.W.J. 'How Green was My Valance: Environmental Arsenic Poisoning and the Myth of Victorian Domesticity', *English Historical Review*, cix (1994)

Bartrip, P.W.J. ' "Petticoat Pestering": the Women's Trade Union League and Lead Poisoning in the Staffordshire Potteries, 1890-1914', *Historical Studies in Industrial Relations*, 2 (1996)

Bartrip, P.W.J. 'Too Little Too Late? The Home Office and the Asbestos Industry Regulations, 1931', *Medical History*, 42 (1998)

Bartrip, P.W.J. 'Nellie Kershaw, Turner and Newall, and Asbestos-Related Disease in 1920s Britain', *Historical Studies in Industrial Relations Historical Studies in Industrial Relation*, 9 (2000)

Bartrip P.W.J. and Fenn, P.T. 'The Administration of Safety: the Enforcement Policy of the Early Factory Inspectorate, 1844-1864', *Public Administration*, 58 (1980)

Bartrip P.W.J. and Fenn, P.T. 'The Conventionalization of Factory Crime—a Re-assessment' Crime', *International Journal of the Sociology of Law*, 8 (1980)

Bartrip P.W.J. and Fenn, P.T. 'The Evolution of Regulatory Style in the Nineteenth Century British Factory Inspectorate', *Journal of Law and Society*, 10 (1983)

Bartrip P.W.J. and Hartwell, R.M. 'Profit and Virtue. Economic Theory and the Regulation of Occupational Health in Nineteenth and Twentieth Century Britain', in Keith Hawkins (ed.), *The Human Face of Law. Essays in Honour of Donald Harris* (Oxford: Clarendon Press, 1997)

Bartrip P.W.J. and Fenn, P.T. 'The Measurement of Safety. Factory Accident Statistics in Victorian and Edwardian Britain', *Historical Research*, 63 (Feb. 1990)

Benson, J. 'Colliery Disaster Funds, 1860-1897', *International Review of Labour History*, XIX (1974)

Benson, J. 'English Coal-Miners' Trade Union Accident Funds, 1850-1900' *Economic History Review,* 2nd. ser 28 (1975)

Benson, J. 'Non-Fatal Coal Mining Accidents', *Bulletin of the Society for the Study of Labour History*, 32 (1976)

Brown J.R. and Thornton, J.L. 'Percivall Pott and Chimney Sweepers' Cancer of the Scrotum', *British Journal of Industrial Medicine,* 14 (1957)

Burnett, J. *Plenty and Want. A Social History of Diet in England from 1815 to the Present Day* (London: Scolar Press, 1979 edn)

Busbey, K. 'The Women's Trade Union Movement in Great Britain', *Bulletin of the Bureau of Labour*, 83 (1909)

Bynum, W.F. '"C'est un Malade": Animal Models and Concepts of Human Diseases', *Journal of the History of Medicine and Allied Sciences*, 45 (1990)

Carmichael A. and Tigertt W. 'Reviews', *Journal of the History of Medicine*, 41 (1986)

Carson, W.G. 'The Conventionalization of Early Factory Crime', *International Journal of the Sociology of Law*, 7 (1979)

Carter, K.C. 'The Koch-Pasteur Dispute on Establishing the Cause of Anthrax', *Bulletin of the History of Medicine*, 62 (1988)

Chaloner, W.H. 'Bibliographical Introduction' to Edward Baines, *History of the Cotton Manufacture of Great Britain* (London: Frank Cass, 1966 edn)

Clark, J.F.M. 'Eleanor Ormerod (1828-1901) as an Economic Entomologist: "Pioneer of Purity even more than of Paris Green"', *British Journal for the History of Science*, xxv (1992)

Clark, J.F.M. 'Beetle Mania: the Colorado Beetle Scare of 1877', *History Today*, xii (1992)

Clayton, E.G. *A Memoir of the late Dr. A.H. Hassall* (London: n.p.,1908)

Cleeland J. and Burt S. 'Charles Turner Thackrah: a Pioneer in the Field of Occupational Health', *Occupational Medicine*, 45 (1995)

Colley, N. G. 'Alfred Swaine Taylor, MD FRS (1806-1880): forensic toxicologist', *Medical History*, 35 (1991)

Concise Medical Dictionary (Oxford, Oxford University Press, 1987)

Conolly, J. 'Biographical Memoir of the Late John Darwall of Birmingham', *Transactions of the Provincial Medical and Surgical Association*, 2 (1834)

Davidson R. and Lowe, R. 'Bureaucracy and Innovation in British Welfare Policy, 1870-1945' in W.J. Mommsen (ed.), *The Emergence of the Welfare State in Britain and Germany, 1850-1950* (London: Croom Helm, 1981)

Davin, A. 'Imperialism and Motherhood', *History Workshop*, 5 (1978)

Dearden, W.F. 'Fragilitas ossium amongst Workers in Lucifer Match Factories', *BMJ*, 29 July 1899

Dyhouse, C. 'Working Class Mothers and Infant Mortality, 1895-1894', *Journal of Social History*, 12 (1978)

Eurich, F.W. 'Anthrax in the Woollen Industry, with Special Reference to Bradford', *Proceedings of the Royal Society of Medicine*, VI (1912-13)

Feurer, R. 'The Meaning of "Sisterhood": The British Women's Movement and Protective Labor Legislation', 1870-1900', *Victorian Studies*, 31 (1988)

Figlio, K. 'How Does Illness Mediate Social Relations? Workmen's Compensation and Medico-Legal Practices, 1890-1940' in P.Wright and A. Treacher (eds), *The Problem of Medical Knowledge* (Edinburgh: Edinburgh University Press, 1982)

Figlio, K. 'What is an Accident' in Paul Weindling (ed.), *The Social History of Occupational Health* (London: Croom Helm, 1985)

Flavell, C.F. 'On Grinders Asthma', *Transactions of the Provincial Medical and Surgical Association*, new ser. vol.2 (1846)

Gilfillan, S. Colum 'Lead Poisoning and the Fall of Rome', *Journal of Occupational Medicine*, 7 (1965)

Godwin, A. 'Early Years in the Trade Unions', in L. Middleton (ed.), *Women in the Labour Movement: the British Experience* (Beckenham: Croom Helm, 1977)

Goldwater, L. J. 'From Hippocrates to Ramazzini: Early History of Industrial Medicine', *Annals of Medical History*, new ser. 8 (1936)

Gray, R. 'Medical Men, Industrial Labour and the State in Britain, 1830-1850', *Social History*, 16 (1991)

Gray, R. 'Factory Legislation and the Gendering of Jobs in the North of England, 1830-1860', *Gender & History*, 5 (1993)

Greenberg, M. 'Knowledge of the Health Hazard of Asbestos Prior to the Merewether and Price Report of 1930', *Social History of Medicine*, 7 (1994)

Guy, W.A. 'Contributions to a Knowledge of the Influence of Employments upon Health', *Journal of the Royal Statistical Society*, (1843)

Guy, W.A. 'Effects of Arsenite of Copper on Paper Stainers', *Archives of Medicine*, I (1857)

Haller J S. Jnr. 'Therapeutic Mule: the Use of Arsenic in Nineteenth Century *Materia Medica*', *Pharmacy in History*, 17 (1975)

Hamer W.H. 'Anthrax' in Thomas Oliver (ed.), *Dangerous Trades. The Historical, Social and Legal Aspects of Industrial Occupations as Affecting Health, by a Number of Experts* (London: John Murray, 1902)

Harrison, B. '"Some of Them gets Lead Poisoned": Occupational Health Exposure in Women, 1880-1914', *Social History of Medicine*, 2 (1989)

Harrison, B. 'Suffer the Working Day. Women in the "Dangerous Trades", 1880-1914', *Women's Studies International Forum*, 13 (1990)

Harrison, B. 'Women's Health or Social Control? The Role of the Medical Profession in Relation to Factory Legislation in Late Nineteenth-Century Britain', *Sociology of Health and Illness*, 13 (1991)

Harrison, B. 'Feminism and Health Consequences of Work in Late Nineteenth and Early Twentieth Century Britain' in S. Platt (*et al*), *Locating Health. Sociological and Historical Explorations* (Aldershot: Avebury, 1993)

Harrison, B. 'The Politics of Occupational Health in Late Nineteenth Century and Early Twentieth Century Britain', *Sociology of Health and Illness*, 13 (1995)

Harrison B. and Mockett, H. 'Women in the Factory: The State and Factory Legislation in Nineteenth Century Britain' in L. Jamieson and H. Corr (eds), *State, Private Life and Political Change* (London: Macmillan, 1990)

Hart, B.H. Liddell *History of the First World War* (London: Cassell, 1970 edn)

Hartwell, R.M. 'Entrepreneurship and Public Inquiry: the Growth of Government in Nineteenth Century Britain', in Thompson, F.M.L. (ed.) *Landowners, Capitalists and Entrepreneurs* (Oxford: Clarendon Press, 1994)

Hawkins, K. ' "FATCATS" and Prosecution in a Regulatory Agency: A Footnote on the Social Construction of Risk', *Law and Policy*, 11 (1989)

Holdsworth, C. 'Women's Work and Family Health: Evidence from the Staffordshire Potteries, 1890-1920', *Continuity and Change*, 12 (1997)

Holdsworth, C. 'Dr John Thomas Arlidge and Victorian Occupational Medicine', *Medical History*, 42 (1998)

Hughes J.P.W. *et al*, 'Phosphorus Necrosis of the Jaw: A Present-Day Study', *British Journal of Industrial Medicine*, 19 (1962)

Hutt, W.H. 'The Factory System in the Early Nineteenth Century' in F.A. Hayek (ed.), *Capitalism and the Historians* (London: Routledge and Kegan Paul, 1954)

Ineson A. and Thom, D. 'T.N.T. Poisoning and the Employment of Women Workers in the First World War' in Weindling Paul (ed.), *The Social History of Occupational Health* (London: Croom Helm, 1985)

Jackson, J. 'On the Influence of the Cotton Manufactories on the Health', *London Medical and Physical Journal*, xxxix (1818)

Jenkins, S. 'Risking our Sanity', *The Times*, 20 Oct. 1999

Jeremy, D. J. 'Corporate Responses to the Emergent Recognition of a Health Hazard in the UK Asbestos Industry: The Case of Turner & Newall, 1920-1960', *Business and Economic History*, 24 (1995)

Johnson, M.P. 'Grinders' Asthma in Sheffield', *Bulletin of the Society for the Social History of Medicine*, 16 (1975)

Johnstone, J. 'Some Account of a Species of Pthisis Pulmonalis, Peculiar to Persons Employed in Pointing Needles in the Needle Manufacture', *Memoirs of the Medical Society of London*, V (1799)

Jones, H. 'Women Health Workers. The case of the First Women Factory Inspectors in Britain', *Social History of Medicine*, 1 (1988)

Kay, J.P. 'Observations and Experiments Concerning Molecular Irritation of the Lungs as One Source of Tubercular Consumption and on Spinners' Pthisis', *North of England Medical and Surgical Journal*, 1 (1830-31)

Knelman, J. 'The Amendment of the Sale of Arsenic Bill', *Victorian Review*, xvii (1991)

Knight, A. 'On the Grinders' Asthma', *North of England Medical and Surgical Journal*, 1 (1830-1)

Knight, P. 'Women and Abortion in Victorian and Edwardian England', *History Workshop*, 4 (1977)

Laforce, F. Marc 'Woolsorters' Disease in England', *Bulletin of the New York Academy of Medicine*, 54 (1978)

Lee W.R. 'Robert Baker: the First Doctor in the Factory Department', *British Journal of Industrial Medicine*, 21 (1964)

Lee, W.R. 'The History of Mercury Poisoning in Great Britain', *British Journal of Industrial Medicine*, 25 (1968)

Legge, T.M. 'The Milroy Lectures on Industrial Anthrax', *British Medical Journal*, 11,18, 25 March, 1905

Legge, T.M. 'Industrial Diseases in the Middle Ages', *Journal of Industrial Hygiene*, I (1919-20)

Lewis J. and Davies, C. 'Protective Legislation in Britain, 1870-1900: Equality, Difference and their Implications for Women', *Policy and Politics*, 1 (1991)

Luckin, B. 'War on the Roads: Traffic Accidents and Social Tension in Britain, 1939-45' in R. Cooter and B. Luckin (eds) *Accidents in History: Injuries, Fatalities and Social Relations* (Amsterdam and Atlanta: Rodopi, 1997)

MacDonagh, O. ' The Nineteenth Century Revolution in Government: a Re-appraisal', *Historical Journal*, I (1958)

Malone, C. 'The Gendering of Dangerous Trades: Government Regulation of Women's Work in the White Lead Trade in England, 1892-1918', *Journal of Women's History*, 8 (1996)

Malone, C. 'Gendered Discourses and the Making of Protective Labor Legislation in England, 1830-1914', *Journal of British Studies*, 37 (1998)

Malone, C. 'Sensational Stories, Endangered Bodies: Women's Work and the New Journalism in England in the 1890s' *Albion*, 31 (1999)

Manchee R.J. *et al* 'Bacillus Anthracis on Gruinard Island' *Nature*, 19 Nov. 1981

McCready, B.W. 'On the Influence of Trades, Professions and Occupations in the United States in the Production of Disease', *Transactions of the Medical Society of the State of New York*, 3 (1836-7)

McEvoy, A.F. 'Working Environments: An Ecological Approach to Industrial Health and Safety', *Technology and Culture Supplement*, 36 (1995)

McIvor, A.J. 'Employers, the Government and Industrial Fatigue in Britain, 1890-1918', *British Journal of Industrial Medicine*, 44 (1987)

McIvor, A.J. 'Manual Work, Technology and Industrial Health, 1918-39', *Medical History*, 31 (1987)

McIvor, A.J. 'Work and Health, 1880-1914. A Note on a Neglected Interaction', *Scottish Labour History Society Journal*, 24 (1989)

McKendrick, N. 'The Victorian View of Midland History: a Historiographical Study of the Potteries', *Midland History*, I (1971)

Meiklejohn, A. 'John Darwall, MD (1796-1833) and Diseases of Artisans', *British Journal of Industrial Medicine*, 13 (1956)

Meiklejohn, A. 'Outbreak of Fever in Cotton Mills at Radcliffe', *British Journal of Industrial Medicine*, 16 (1959)

Morton, L.T. *A Medical Bibliography (Garrison and Morton). An Annotated Check-List of Texts Illustrating the History of Medicine* (Aldershot: Gower, 1983)

Noble, D. 'On the Influence of the Factory System in the Development of Pulmonary Consumption', *Journal of the Statistical Society of London*, V, 1832

'One of the Evils of Match-Making', *Household Words*, (1 May 1852)

Owen, R. 'On the Employment of Children in Manufactories' (1818) in Robert Owen, *A New View of Society and Other Writings* (London: Everyman, 1927)

Pearce F. and Tombs, S. 'Ideology, Hegemony and Empiricism—Compliance Theories of Regulation', *British Journal of Criminology*, 30 (1990)

Posner, E. 'Thomas Arlidge (1822-1899) and the Potteries', *British Journal of Industrial Medicine*, xxx (1973)

Posner, E. 'Dr John Thomas Arlidge and Victorian Occupational Medicine', *Medical History*, 42 (1998)

Pott, P. 'Cancer Scroti' in Sir James Earle (ed.), *The Chirurgical Works of Percivall Pott FRS Surgeon to St. Bartholomew's Hospital* (London: Wood & Innes, 1808)

Priestman, G. 'Frederick William Eurich and Anthrax—the Woolsorters' Disease', *Journal of the Bradford Textile Society*, (1956-7)

Proskauer, C. 'A Civil Ordinance of the Year 1846 to Combat Phosphorus Necrosis', *Bulletin of the History of Medicine*, xi (1942)

Roberts, D. 'Lord Palmerston at the Home Office', *The Historian*, xxi (1958)

Rose, M. 'The Doctor in the Industrial Revolution', *British Journal of Industrial Medicine*, 28 (1971)

Rose, S. 'Gender Antagonism and Class Conflict: Exclusionary Strategies of Male Trade Unionists in Nineteenth Century Britain', *Social History*, 13 (1988)

Rose, S. '"From Behind the Women's Petticoats": Factory Act Reform and the Politics of Motherhood in Britain, 1870-1878', *Journal of Historical Sociology*, 4 (1991)

Rosen, G. 'Occupational Diseases of English Seamen during the Seventeenth and Eighteenth Centuries', *Bulletin of the History of Medicine*, 7 (1939)

Satre, L.J. 'After the Match Girls' Strike: Bryant and May in the 1890s', *Victorian Studies*, 26 (1982)

Selikoff I.J. and Greenberg, M. 'A Landmark Case in Asbestosis', *JAMA*, 265 (20 Feb. 1991)

Sellers, C. 'Working Disease In: Silicosis, Science and the Social History of Medicine. An Essay Review', *Journal of the History of Medicine and Allied Sciences*, 48 (1993)

Sigerist, H.E. 'Historical Background of Industrial and Occupational Diseases', *Bulletin of the New York Academy of Medicine*, 12 (1936)

Smith, M. 'Lead in History', in Richard Lansdown and William Yule (eds), *The Lead Debate: The Environment, Toxicology and Child Health* (London: Croom Helm, 1986)

Szreter, S. 'The Importance of Social Intervention in Britain's Mortality Decline c.1850-1914: a Re-interpretation of the Role of Public Health', *Social History of Medicine*, I (1988)

Tennant, H.J. 'Dangerous Trades. A Case for Legislation', *Fortnightly Review*, (Feb. 1899)

Tennant, H.J. 'Principles of Prospective Legislation for Dangerous Trades' in Thomas Oliver (ed.), *Dangerous Trades. The Historical, Social and Legal Aspects of Industrial Occupations as Affecting Health, by a Number of Experts* (London: John Murray, 1902)

Theodorides, John 'Casimir Davaine (1812-1882): a precursor of Pasteur', *Medical History*, 10 (1966)

Thompson, F.M.L. 'Nineteenth Century Horse Sense', *Economic History Review*, 29 (1976)

Tigertt, W.D. 'Anthrax. William Smith Greenfield, MD FRCP, Professor Superintendent the Brown Animal Sanctuary Institution (1878-1881) Concerning the Priority Due to him for the Production of the First Vaccine against Anthrax', *Journal of Hygiene*, 85 (1980)

Travis, A.S. 'Science's Powerful Companion: A.W. Hofmann's Investigation of Aniline Red and its Derivatives', *British Journal of the History of Science*, xxv (1992)

Tuckwell, G. 'Commercial Manslaughter', *Nineteenth Century*, 44 (1898)

Tuckwell, Miss Gertrude 'The More Obvious Defects in our Factory Code', in Mrs S. Webb (ed.) *The Case for the Factory Acts* (London: Grant Richards, 1901)

Tweedale G. and Hansen, P. 'Protecting the Workers: the Medical Board and the Asbestos Industry, 1930s-1960s', *Medical History*, 42 (1998)

Waldron, H.A. 'A Brief History of Scrotal Cancer', *British Journal of Industrial Medicine*, 40 (1983)

Waldron, H.A. 'Occupational Health during the Second World War: Hope Deferred or Hope Abandoned?', *Medical History*, 41 (1997)

Watterson, A. 'Occupational Health Education in the United Kingdom Workplace: Looking backwards and Going Forwards? The Industrial Health Education Society at Work, 1922-40', *British Journal of Industrial Medicine*, 47 (1990)

Webster, C. 'Two-Hundredth Anniversary of the 1784 Report on Fever at Radcliffe Mill', *Bulletin of the Society for the Social History of Medicine*, 36 (1985)

Webster C. and Barry, J. 'The Manchester Medical Revolution' in Barbara Smith (ed.), *Truth, Liberty and Religion. Essays Celebrating Two Hundred Years of Manchester College* (Oxford: Manchester College, 1986)

Weindling, P. 'Linking Self Help and Medical Science: the Social History of Occupational Health' in P. Weindling (ed.) *The Social History of Occupational Health* (London: Croom Helm, 1985)

Wikeley, N.J. 'The Asbestos Regulations 1931: A Licence to Kill?', *Journal of Law and Society*, 19 (1992)

Wikeley, N.J. 'Turner & Newall: Early Organizational Responses to Litigation Risk', *Journal of Law and Society*, 24 (1997)

Wilkinson, L. 'Review', *Medical History*, 29 (1985)

Wilks, S. 'Report of the Clinical Society from March 1846 to April 1847: Part ii. Surgical Division', *Guy's Hospital Reports*, 2nd. ser. v (1847)

Wilson, Sir G. 'The Brown Animal Sanitary Institution', *Journal of Hygiene*, 82 (1979)

Theses

Bledington, R.H. 'The Growth in Awareness of Health and Safety at Work, 1780-1900', University of Aston M.Phil. (1983)

Donajgrodski, A.P. 'The Home Office, 1822-48', University of Oxford D.Phil. (1974)

Holdsworth, C. 'Potters' Rot and Plumbism: Occupational Health in the North Staffordshire Pottery Industry', Liverpool University Ph.D. (1995)

Huzzard, S. 'The Role of the Certifying Surgeon in the State Regulation of Child Labour and Industrial Health, 1833-1973', Manchester University, M.A. (1976)

Jones, H. 'The Home Office and Working Conditions, 1914-1940', University of London Ph.D. 1983

Malone, C. 'Sex in Industry: Protective Labor Legislation in Engand, 1891-1914', University of Rochester Ph.D. (1991)

Novels

Collins, W. *The Moonstone* (1868)

Gaskell, E. *North and South* (1855)

Tonna C. *Helen Fleetwood* (1841)

Tressell, R. *The Ragged Trousered Philanthropists* (London: Lawrence & Wishart, 1955 edn),

Newspapers and Periodicals

All the Year Round

Birmingham Post

Bradford Telegraph and Argus

British and Foreign Medical and Chirurgical Review

British Clayworker

British Medical Journal

Critic

Daily Chronicle

Daily News

Daily Telegraph

Dorset County Chronicle and Somerset Gazette

Dublin Quarterly Journal of Medical Science

Edinburgh Medical and Surgical Journal

Englishwoman's Journal

Household Words

Independent

Journal of the Society of Arts

Justice
Lancet
Leeds Mercury
Medical Times
Medical Times and Gazette
Morning Leader
Pall Mall Gazette
Pharmaceutical Journal
Potter
Practitioner
Reynold's Newspaper
ProvinciaL Medical and Surgical Journal
Provincial Medical Journal and Retrospect of the Medical Sciences
St James's Gazette
Staffordshire Sentinel
Star
Times
Times and Echo
Transactions of the National Association for the Promotion of Social Science
Transactions of the Society of Arts
Truth
Westminster Gazette
Women's Trade Union Review
Yorkshire Observer

Legal Cases

Brintons Ltd. *v.* Turvey [1905] A.C. 230
Fenton v. Thorley & Co. Ltd. [1903] A.C. 443

On-Line, Radio and Television

BBC Radio 4, 'Bookshelf', 20 Oct. 1985
BBC Television Documentary, 'Dust to Dust', 17 Aug. 1982
Oxford English Dictionary On-Line
Palmers Index to *The Times* on CD-ROM

Unpublished Papers and Reports

Clark, A.R.L. 'Industrial Plumbism. A Study of Theories and Attitudes which Inhibited its Control in the Nineteenth Century', (unpublished essay presented for the Diploma in the History of Medicine of the Society of Apothecaries, 1984).

Irwin, K. 'Reproductive Hazards in the Victorian Lead Trades: Blessing or Curse', (unpublished paper dated 18 March 1983)

Martin B. 'The Development of the Factory Office up to 1878: Administrative Evolution and the Establishment of a Regulatory Style in the early Factory Inspectorate', (unpublished and undated paper)

Index

Abbreviations: OH, occupational health. Names of persons are largely confined to those of historical persons apart from those contributing to the historiography of occupational health.

A

B

E

M

Q

R